Novel Biocomposite Engineering and Bio-Applications

Novel Biocomposite Engineering and Bio-Applications

Special Issue Editor

Gary Chinga Carrasco

MDPI • Basel • Beijing • Wuhan • Barcelona • Belgrade

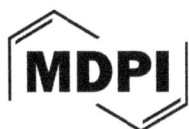

MDPI

Special Issue Editor
Gary Chinga Carrasco
Lead Scientist—Biocomposites RISE PFI
Norway

Editorial Office
MDPI
St. Alban-Anlage 66
4052 Basel, Switzerland

This is a reprint of articles from the Special Issue published online in the open access journal *Bioengineering* (ISSN 2306-5354) from 2017 to 2018 (available at: https://www.mdpi.com/journal/bioengineering/special_issues/novel_biocomposite)

For citation purposes, cite each article independently as indicated on the article page online and as indicated below:

LastName, A.A.; LastName, B.B.; LastName, C.C. Article Title. *Journal Name* **Year**, *Article Number*, Page Range.

ISBN 978-3-03897-382-9 (Pbk)
ISBN 978-3-03897-383-6 (PDF)

Cover image courtesy of Gary Chinga Carrasco.

Contents

About the Special Issue Editor

Gary Chinga Carrasco is the lead scientist of the Biocomposites area at RISE PFI, Norway, with background from cell biology (Cand. Scient. degree) and chemical engineering (Dr. Ing. degree). Dr. Chinga Carrasco has published more than 90 peer-reviewed articles, in addition to 4 critical reviews, 6 book chapters and over 90 conference contributions and invited talks. He has extensive project manager experience and during the last years he has been coordinating various major international and multidisciplinary projects regarding; processing technology for production of biomaterials and biocomposites, including production of ultrapure nanocellulose, characterization and application as a biomaterial for bio-medical applications. His recent research activities focus on additive manufacturing, and development of biobased inks for various 3D printing technologies.

Preface to "Novel Biocomposite Engineering and Bio-Applications"

The engineering and utilization of biocomposites is a research field of major scientific and industrial interest worldwide. Biocomposites include materials that contain at least one biocomponent. The biocomposite area is extensive and spans from structured and solid biocomposites (e.g., reinforced bioabsorbable polymers), films (e.g., antimicrobial barriers), to soft biocomposites (e.g., scaffolds for tissue engineering). Key aspects in this respect are the appropriate engineering and production of biomaterials, nanofibres, bioplastics, their functionalization enabling intelligent and active materials, processes for effective manufacturing of biocomposites and the corresponding characterization for understanding their properties.

The current Special Issue Book emphasizes the bio-technological engineering of novel biomaterials and biocomposites, considering also important safety aspects in the production and use of bio- and nanomaterials. It includes:

- Synthesis, production, surface modification and applications of novel biomaterials

- Hydrogels, films, solid materials

- Safety aspects, including cytotoxicity, genotoxicity, immunogenic properties

- Microbiological aspects

- Scaffolds for tissue engineering

- New processing methods, including 3D printing

- Encapsulation for controlled release

- Characterisation, including structural, physical, chemical, biological and mechanical properties

Gary Chinga Carrasco
Special Issue Editor

bioengineering

MDPI

Editorial

Novel Biocomposite Engineering and Bio-Applications

Gary Chinga-Carrasco

RISE PFI, Høgskoleringen 6b, 7491 Trondheim, Norway; gary.chinga.carrasco@rise-pfi.no; Tel.: +47-908-36-045

Academic Editor: Liang Luo
Received: 14 September 2018; Accepted: 25 September 2018; Published: 28 September 2018

The engineering and utilization of biocomposites is a research field of major scientific and industrial interest worldwide. Biocomposites include materials composed of at least two components with a distinct morphology and chemistry, where at least one component is bio-based. Furthermore, biocomposites can be classified into different areas depending on their specific application. Hence, in this special issue, various research groups were invited to contribute and cover several aspects and applications of biocomposite materials, spanning from solid biocomposites for structural applications, films such as antimicrobial barriers, to soft biocomposites for specific biomedical purposes, e.g., drug delivery and scaffolds for tissue regeneration.

During recent years, bio-based polymers have attracted major attention due to growing environmental concerns, e.g., ocean littering. There are various types of bio-based polymers or bioplastics, including durable, compostable, and biodegradable materials, suited for specific applications [1,2]. Bioplastics such as polylactic acid (PLA) can be derived from a series of biomass resources, including corn, sugar beet, and sugar cane. PLA has several advantages and can degrade in industrial compostable conditions. The mechanical properties of PLA may be improved by the addition of cellulose nanofibres, provided that the interfacial adhesion between the nanofibers and the PLA matrix is optimized. This has been addressed by Immonen et al. [3], where various types of cellulosic materials were tested for the reinforcement of PLA. Both the type of cellulosic material and the additives used for better dispersion in the PLA matrix were found to affect the mechanical properties of the biocomposites.

PLA is a versatile polymer, which can be used for encapsulation purposes with a range of applications, e.g., within cosmetics. The study conducted by Kesente et al. [4], demonstrated the potential of PLA nanoparticles for encapsulating olive leaves' extract. The loaded nanoparticles were incorporated in cosmetic formulations. The encapsulated olive leaves' extract showed a higher stability compared to pure extract and opens the possibility to better exploit the potential of plant and herb extracts rich in natural antioxidants. This can be used in topical formulations to enhance the skin's endogenous protection system against oxidative damage [4]. Furthermore, encapsulation is an attractive approach for various products [5]. The potential of cyclic water-soluble oligosaccharides (cyclodextrins) to encapsulate oregano essential oil was demonstrated [5]. The authors suggested a range of applications for the cyclodextrin capsules, such as in the preparation of films for active packaging of food products, in personal care products, and for the improvement of their properties, e.g., antioxidant and antimicrobial [5].

Biopolymers such as PLA and polyhydroxyalkanoates (PHA) are polyesters which have a range of applications within biomedicine, e.g., for the fabrication of artificial tissue or scaffolds for bone regeneration [6]. This is facilitated by three-dimensional (3D) printing technology. 3D printing has gained major attention in recent years due to the capability of technology to create personalized and complex devices. Fused deposition modeling (FDM) is perhaps the most used technology for 3D printing of PLA-based constructs with potential applications within biomedicine, e.g., scaffolds and prosthetics. Additionally, PHA is also printable by FDM technology. According to the authors, PLA and PHA are suitable materials for in vivo applications due to their biocompatibility, biodegradability, good mechanical strength, and processability [6].

Natural polymers such as bacterial cellulose have been a focus for years and a range of applications have been proposed, including food packaging, biomedical devices, cosmetics, and as a barrier for degraded paper restoration. Bacterial cellulose consists of pure cellulose, with high crystallinity and a high degree of polymerization. The composition of bacterial cellulose can be modified with additional polysaccharides such as xylans, to form biocomposites with tailored properties [7]. Comprehensive characterization and understanding of the effect of xylan on the properties of bacterial cellulose were performed and shed more light on the potential of the formed biocomposite material [7]. Cotton is another cellulose-rich fiber applied to form textiles. Additionally, cotton fabrics can be functionalized with metal-organic frameworks to form substrates for the filtration of wastewater, allowing photocatalytic activity, decontamination, and micropollutant degradation as demonstrated by Schelling et al. [8]. Surface functionalization of materials to introduce new properties is also promising for biomedical devices. Villegas et al. [9] reported an interesting approach where bioceramics were modified with a lysine amino acid with a zwitterionic function that provides resistance to bacterial biofilm formation. The modified biomaterial was tested against *E. coli* and *S. Aureus*, thus demonstrating the effect of the surface modification on limiting the biofilm formation of the assessed microorganisms.

Polymers intended for biomedical use (biomaterials) are a timely topic of research. Biomaterials have potential in e.g., regenerative medicine, as drug delivery vehicles, and wound dressings, provided that the biomaterials are biocompatible with the human organism. Cellulose and chitosan are two major natural polymers that have been combined to design biocomposite hydrogel beads proposed as scaffolds for bone tissue engineering [10]. The study demonstrated the potential of natural polymers and a facile chemical approach to design hydrogel beads that were tested for cytocompatibility and cell attachment, important initial aspects to consider if the biomaterial is intended for tissue engineering applications. In addition to natural polymers to fabricate scaffolds for bone tissue engineering [10], repair of bone tissue using hypertrophic cartilage grafts has been demonstrated in this issue [11]. The authors explored the development of a devitalized hypertronic cartilage matrix in amounts that were clinically relevant and assessed its effect on chondrogenic differentiation in vivo [11].

Tissue engineering includes a series of biomaterials and applications with the potential to improve people's quality of life, of which the regeneration of neural tissue is a specific example. Hence, biomaterials that counteract neurodegenerative disorders by repairing damaged tissue and promoting the growth of healthy tissue pose great societal benefits. Biocomposite scaffolds are necessary to mimic the properties of healthy tissue. In this issue, self-assembled nanoribbon combined with conductive polymers were the basis to form biocomposite scaffolds which promoted growth and proliferation of cortical cells and axonal outgrowth [12]. Provided that the scaffolds are biodegradable to promote cell proliferation and that biocompatibility is secured, the approach seems promising for neural tissue engineering. Additionally, biomaterials based on proteins are interesting for biomedical devices due to their biodegradability and biocompatibility [13]. This paper provides a clear example of advanced bioengineering processes for the biosynthesis of proteins containing non-canonical amino acids. The chemical functionalities of proteins can thus be tailored, expanding their characteristics and applications within biomaterial science [13]. Importantly, the use of biomaterials as scaffolds for tissue engineering requires a thorough understanding of the mechanical properties of the biomaterials and how these properties affect cellular behavior such as proliferation and differentiation. It is thus of great importantance to have adequate methods to measure and understand the cell-cell interactions and the mechanotransduction between cells and the surrounding matrix. These physiological processes were extensively reviewed by Zhang et al. [14], focusing on the detailed understanding of the mechanosensory responses of cells by using e.g., cell traction force microscopy techniques. Assessment of the cascade of signals involved in mechanotransduction in 3D microenvironments is expected to facilitate the design of tailored scaffolds for tissue engineering [14].

Bioengineering **2018**, *5*, 80

Finally, during recent years there has been an extensive development of bio-based materials intended for biomedical applications (e.g., scaffolds for tissue engineering or wound dressings). Although these bio-based materials are derived from natural biomass resources and are generally considered to be non-toxic, some of the materials have nano-dimensions and surface chemistries that differ from the original and natural state. It is thus of utmost importance to ensure that such nano-dimensions and surface modifications do not compromise the biocompatibility. These aspects, in addition to relevant endpoints, should be evaluated in every case to secure safety and human health [15].

Funding: Part of this work was funded by the MedIn project, MNET17/NMCS-1204—"New functionalized medical devices for surgical interventions in the pelvic cavity", Research Council of Norway, Grant: 283895.

Conflicts of Interest: The author declares no conflict of interest.

References

1. Brodin, M.; Vallejos, M.; Opedal, M.T.; Area, M.C.; Chinga-Carrasco, G. Lignocellulosics as sustainable resources for production of bioplastics—A review. *J. Clean. Prod.* **2017**, *162*, 646–664. [CrossRef]
2. Albertsson, A.-C.; Hakkarainen, M. Designed to degrade. *Science* **2017**, *358*, 872–873. [CrossRef] [PubMed]
3. Immonen, K.; Lahtinen, P.; Pere, J. Effects of Surfactants on the Preparation of Nanocellulose-PLA Composites. *Bioengineering* **2017**, *4*, 91. [CrossRef] [PubMed]
4. Kesente, M.; Kavetsou, E.; Roussaki, M.; Blidi, S.; Loupassaki, S.; Chanioti, S.; Siamandoura, P.; Stamatogianni, C.; Philippou, E.; Papaspyrides, C.; et al. Encapsulation of Olive Leaves Extracts in Biodegradable PLA Nanoparticles for Use in Cosmetic Formulation. *Bioengineering* **2017**, *4*, 75. [CrossRef] [PubMed]
5. Kotronia, M.; Kavetsou, E.; Loupassaki, S.; Kikionis, S.; Vouyiouka, S.; Detsi, A. Encapsulation of Oregano (*Origanum onites* L.) Essential Oil in β-Cyclodextrin (β-CD): Synthesis and Characterization of the Inclusion Complexes. *Bioengineering* **2017**, *4*, 74. [CrossRef] [PubMed]
6. Chiulan, I.; Frone, A.N.; Brandabur, C.; Panaitescu, D.M. Recent Advances in 3D Printing of Aliphatic Polyesters. *Bioengineering* **2018**, *5*, 2. [CrossRef] [PubMed]
7. Santos, S.M.; Carbajo, J.M.; Gómez, N.; Ladero, M.; Villar, J.C. Modification of Bacterial Cellulose Biofilms with Xylan Polyelectrolytes. *Bioengineering* **2017**, *4*, 93. [CrossRef] [PubMed]
8. Schelling, M.; Kim, M.; Otal, E.; Hinestroza, J. Decoration of Cotton Fibers with a Water-Stable Metal–Organic Framework (UiO-66) for the Decomposition and Enhanced Adsorption of Micropollutants in Water. *Bioengineering* **2018**, *5*, 14. [CrossRef] [PubMed]
9. Villegas, M.F.; Garcia-Uriostegui, L.; Rodríguez, O.; Izquierdo-Barba, I.; Salinas, A.J.; Toriz, G.; Vallet-Regí, M.; Delgado, E. Lysine-Grafted MCM-41 Silica as an Antibacterial Biomaterial. *Bioengineering* **2017**, *4*, 80. [CrossRef] [PubMed]
10. Trivedi, P.; Saloranta-Simell, T.; Maver, U.; Gradišnik, L.; Prabhakar, N.; Smått, J.-H.; Mohan, T.; Gericke, M.; Heinze, T.; Fardim, P. Chitosan–Cellulose Multifunctional Hydrogel Beads: Design, Characterization and Evaluation of Cytocompatibility with Breast Adenocarcinoma and Osteoblast Cells. *Bioengineering* **2018**, *5*, 3. [CrossRef] [PubMed]
11. Le, B.Q.; Van Blitterswijk, C.; De Boer, J. An Approach to In Vitro Manufacturing of Hypertrophic Cartilage Matrix for Bone Repair. *Bioengineering* **2017**, *4*, 35.
12. Smith, A.M.; Pajovich, H.T.; Banerjee, I.A. Development of Self-Assembled Nanoribbon Bound Peptide-Polyaniline Composite Scaffolds and Their Interactions with Neural Cortical Cells. *Bioengineering* **2018**, *5*, 6. [CrossRef] [PubMed]
13. Crnković, A.; Vargas-Rodriguez, O.; Merkuryev, A.; Söll, D. Effects of Heterologous tRNA Modifications on the Production of Proteins Containing Noncanonical Amino Acids. *Bioengineering* **2018**, *5*, 11. [CrossRef] [PubMed]

14. Zhang, Y.; Liao, K.; Li, C.; Lai, A.C.K.; Foo, J.-J.; Chan, V. Progress in Integrative Biomaterial Systems to Approach Three-Dimensional Cell Mechanotransduction. *Bioengineering* **2017**, *4*, 72. [CrossRef] [PubMed]
15. Catalán, J.; Norppa, H. Safety Aspects of Bio-Based Nanomaterials. *Bioengineering* **2017**, *4*, 94. [CrossRef] [PubMed]

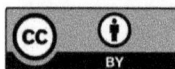

bioengineering

MDPI

Article

Effects of Surfactants on the Preparation of Nanocellulose-PLA Composites

Kirsi Immonen [1,*], Panu Lahtinen [2] and Jaakko Pere [3]

1   Biocomposites and Processing, VTT Technical Research Centre of Finland, 33101 Tampere, Finland
2   Biomass Processing Technologies, VTT Technical Research Centre of Finland, 02150 Espoo, Finland; panu.lahtinen@vtt.fi
3   High Performance Fibre Products, VTT Technical Research Centre of Finland, 02150 Espoo, Finland; jaakko.pere@vtt.fi
*   Correspondence: kirsi.immonen@vtt.fi; Tel.: +358-40-5185351

Academic Editor: Gary Chinga Carrasco
Received: 29 September 2017; Accepted: 15 November 2017; Published: 17 November 2017

Abstract: Thermoplastic composite materials containing wood fibers are gaining increasing interest in the manufacturing industry. One approach is to use nano- or micro-size cellulosic fibrils as additives and to improve the mechanical properties obtainable with only small fibril loadings by exploiting the high aspect ratio and surface area of nanocellulose. In this study, we used four different wood cellulose-based materials in a thermoplastic polylactide (PLA) matrix: cellulose nanofibrils produced from softwood kraft pulp (CNF) and dissolving pulp (CNFSD), enzymatically prepared high-consistency nanocellulose (HefCel) and microcellulose (MC) together with long alkyl chain dispersion-improving agents. We observed increased impact strength with HefCel and MC addition of 5% and increased tensile strength with CNF addition of 3%. The addition of a reactive dispersion agent, epoxy-modified linseed oil, was found to be favorable in combination with HefCel and MC.

Keywords: wood fibers; nanocellulose; composites; wood fiber composites; wood polymer composites; PLA

---

1. Introduction

The growing awareness of environmental issues has directed a focus towards the use of more sustainable materials. Thermoplastic materials and thermoplastic composites are used as building materials in an increasing number of products due to their easy processing, free forms of design and the possibility to create products with lighter weight compared to metals or composites containing glass fiber [1]. Among polymer matrices, polylactide (PLA) is a good choice, being derived from renewable sources such as corn, sugar beet, sugar cane, cassava, but also from non-food cellulosic feedstocks such as bagasse, wheat straw or wood chips [2]. Those are natural glucose sources from which lactic acid, the monomer of PLA, can be produced by fermentation [3]. PLA has high strength and modulus compared to e.g., polyolefins, and is biodegradable, if only in industrial composting conditions. The disadvantages of PLA polymer are its low temperature resistance including low heat deflection temperature (HDT) (below 60 °C), low moisture resistance and low flexibility. However, for fiber composite materials PLA is an attractive matrix. When ligno-cellulosic fibers are added to PLA, they usually improve the tensile properties, but impact properties are weakened and the material becomes brittle if no coupling agents are added [4]. This is due to poor interaction between fiber and polymer, which has also been demonstrated in other studies [5–7].

Microcrystalline cellulose is an interesting reinforcement material for PLA, because it contains mainly crystalline cellulose and no weaker amorphous regions [8]. The crystallinity and low aspect ratio are expected to provide better dispersion to PLA than cellulose materials with a high aspect ratio. Microcrystalline celluloses are typically available in powder form and are much more easily applied in thermoplastic processes than nanocelluloses or cellulose pulp. The high specific surface area (>0.5 m^2/g) and crystalline structure of microcellulose may also offer a greater reinforcing effect when compared to conventional cellulose fibers [9].

The use of nanocellulose in different forms and from different origins has been the focus in the composite research work of several authors [10,11]. Due to their advantageous mechanical properties and high surface area, nanocellulose fibers have good potential for utilization in load-bearing composites. The theoretical tensile strength values for nanocellulose crystals are in the range of 0.3–22 GPa and modulus values for a single cellulose nanofiber between 100 and 160 GPa. The specific surface area of nanocellulose is estimated to range between tens to hundreds of square meters per gram [12]. Improved composite properties have been demonstrated even with a very low degree of filling of nanocellulose, below 5% [13]. The most effective way for production of nanocellulose-reinforced composites is to use solvent casting, but from the manufacturing point of view thermoplastic processing is a more cost-effective method. Jonoobi et al. presented a combined thermoplastic extrusion process and solvent casting. PLA-CNF masterbatch was prepared by dissolving PLA in acetone-chloroform mixture and solvent-exchanged kenaf CNF from aqueous mixture to acetone, followed by mixing those two solutions and evaporating the solvent. This PLA-CNF blend was then mixed with PLA using extrusion, and injection molded to test specimens. The authors reported significant improvements in modulus and tensile strength of compounds, but also clearly visible aggregates of nanofibers in PLA [14].

Several approaches have been reported in literature to improve the compatibility of hydrophilic cellulose with hydrophobic PLA and to break the strong interaction between cellulose fibers. These include different fiber modifications (e.g., acetylation, esterification, silylation, silanization, oxidation, grafting, surfactants, coupling agents, plasticizers and physical modifications) [15–19]. Lu et al. modified cellulose nanofibrils to be more hydrophobic using amine-functionalization and gained improved strength properties for PLLA using solvent casting method and quite high nanomaterial addition (5–15%) [20]. Bulota et al. introduced acetylated microfibrillous cellulose to PLA with solvent casting method using fiber contents 2–20%. He had the best tensile strength results with fiber content over 10%. At 10% fiber content the Young's modulus increased by approximately 15% and tensile strength remained the same. However, the strain at break increased from 8.4% to 76.1% with 5% fiber loading and DS 0.43 [21]. The review article from Oksman presents comprehensively several techniques for nanocellulose PLA composite manufacturing and mentions the use of plasticizers together with nanocellulose in addition to improve nanocellulose dispersion to PLA [22]. One group of additives also giving potential plasticizing effect is fiber de-bonders that enable cellulosic fibers to disperse more evenly on polymeric materials in a variety of absorbent products [23]. Our assumption was that a blend of non-ionic and cationic surfactants on cellulose fiber could improve the fiber dispersion in PLA, thus improving its strength properties. Another group of additives are epoxidized vegetable oils, which are bio-based plasticizer-stabilizers mainly used in PVC applications. They can also be used as plasticizers with other polymers such as PLA [24]. Miao et al. also prepared composites using only cellulose (paper) and epoxidized soy oil (ESO), which demonstrated the compatibility of ESO and cellulose [25]. For coupling they used a catalyzer, which is assumed not to be needed in this thermal molding process, due to the high temperature (>180 °C) in the process. When introduced on the surface of the fibers, ESO is assumed to improve fiber dispersion in PLA due to the long alkyl chain. The reaction between the OH group of cellulose and epoxies has been confirmed to proceed through the opening of the epoxide ring in acidic conditions, caused by residual moisture in cellulose [26]. Nanocellulose, having a high specific surface area, also has a large number of OH-groups enabling the reaction with epoxy groups even in lower temperature, which has been proven by Ansari et al. [27].

In this study, we prepared CNFs from three different wood-based raw materials and studied the effect of the raw material in thermoplastic PLA composites using thermoplastic compounding and injection molding as processing methods. There are certain challenges related to the thermoplastic processing and to achieving proper dispersion of the hydrophilic cellulosic material into the hydrophobic polymer. In order to minimize this effect we used two-stage compounding. For material comparison, we used microcellulose, which was easier to disperse into PLA than fibrous nanocelluloses. Our approach was also to treat the cellulose fibers with two different commercial long alkyl chain dispersion additives before compounding fibrils with PLA.

2. Materials and Methods

2.1. Polymer

Bio-based polylactide PLA 3052D (NatureWorks, Minnetonka, USA) was used as matrix polymer in this study. The polymer content in the studied materials was between 95% and 97%. PLA 3052D is a semi-crystalline polymer. It has melt flow index of 14 g/10 min (210 °C, 2.16 kg), specific gravity 1.24 and relative viscosity 3.3 [28]. It has an average molecular weight M_w 228.2 kg/mol and M_n 154.8 kg/mol determined in conjunction with this study by Virtanen et al. [29].

2.2. Nanocellulose Preparation

Cellulose nanofibrils (CNF) were produced using once dried bleached softwood kraft pulp from a Finnish pulp mill (MetsäFibre, Äänekoski, Finland) and softwood dissolving pulp from Domsjö Fabriker (CNFSD) (Örnsköldsvik, Sweden) followed by mechanical treatment with a high-shear grinder as described in the following. The pulps were first soaked at 1.8% consistency for one day and dispersed using a high shear Ystral Dispermix (Ystral, Markgräflerland, Germany) for 10 minutes at 2070 rpm. Suspension was then fed into a Masuko Supermasscolloider (Masuko Sangyo Co., Kawaguchi-city, Japan) type MKZA10-15J. The kraft pulp was ground with six passes and the dissolving pulp was ground seven passes in order to obtain the CNF. The rotation speed was fixed at 1500 rpm. The gap width was approximately 0.14–0.25 mm depending on the fibrillation cycle. The production yield of ground material was 95% based on mass balance calculation. The material was stored at +5 °C until used.

2.3. High-Consistency Nanocellulose Preparation

Bleached softwood pulp from a Finnish pulp mill (MetsäFibre, Äänekoski, Finland) was used as the raw material for producing CNF at high consistency (HefCel). The enzymatic treatment was carried out at a consistency of 25 w-% for 6 h at 70 °C using a two shaft sigma mixer (Jaygo Incorporated, NJ, USA) running at 25 rpm. The pulp batch size was 300 g on dry basis. After the treatment enzyme activity was stopped by increasing temperature of the mixer to 90 °C for 30 min. The fibrillated material was diluted with deionized water, filtered and washed thoroughly with deionized water. Finally, the fibrillated material was dewatered to a consistency of ~20% by filtration. The gravimetric yield of the fibrillated material was 90%. The material was stored at +4 °C until used.

2.4. Microcellulose

Powdery microcellulose (MC), Arbocel B600 was obtained from Rettenmeier and Söhne GmbH (Rosenberg, Germany). Typical topological polar surface area according to Chemical trading guide is 40.8 m^2/g [30].

2.5. Nanocellulose Modification and Surface Treatments

In order to improve the dispersion of hydrophilic cellulosic fibers to hydrophobic PLA two different dispersion additives were used. Arosurf PA780, obtained from Evonik (Essen, Germany), is according to the manufacturer a fatty quarternary blend of non-ionic and cationic surfactants [31]. Referred to here as DA. It contains <20% imidazolium compounds, 2-C17-unsaturated-alkyl-1-(2-C18-unsaturated amidoethyl)-4,5-dihydro-N-methyl, Me sulfates [32].

Arosurf PA780 is a fiber de-bonder used in fluff pulp manufacturing [23]. In composites it was assumed mainly to increase hydrophobicity on fiber surface and to improve fiber dispersion to the polymer.

The second dispersion additive was epoxydized linseed oil Vikoflex 7190 from Arkema (Colombes, France), referred to here as VF (Vikoflex). It is recommended for plasticization and stabilization for polymers such as PVC and limits color formation during processing [33]. It has minimum 9.0% oxirane oxygen, capable of effecting a ring opening reaction in elevated temperature [34].

The introduction of both dispersing additives was carried by mixing the additives to CNF and HefCel water dispersions and MC powder in a dough mixer. DA was added to 20 w-% of fiber amount and VF to 10 w-% of fiber amount.

2.6. Drying

Before compounding with PLA HefCel and CNF were dried using a freeze-drying method. Freeze drying agglomerated fibrils to some extent, but it was the best available methods for this purpose. The water-containing slurry was frozen at −40 °C followed by freeze drying in a Supermodulyo 12K Freeze Dryer (Edwards High Vacuum International, Crowley, UK). The modified MC was oven dried at 50 °C overnight.

For plastic processing the PLA was dried in an oven at 50 °C overnight and nanomaterials were added directly from the freeze-drying process.

2.7. Plastic Processing

The compounding of materials to total cellulose contents of 3% or 5% in PLA was performed using a co-rotating Berstorff ZE 25x33D compounder (Berstorff GmbH, Hanover, Germany) and the compounds were injection molded to standard (ISO 527) dog bone shaped test pieces with an Engel ES 200/50 HL injection-molding machine (Engel Maschinenbau Geschellschaft m.b.H, Schwefberg, Austria). In order to ensure proper dispersion of fibrous material the compounding stage was performed twice. The reference PLA was also compounded as such before injection molding, in order to ensure the same thermal stress on materials. In compounding the temperature profile was from 165 °C in the feeding zone to 200 °C in the nozzle and the screw speed was 100 rpm. The temperature profile in injection molding was from the feed 180 °C to the nozzle 200 °C and the mold temperature was 25 °C.

2.8. Mechanical Testing

Tensile testing was performed according to ISO 527 using Instron 4505 Universal Tensile Tester (Instron Corp., Canton, MA, USA) mechanical test equipment. The results are the average of a minimum of five replicate samples with thickness 4 mm, total length 170 mm, in measurement point the test specimen length is 85 mm and width 10 mm.

Charpy impact strength was tested according to ISO 179 using unnotched samples flatwise and using a Charpy Ceast Resil 5.5 Impact Strength Machine (CEAST S.p.a., Torino, Italy). Sample size was 4 mm × 10 mm × 100 mm and the result is the average of 10 samples.

All the tested samples were conditioned at 23 °C and 50% relative humidity for a minimum of five days before testing.

2.9. SEM and Optical Microscopy

The morphologies of fibers and injection-molded samples were studied by scanning electron microscopy (SEM). The sample surface was coated with gold to prevent surface charging. In the case of injection-molded samples the scanning was made on cross-cut surfaces. Analyses were performed using JEOL JSM T100 (JEOL ltd., Tokyo, Japan) with a voltage of 25 kV.

Optical microscopy pictures were taken according to Kangas et al. [35].

3. Results and Discussion

3.1. Characterisation of Micro- and Nanocellulose Fibers

Optical microscopy images of micro- and nanocelluloses are presented in Figure 1. According to the microscopic images only a few fibril bundles still existed in the CNF samples, but the amount of residual fibers was low. No clear differences were observed between CNF and CNFSD. MC appeared as round particles together with some long fibrous particles about 100 μm long (Figure 1 down right). The SEM images presented in Figure 2 provide a closer view of CNF and HefCel. Both CNF made of softwood pulp and HefCel appear as a network of slender fibrils and fibril aggregates. During the sample preparation HefCel had a high tendency to film formation, which partly covered the fibrillar network beneath. Morphological characteristics were evaluated based on optical microscopy and SEM. The average fiber dimensions of CNF, HefCel and MC are presented in Table 1.

Table 1. Fiber dimension of cellulosic materials used in PLA composites.

Fiber	Fiber Length, μm	Mean Fiber Width, nm
CNF/CNFSD	<10	15–40
HefCel	0.2–0.5	15–20
MC	Average 60 [36]	n.a.

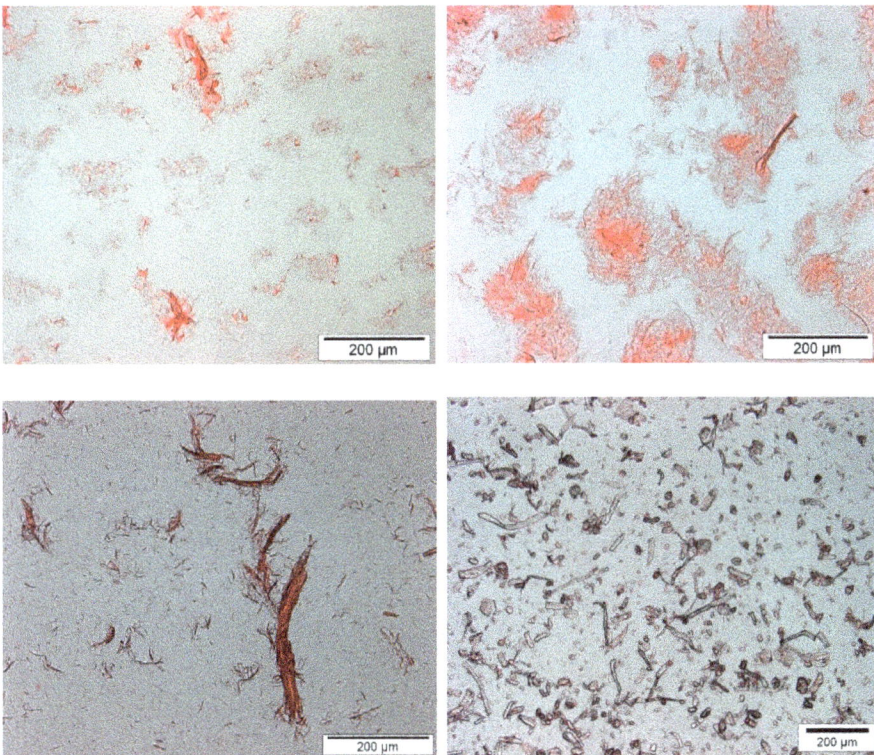

Figure 1. Images of fibrillated samples. CNF made of dissolving pulp CNFSD (**upper left**), kraft pulp CNF (**upper right**), HefCel CNF (**lower left**) and microfiber MC (**lower right**).

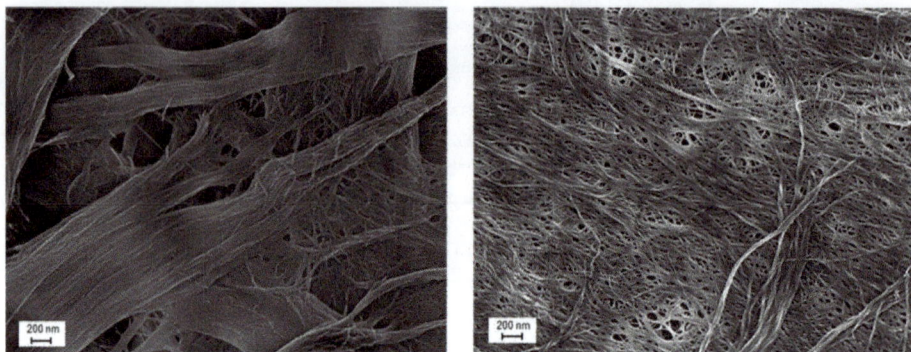

Figure 2. SEM images of fibrillated samples. HefCel CMF (**left**) and CNF kraft pulp (**right**).

3.2. Characterisation of Injection Moulded Test Bars

Injection molded test bars are shown in Figure 3. The dispersion of CNFs and HefCel into PLA was poorer than with MC and fibril aggregates, as observed in test bars containing CNF and HefCel. The addition of both the dispersion additives DA and VF improved the dispersion of all cellulosic materials to PLA. In composites containing MC the effect of dispersion agent cannot be seen due to the better dispersion capacity of MC as such, which may be due to its content of individual particles, without aggregates.

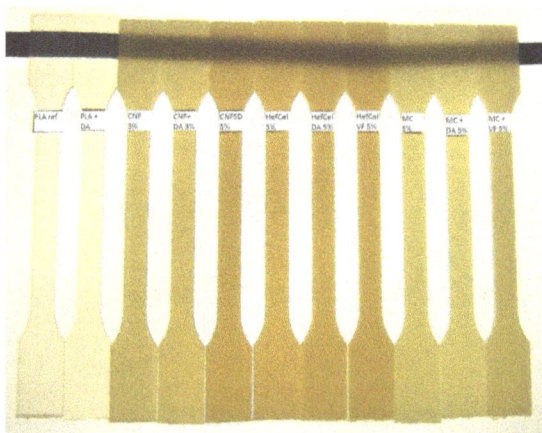

Figure 3. Injection molded test bars.

3.2.1. SEM

Although the injection molded test bars contained visible cellulose aggregates, individual well-dispersed fibers were detected within the PLA matrix in SEM images (Figure 4). A closer look with a higher magnification shows a small orbicular area between fiber and polymer in all the composite samples indicating a poor connection between the PLA polymer matrix and the embedded cellulose fibrils and particles (Figure 5).

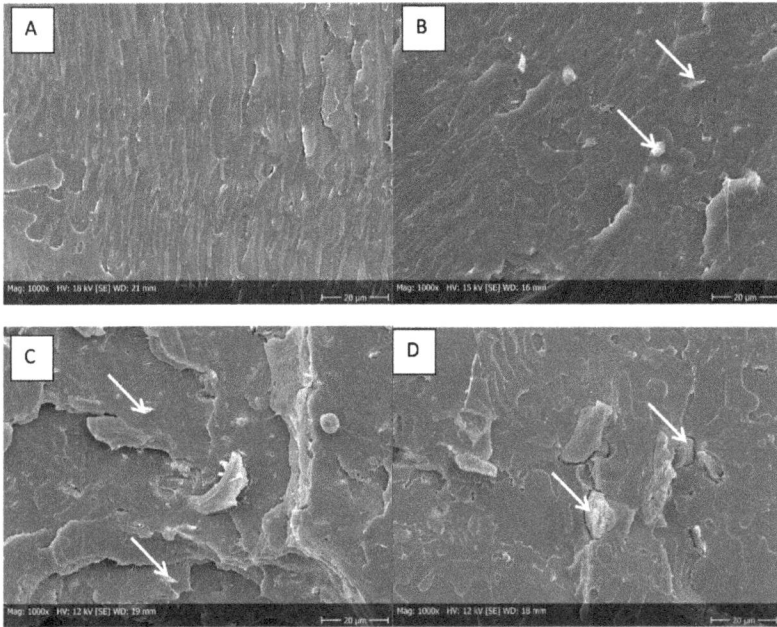

Figure 4. SEM image of injection molded test bars. (**A**) PLA matrix, (**B**) PLA with CNF, (**C**) PLA with HefCel CMF and (**D**) PLA with MC. Arrows are indicating fibers.

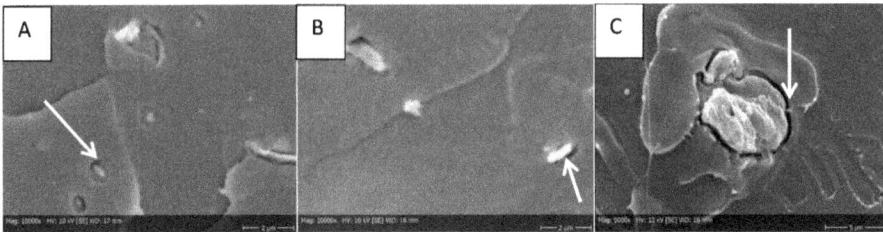

Figure 5. SEM image of injection molded test bars. (**A**) PLA with CNF, (**B**) PLA with HefCel CMF and (**C**) PLA with MC. Fiber loading 5%. Arrows are indicating a gap between the fiber and polymer.

3.2.2. Mechanical Results

Mechanical tests such as tensile strength and Charpy impact strength were performed for injection molded composite samples containing 3% or 5% cellulosic fibers in PLA. The tensile test results are presented in Figure 6 and the Charpy impact strength (unnotched) results in Figure 7. In the results, PLA 3052 is presented after injection molding and PLA ref., after going through the same compounding and injection molding processes as the fiber containing materials.

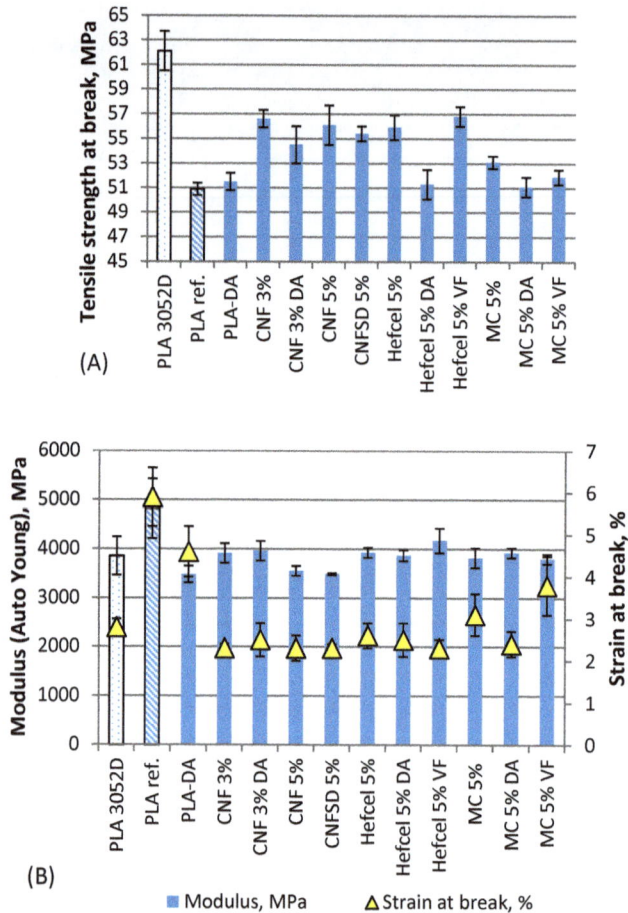

Figure 6. Tensile strength results (**A**), and modulus and strain at break (**B**) for injection molded PLA composites.

Reduced tensile strength and increased elongation and modulus can be seen for neat PLA after an additional compounding stage (Figure 6). The increase in modulus in twice compounded PLA ref compared to PLA 3052D may be related to increased crystallinity of PLA due to additional processing cycles. For example Tábi et al. observed increased crystallization in PLA sheets due to heat treatment [37]. The tensile strength reduction indicates PLA degradation due to additional thermal stress, which has also been found by other authors [38–40]. The effect of compounding on PLA 3052D molecular weight was determined in study by Virtanen et al. [29]. The same compounding method was used in this study and the current composite results can be compared to the PLA ref. and PLA-DA, which is PLA ref with DA. The addition of 1% of dispersion additive DA to PLA is able to plasticize the PLA and the effect can be seen as a 39% decrease in the modulus (PLA-DA).

When comparing the results without any dispersion additives, the PLA compounds with CNF, CNFSD, HefCel and MC gave very similar response in the tensile strength results; reduced strain at break, 19–27% decrease to modulus, but 4–11% increase in tensile strength at break value. Comparing the CNF addition in levels of 3% and 5% the CNF amount of 3% gave better tensile modulus (3910 MPa vs. 3550 MPa) and slightly better tensile strength value (56.6 MPa vs. 56.1 MPa). This can also be seen in the impact strength values (Figure 7) for CNF and CNFSD, which may indicate that the optimum value for CNF addition to PLA is below 5%. The lowest effect on tensile strength results was obtained with MC, which result is supported also by Bulota et al. [21]. The low optimum, below 5% of cellulosic nanomaterial to PLA, is supported by the results of other studies [19,41].

The dispersion additive DA appears to provide no additional improvements to tensile strength values with CNF, HefCel or MC compared to materials without dispersion additive. The presence of 3% CNF gave about 6% increase in tensile strength at break compared to PLA-DA without fibers (54.5 MPa vs. 51.5 MPa). 5% of HefCel-DA and MC-DA decreased the tensile strength by 4–6% compared to composite materials without DA. When the modulus of fiber materials with DA is compared to PLA-DA, there is an 11% to 13% increase in results with all fibers from 3480 MPa to over 3800 MPa, which indicates the stiffening effect of DA-containing materials due to the fibers. The same effect on the modulus was also observed when dispersion additive VF was used in combination with HefCel and MC. A 20% increase in modulus was observed with HefCel-VF and a 9% increase with MC-VF compared to PLA-DA. High modulus with HefCel-VF (4179 MPa) may indicate a reaction between fiber and polymer in addition to the improved dispersion presented in Figure 3. The strengthening of the dispersing additive VF containing HefCel can also be seen as an 8% higher tensile strength at break compared to HefCel-DA. The different effect of VF in HefCel and MC may be due to different surface area of fibers. HefCel has more surface area compared to MC thus providing more space for VF to react when applied on the fiber surface. The actual surface area of HefCel nanofibrillar material was not measured. Literature represents surface area for bleached softwood-based cellulose nanofibrils prepared with enzymatic method 304 m^2/g [42] and without enzymes 195 m^2/g [43]. According to SEM-pictures and fiber length, HefCel is nano-size material and is assumed to have larger specific surface area than MC (40.8 m^2/g) [30]. Due to the small amount of fibers and additives in the polymer, also the actual reaction of VF between fibrils and polymer could not be verified by FTIR and only secondary indication through the mechanical results was used.

No significant difference between dissolving pulp CNF or kraft pulp CNF was observed in the tensile strength results in PLA composites. There was only a slight indication that kraft pulp CNF could be better for this purpose. Furthermore, no significant difference between CNF and HefCel was found in the tensile strength results.

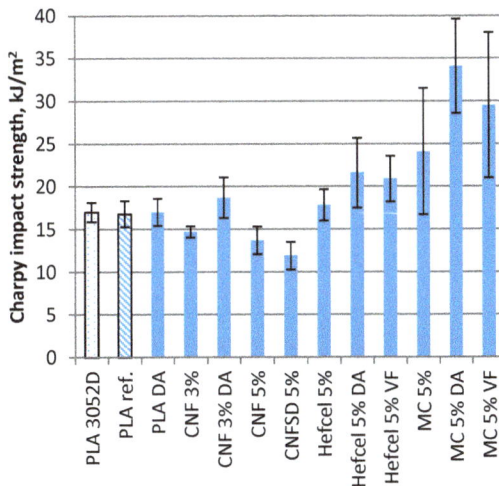

Figure 7. Charpy impact strength (unnotched) results for injection molded PLA composites with cellulosic fiber content of 3% or 5%.

The Charpy impact strength results in Figure 7 show no difference for neat PLA, after compounding (PLA ref.) or for PLA with DA. The addition of CNF (3% or 5%) and CNFSD (5%) caused 14–30% reduction in impact strength in comparison to PLA ref., which may be due to poor fibril dispersion. However the addition of pure HefCel increased the impact strength by 5% (from 16.8 to 17.8 kJ/m^2) even with poor fibril dispersion. Pure MC addition had a clear positive effect on impact strength, as indicated by a 42% increase (from 16.8 to 24.1 kJ/m^2), which may also have been partly due to better fiber dispersion of MC to PLA compared to nanofibers. The DA addition had a small positive effect on the CNF results probably due to improved dispersion. The same effect of DA can be seen for HefCel as a 27% increase in impact strength and for MC as a 100% increase in impact strength (from 17.0 to 34.1 kJ/m^2). VF addition has a 17% positive effect on impact strength with HefCel (from 17.8 to 20.9 kJ/m^2) and a 74% increase with MC (from 17.0 to 29.5 kJ/m^2). The smaller effect of VF may also be due to the fact that DA addition to fiber was double compared to VF. Part of this impact strength increase may come from improved dispersion, and it appears that the aspect ratio also has an impact on dispersion effectiveness. The highest impact strength was obtained with MC with very good dispersion to PLA, and the second best was with HefCel with improved dispersion due to dispersing agents. DA improved the dispersion of CNF and gave slightly better impact strength results compared to composite without DA. However, there are still challenges to disperse the hydrophilic nanofibrillous material in hydrophobic PLA polymer.

The higher variance in impact strength results of MC containing composites may be due to their lower aspect ratio compared to nanomaterials and poor connection to the polymer matrix, which can be seen in Figure 5C.

4. Conclusions

In this study, cellulose nanofibrils (CNF and CNFSD) and high-consistency HefCel nanocellulose were prepared and their effects on PLA–cellulose composites were studied. Commercial microcellulose (MC) was used as comparison for nanocelluloses. The target was to explore the effects of these nanomaterials in thermoplastic PLA composites when used in small amounts of 3% to 5%. In the processing we used thermoplastic processes such as compounding and injection molding. We appreciated the challenges that may occur during the thermoplastic processing and in obtaining efficient dispersion of hydrophilic cellulosic material to hydrophobic polymer. A two-stage compounding process was used to improve the cellulosic material dispersion into polymer matrix. In addition, in order to improve the fiber dispersion to PLA, two different long alkyl chain dispersion-improving additives were introduced on the fiber before compounding with PLA. One of them, VF, was also able to cross-link fibers and polymers.

As a result it was found that the introduction of 3% to 5% cellulosic nanomaterial to PLA without dispersing additives provided no improvement in tensile strength at yield, modulus or elongation of PLA. However the tensile strength at break was improved 4%–11%. The best result without dispersing additives was obtained using 3% CNF in PLA. There was a 4%–28% reduction in the modulus compared to reference PLA. The highest reduction in modulus occurred when the dispersing additive DA was used without fibers. However when the dispersing additive was changed to a more reactive additive, VF, and the matrix was loaded with HefCel, the modulus increased by 20% compared to PLA-DA. This indicated toughening of fiber-PLA composites and a reaction between the fiber and the polymer matrix. A higher effect on modulus was observed with HefCel due to its greater surface area compared to MC.

The impact strength results showed 14–30% reduction when CNF and CNFSD were used without additives. No clear effect was observed with HefCel without additives. MC dispersed most easily on PLA and gave significantly better impact strength results compared to nanocellulose material. A 42% increase with MC was observed indicating the positive effect of good dispersion, but also indicating the effect of fiber dimensions on strength properties. The filler type fiber, MC, with its low aspect ratio, gave the best results for impact strength and even HefCel, with its wide variation of fiber lengths and fibrillation degree, gave better results than CNF. The improved dispersion due to the dispersion additives DA and VF improved impact strength with all the fibers. The reactive additive VF was able to increase impact strength when used at only 10 w-% on the fiber surface. This also indicates that the reactive additive VF is the more effective additive for cellulosic fiber in PLA composites than pure dispersing agents without the ability to cross-link fibers and polymers.

According to these results, there were no significant differences between dissolving pulp CNF and kraft pulp CNF in the tensile strength results in PLA composites. There was only slight indication that kraft pulp CNF could be better for this purpose. We observed that HefCel was easier to process and disperse in PLA than CNF, and that HefCel gave slightly better overall mechanical results than CNF. However, when the surface of nanocellulose can be modified for improved dispersion to polymers, there is more potential to further improve the PLA properties even at low dosages below 5%. This opens new potential uses for PLA in biomedical devices and implants in applications in which improved strength is needed. Especially in 3D-printing with PLA filament, there are challenges in the strength properties of thin-walled and structured parts due to the lack of pressure in manufacturing. Thus, improvements in inherent material strength are needed.

Acknowledgments: The authors thank Upi Anttila, Mirja Nygård, Ulla Salonen and Katja Pettersson for performing the characterization and processing work. This research received no specific grant from any funding agency in the public, commercial or not-for-profit sectors.

Author Contributions: Jaakko Pere was responsible for the HefCel nanocellulose and characterization. Panu Lahtinen was responsible for the production of the other nacellulose grades and their characterization. Kirsi Immonen was responsible of the plastic processing and composite testing as well main responsible for writing of this paper.

Conflicts of Interest: The authors declare no conflict of interest.

References

1. Mohanty, A.K.; Misra, M.; Drzal, L.T. Sustainable Bio-Composites from Renewable Resources: Opportunities and Challenges in the Green Materials World. *J. Polym. Environ.* **2002**, *10*, 19–26. [CrossRef]
2. Lovett, J.; de Bie, F. Corbion Whitepaper Sustainable Sourcing of Feedstocks for Bioplastics. 2016. Available online: www.corbion.com/bioplastics (accessed on 8 November 2017).
3. Masutani, K.; Kimura, Y. PLA Synthesis. From the Monomer to the Polymer. In *Poly(Lactic Acid) Science and Technology: Processing, Properties, Additives and Applications*; RSC Polymer Chemistry Series No. 12; The Royal Society of Chemistry: Cambridge, UK, 2015; Chapter 1.
4. Sahari, J.; Sapuan, S.M. Natural fibre reinfroced biodegradable polymer composites. *Rev. Adv. Mater. Sci.* **2011**, *30*, 166–174.
5. Oksman, K.; Skrivfars, M.; Selin, J.-F. Natural fibres as reinforcements in polylactic acid (PLA) composites. *Compos. Sci. Technol.* **2003**, *63*, 1317–1324. [CrossRef]
6. Tawakkal, I.S.M.A.; Talib, R.A.; Abdan, K.; Ling, C.N. Mechanical and physical properties of Kenaf-derived cellulose (KDC)-filled polylactic acid (PLA) composites. *BioResources* **2012**, *7*, 1643–1655. [CrossRef]
7. Huda, M.S.; Drzal, L.T.; Misra, M.; Mohanty, A.K. Wood-Fiber-Reinforced Poly(lactic acid) Composites: Evaluation of the Physicomechanical and Morphological Properties. *J. Appl. Polym. Sci.* **2006**, *102*, 4856–4869. [CrossRef]
8. Mathew, A.P.; Oksman, K.; Sain, M. Mechanical Properties of Biodegradable Composites from Poly Lactic Acid (PLA) and Microcrystalline Cellulose (MCC). *J. Appl. Polym. Sci.* **2005**, *97*, 2014–2025. [CrossRef]
9. Vehovec, T.; Gartner, A.; Planinšek, O.; Obreza, A. Influence of different types of commercially available microcrystalline cellulose on degradation of perindopril erbumine and enalapril maleate in binary mixtures. *Acta Pharm.* **2012**, *62*, 515–528. [CrossRef] [PubMed]
10. Kalia, S.; Dufresne, A.; Cherian, B.M.; Kaith, B.S.; Avérous, L.; Njuguna, J.; Nassiopoulus, E. Cellulose-Based Bio- and nanocomposites: A Review. *Int. J. Polym. Sci.* **2011**, *2011*, 837875. [CrossRef]
11. Lee, K.-Y.; Aitomäki, Y.; Berglund, L.A.; Oksman, K.; Bismarck, A. On the use of nanocellulose as reinforcement in polymer matrix composites. *Compos. Sci. Technol.* **2014**, *105*, 15–27. [CrossRef]

12. Henze, H.-P. *From Nanocellulose Science toward Applications PulPaper 2010*; Conference presentation VTT Technical Research Center of Finland: Helsinki, Finland, 2010.
13. Ketabchi, M.R.; Khalid, M.; Ratnam, C.T.; Walwekar, R. Mechanical and thermal properties of polylactic acid composites reinforced with cellulose nanoparticles extracted from kenaf fibre. *Mater. Res. Express* **2016**, *3*, 125301. [CrossRef]
14. Jonoobi, M.; Harun, J.; Mathew, A.P.; Oksman, K. Mechanical properties of cellulose nanofiber (CNF) reinforced polylactic acid (PLA) prepared by twin screw extrusion. *Compos. Sci. Technol.* **2010**, *70*, 1742–1747. [CrossRef]
15. Islam, M.T.; Alam, M.M.; Zoccola, M. Review on modification of nanocellulose for application in composites. *Int. J. Innov. Res. Sci. Eng. Technol.* **2013**, *2*, 5444–5451.
16. Song, Z.; Xiao, H.; Zhao, Y. Hydrophobic-modified nano-cellulose fiber/PLA biodegradable composites for lowering water vapor transmission rate (WVTR) of paper. *Carbohydr. Polym.* **2014**, *111*, 442–448. [CrossRef] [PubMed]
17. Robles, E.; Urruzola, I.; Labidi, J.; Serrano, L. Surface-modified nano-cellulose as reinforcement in poly(lactic acid) to conform new composites. *Ind. Crops Prod.* **2015**, *71*, 44–53. [CrossRef]
18. Lönnberg, H.; Zhou, Q.; Brumer, H.; Teeri, T.T.; Malmström, E.; Hult, A. Grafting of Cellulose Fibers with Poly(ε-caprolactone) and Poly(L-lactic acid) via Ring-Opening Polymerization. *Biomacromolecules* **2006**, *7*, 2178–2185. [CrossRef] [PubMed]
19. Ng, H.-M.; Sin, L.T.; Bee, S.-T.; Tee, T.T.; Rahmat, A.R. A Review of Nanocellulose Polymer Composites Characteristics and Challenges. *Polym. Plast. Technol. Eng.* **2016**, *56*, 687–731. [CrossRef]
20. Lu, Y.; Calderón, C.M.; Lara-Curzio, E.; Ozcan, S. Improved mechanical properties of polylactide nanocomposites-reinforced with cellulose nanofibrils through interfacial engineering via amine-functionalization. *Carbohydr. Polym.* **2015**, *131*, 208–217. [CrossRef] [PubMed]
21. Bulota, M.; Kreitsmann, K.; Hughes, M.; Paltakari, J. Acetylated mcrofibrillated cellulose as a toughening agent in poly(lactic acid). *J. Appl. Polym. Sci.* **2012**, *126*, E448–E457. [CrossRef]
22. Oksman, K.; Aitomäki, Y.; Mathew, A.P.; Siqueira, G.; Zhou, Q.; Butylina, S.; Tanpichai, S.; Zhou, X.; Hooshmand, S. Review of the recent developments in cellulose nanocomposite processing. *Compos. Part A* **2016**, *83*, 2–18. [CrossRef]
23. Evonik AROSURF PA 780: Highly Absorbent, VOC-Free, Cuts Impact on Fluff Pulp Absorbency, Capacity. Available online: http://www.paperindustrymag.com/issues/Feb11/evonik.html (accessed on 26 November 2017).
24. Buong, W.C.; Nor, A.I.; Yoon, Y.T.; Yuet, Y.L. Epoxidized Vegetable Oils Plasticized Poly(lactic acid) Biocomposites: Mechanical, Thermal and Morphology Properties. *Molecules* **2014**, *19*, 16024–16038. [CrossRef]
25. Miao, S.; Liu, K.; Wang, P.; Su, Z.; Zhang, S. Preparation and Characterization of Epoxidized Soybean Oil-Based Paper Composite as Potential Water-Resistant Materials. *J. Appl. Polym. Sci.* **2015**, *132*, 41575. [CrossRef]
26. May, C.A. (Ed.) *Epoxy Resins, Chemistry and Technology*, 2nd ed.; Cellulose Fibres; CRC Press: New York, NY, USA, 1988; Chapter 11; p. 960.
27. Ansari, F.; Galland, S.; Johansson, M.; Plummer, C.J.G.; Berglund, L.A. Cellulose nanofiber network for moisture stable, strong and ductile biocomposites and increased epoxy curing rate. *Compos. Part A* **2014**, *63*, 35–44. [CrossRef]
28. Ingeo PLA 3052D Technical Data Sheet. Available online: http://www.natureworksllc.com/~/media/Files/NatureWorks/Technical-Documents/Technical-Data-Sheets/TechnicalDataSheet_3052D_injection-molding_pdf.pdf (accessed on 26 October 2017).
29. Virtanen, S.; Wikström, L.; Immonen, K.; Anttila, U.; Retulainen, E. Cellulose kraft pulp reinforced polylactic acid (PLA) composites: Effect of fibre moisture content. *AIMS Mater. Sci.* **2016**, *3*, 756–769. [CrossRef]
30. Chemical Trading Guide. Available online: http://www.guidechem.com/reference/dic-15945.html (accessed on 20 September 2017).
31. Arosurf Softness Solutions for Tissue and Fluff Pulp, Product Overwiev, Evonik. Available online: http://www.tissueadditives.com/product/tissue-additives/Documents/Softness-solutions-for-tissue-and-fluff-pulp-EN.pdf (accessed on 15 February 2017).
32. *Arosurf PA 780 MSDS from Evonik*; Manufacturer Evonik: Essen, Germany.

33. Vikoflex 7190 Product Description, Arkema. Available online: http://www.arkemaepoxides.com/export/sites/epoxides/.content/medias/downloads/literature/vikoflex-7190.pdf (accessed on 26 October2017).

34. Lee, C.S.; Ooi, T.L.; Chuah, C.H. The Effect of Reaction Temperature on Retaining Oxirane Oxygen Contents in the Synthesis of Epoxidized Diethanolamides. *Am. J. Appl. Sci.* **2009**, *6*, 72–77. [CrossRef]

35. Kangas, H.; Lahtinen, P.; Sneck, A.; Saariaho, A.-M.; Laitinen, O.; Hellen, E. Characterization of fibrillated celluloses. A short review and evaluation of characteristics with a combination of methods. *Nordic Pulp Pap. Res. J.* **2014**, *29*, 129–143. [CrossRef]

36. J. Rettenmeier & Söhne. *Fibres for Construction Chemical Products 02/2014*; Product brochure. JRS Pharma, 2014. Available online: http://www.jrspharma.com (accessed on 2 February 2014).

37. Tábi, T.; Sajó, I.E.; Szabó, F.; Luyt, A.S.; Kovács, J.G. Crystalline structure of annealed polylactic acid and its relation to processing. *eXPRESS Polym. Lett.* **2010**, *4*, 659–688. [CrossRef]

38. Martin, C. Compounding PLA on Twin-screw: What Testing Reveals. *Plastics Technology*, 21 March 2014. Available online: http://www.ptonline.com/articles/compounding-pla-on-twin-screws-what-testing-reveals (accessed on 11 September 2017).

39. Courgneau, C.; Rusu, D.; Henneuse, C.; Ducruet, V.; Lacrampe, M.-F.; Krawczak, P. Characterisation of low-odour emissive polylactide/cellulose fibre biocomposites for car interior. *eXPRESS Polym. Lett.* **2013**, *7*, 787–804. [CrossRef]

40. Wang, Y.; Steinhoff, B.; Brinkmann, C.; Alig, I. IN-line monitoring of the thermal degradation of poly(L-lactic acid) during melt extrusion by UV-vis spectroscopy. *Polymer* **2008**, *49*, 1257–1265. [CrossRef]

41. Arjmandi, R.; Hassan, A.; Haafiz, M.K.M.; Zakaria, Z. Effects of Micro- and Nano-cellulose on Tensile and Morphological Properties of Montmorillonite Nanoclay Reinforced Polylactic Acid Nanocomposites. In *Nanoclay Reinforced Polymer Composites*; Jawaid, M., Qaiss, A., Bouhfid, R., Eds.; Engineering Materials; Springer: Singapore, 2016; pp. 103–125, ISBN 978-981-10-0950-1. [CrossRef]

42. Sehaqui, H.; Zhou, Q.; Ikkala, O.; Berglund, L.A. Strong and Tough Cellulose Nanopaper with High Specific Surface Area and Porosity. *Biomacromolecules* **2011**, *12*, 3638–3644. [CrossRef] [PubMed]

43. Spence, K.L.; Venditti, R.A.; Rojas, O.J.; Habibi, Y.; Pawlak, J.J. The effect of chemical composition on microfibrillar cellulose films from wood pulps: Water interactions and physical properties for packaging applications. *Cellulose* **2010**, *17*, 835–848. [CrossRef]

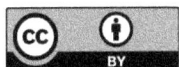

bioengineering

MDPI

Article

Encapsulation of Olive Leaves Extracts in Biodegradable PLA Nanoparticles for Use in Cosmetic Formulation

Maritina Kesente [1], Eleni Kavetsou [1], Marina Roussaki [1], Slim Blidi [2], Sofia Loupassaki [2], Sofia Chanioti [3], Paraskevi Siamandoura [3], Chrisoula Stamatogianni [4], Eleni Philippou [4], Constantine Papaspyrides [5], Stamatina Vouyiouka [5] and Anastasia Detsi [1,*

[1] Laboratory of Organic Chemistry, School of Chemical Engineering, National Technical University of Athens, Zografou Campus, 15780 Athens, Greece; maritina.kesente@gmail.com (M.K.); eleni29@hotmail.com (E.K.); mroussaki@outlook.com (M.R.)

[2] Department of Food Quality and Chemistry of Natural Products, Mediterranean Agronomic Institute of Chania (Centre International de Hautes Etudes Agronomiques Mediterraneennes), 73100 Chania, Crete, Greece; slim.blidi@maich.gr (S.B.); sofia@maich.gr (S.L.)

[3] Laboratory of Food Chemistry and Technology, School of Chemical Engineering, National Technical University of Athens, Zografou Campus, 15780 Athens, Greece; schanioti@gmail.com (S.C.); psiamandoura@hotmail.com (P.S.)

[4] Korres Natural Products, Drosini 3, 14452 Athens, Greece; chrisoula.stamatogianni@korres.com (C.S.); lena.philippou@korres.com (E.P.)

[5] Laboratory of Polymer Technology, School of Chemical Engineering, National Technical University of Athens, Zografou Campus, 15780 Athens, Greece; kp@cs.ntua.gr (C.P.); mvuyiuka@central.ntua.gr (S.V.)

* Correspondence: adetsi@chemeng.ntua.gr; Tel.: +30-210-772-4126

Academic Editor: Gary Chinga Carrasco
Received: 11 July 2017; Accepted: 7 September 2017; Published: 12 September 2017

Abstract: The aim of the current work was to encapsulate olive leaves extract in biodegradable poly(lactic acid) nanoparticles, characterize the nanoparticles and define the experimental parameters that affect the encapsulation procedure. Moreover, the loaded nanoparticles were incorporated in a cosmetic formulation and the stability of the formulation was studied for a three-month period of study. Poly(lactic acid) nanoparticles were prepared by the nanoprecipitation method. Characterization of the nanoparticles was performed using a variety of techniques: size, polydispersity index and ζ-potential were measured by Dynamic Light Scattering; morphology was studied using Scanning Electron Microscopy; thermal properties were investigated using Differential Scanning Calorimetry; whereas FT-IR spectroscopy provided a better insight on the encapsulation of the extract. Encapsulation Efficiency was determined indirectly, using UV-Vis spectroscopy. The loaded nanoparticles exhibited anionic ζ-potential, a mean particle size of 246.3 ± 5.3 nm (Pdi: 0.21 ± 0.01) and equal to 49.2%, while olive leaves extract release from the nanoparticles was found to present a burst effect at the first 2 hours. Furthermore, the stability studies of the loaded nanoparticles' cosmetic formulation showed increased stability compared to the pure extract, in respect to viscosity, pH, organoleptic characteristics, emulsions phases and grid.

Keywords: olive leaves; encapsulation; nanoparticles; delivery; biodegradable polymers; poly(lactic acid); natural antioxidants; cosmetics

---

1. Introduction

Oxidative stress is one of the main factors which cause skin aging [1–9]. For its defence, skin is equipped with enzymes and endogenous antioxidants in order to control the reactive oxygen species

(ROS) in balance and repair the damage caused by them. However, over time this defensive mechanism of the skin weakens [2,7]. Plant and herb extracts, rich in natural antioxidants, have been widely used in topical formulations to help skin's endogenous protection system from oxidative damage [2–4,6,8–12].

From ancient times in the regions around the Mediterranean Sea and the islands therein, olive leaves extract (OLE) has been widely used in folk medicine [13–16]. The main components of the leaves of the olive tree (*Olea europea*) are secoiridoids like oleuropein, ligostroside and dimethyloleuropein. Furthermore, they contain flavonoids (such as luteolin-7-glucoside, apigenin, diosmetin, rutin) as well as phenolic compounds (such as tyrosol, caffeic acid, vanillin, vanillic acid, hydrotyrosol) [15–17].

Among this plethora of active components, oleuropein is the main constituent of olive leaves extract, and presents a very broad variety of properties; anti-inflammatory, antimicrobial, antioxidant, cardio protective, antiviral, anti-ischemic and hypolipimedic [15–17]. Oleuropein can be hydrolysed to hydroxytyrosol and elenolic acid or to oleuropein aglycon and glucose [15,18].

In spite of this wide spectrum of properties, the use of olive leaves extract is limited due to its sensitivity to temperature, light and oxidation, while it presents low aqueous solubility and a bitter taste [19]. A way to overcome these limitations is to encapsulate the extract into biodegradable polymeric nanoparticles (NPs) [20–26]. In general, encapsulation strategies are being constantly developed in order to face a significant number of drawbacks when using pure active compounds systemically or topically. The main benefits are: (i) protection of encapsulated compounds from degradation and adverse environments; (ii) improvement of active compound physicochemical characteristics; (iii) controlled release; and (iv) precision targeting, all resulting in enhanced effectiveness and bioavailability.

Especially for the cosmetics and personal care markets, the topical application of the relevant formulations requires the successful delivery of active ingredients through the skin's lipid barrier, that is, *stratum corneum*; it is the upper 10–20 µm layer of the skin, being the first barrier in dermic diffusion with a structure similar to "plastic wrap" [20]. Transport through the *stratum corneum* is restricted to molecules of low molecular mass (<500 Da) and moderate lipophilicity (partition coefficients, log $K_{o/w}$ values between 1 and 3), having enough solubility in the liquid domain of the *stratum corneum* while still having sufficient hydrophilic nature to allow partitioning into the epidermis [27]. In healthy skins, loaded micro/nanocarriers penetrate into the *stratum corneum* and hair follicle canals, releasing the encapsulated ingredients there, with no evidence for the translocation of the entire particles [20,22,28–32].

In this study, the aim was to encapsulate the olive leaves extract in polymeric NPs, characterize the nanoparticles and define the experimental parameters that affect the encapsulation procedure. Moreover, the loaded nanoparticles were incorporated in a cosmetic formulation and the stability of the formulation was studied for a three-month period study. The polymer selected was poly(lactic acid) (PLA), which is an aliphatic polyester, lipophilic, biodegradable, biocompatible, commonly used in several clinical trials and approved by European regulatory authorities as well as FDA [24,26,29,33,34]. Finally, the emulsification-solvent evaporation technique was the chosen method for the preparation of the nanoparticles.

2. Materials and Methods

2.1. Materials

Olive tree (*Olea europaea*) leaves (1 kg) were collected from pesticide-free olive trees in the "Afidnes" region, belonged to the "Megaritiki" cultivar and were dried at room temperature, in the dark, for nine days. The dried leaf material obtained was 670.4 g. The PLA used presented viscosity-average molecular weight ($\overline{M_v}$) of 46,000 g/mol and was obtained from solid state hydrolysis of a commercial resin (PLI005, NaturePlast, Ifs, France) at 60 °C under acidic conditions (pH 3) [35]. Poly(vinyl alcohol) (PVA) (Alfa Aesar, Ward Hill, MA, USA), which was used as emulsion stabilizer, was of average molecular weight 88,000–97,000, 87–89% hydrolysed. All the organic solvents used were of analytical grade.

2.2. Methods

2.2.1. Preparation of Olive Leaves Extract (OLE)

The dried olive leaves were extracted with organic solvents of different polarity [15]. Briefly, dried leaves (100 g) were chopped and extracted with methanol (500 mL) for 3 days, in the dark, at room temperature. Afterwards the methanol extract was filtered and concentrated under reduced pressure. The residue was re-dissolved in an acetone-water solution (100 mL, 1:1) and washed with hexane (4 × 25 mL), chloroform (4 × 25 mL) and ethyl acetate (4 × 25 mL). The ethyl acetate extracts were combined and concentrated in vacuo (Figure 1). The solid residue (2.2 g) was collected and kept at 4 °C, in dark-coloured glass vials. The procedure was repeated for the rest of the dried material. Finally, from the 670.4 g of dried olive leaves a total amount of 14.8 g of extract was obtained (yield 2.2%).

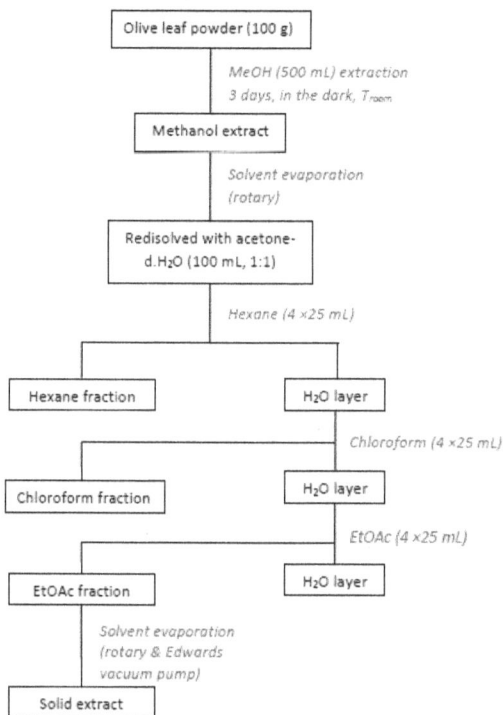

Figure 1. Experimental procedure for the preparation of olive leaves extract (OLE).

2.2.2. High-Performance Liquid Chromatography Analysis of Olive Leaves Extract

HPLC-analysis was performed on a HP 1100 Series gradient HPLC system (Agilent Technologies, Santa Clara, CA, USA) equipped with Class VP chromatography data station software, a SIL-10AF autosampler, a CTO-10AS column oven (251 °C), an SPD-10AV UV Visible detector and a diode array detector (DAD) (Hewlett-Packard, Waldbronn, Germany). A column (250 × 4.6 mm) packed with 5 μm particles Hypersil C18 (MZ 156 Analysentechnik, Mainz, Germany) was used. The elution solvents consisted of aqueous 6% acetic acid and 2 mM sodium acetate (solvent A) and acetonitrile (solvent B). Gradient elution: 0–25 min, 100–50% A and 0–50% B, flow rate 0.8 mL/min; 25–26 min, 50–0% A and 50–100% B, flow rate 0.8 mL/min; 26–27 min, 0% A and 100% B, flow rate 0.8–1.2 mL/min; 27–40 min, 0% A and 100% B, flow rate 1.2 mL/min; 40–41 min, 0–100% A and 100–0% B, flow rate

1.2–0.8 mL/min, 41–45 min, 100% A and 0% B, flow rate 0.8 mL/min The injection volume was 20 μL and DAD signals were recorded at 280 nm (oleuropein) and 330 nm (vanillin and rutin) [36].

The identification of polyphenols in olive leaves extract was performed by comparison of retention times of standard solutions and confirmed with characteristic spectra using the diode array detector.

The quantification of identified phenolic compounds was carried out by external 6-point calibration pure standards. The linearity of the calibration curves was verified in each case by analysis in triplicate of standard solutions containing 100–1000 μg/mL for oleuropein, 0.08–0.8 μg/mL for vanillin and 152–1520 μg/mL for rutin. The concentration of polyphenols was expressed in mg/mL.

2.2.3. Luminol Chemiluminescence Assay

A chemiluminescence method was used as described by [37]. One millilitre of borate buffer solution (50 mM, pH 9) containing $CoCl_2 \cdot 6H_2O$ (8.4 mg/mL) and EDTA (2.63 mg/mL) was first mixed with 0.1 mL of luminol solution (0.56 mM in borate buffer 50 mM, pH 9) and vortexed for 15 s. All samples were dissolved in DMSO. An aliquot of 0.025 mL of sample and 0.025 mL of H_2O_2 aqueous solution (5.4 mM) were then added into the test tube, the mixture was rapidly transferred into a glass cuvette, and the CL intensity (Io) was recorded. The instantaneous reduction in Io elicited by the addition of the sample was recorded as I and the ratio (Io/I) was calculated and plotted vs. concentration (mg/mL) of the sample. The concentration of sample (IC_{50}), which is required to decrease Io intensity by 50%, was also calculated. For all measurements, a LS55 Luminescence Spectrometer-Perkin Elmer was used, keeping the lamp off and using only the photomultiplier of the apparatus. All determinations were carried out at least in triplicate and values were averaged and given along with the standard deviation (±SD).

2.2.4. Preparation of PLA Nanoparticles (PLA NPs)

PLA nanoparticles were prepared by the nanoprecipitation method. For a 20% drug loading (mass of OLE per mass of polymer used, w/w) PLA (20 mg) was dissolved in acetone (2 mL), and then mixed with an OLE-MeOH solution (4 mg of OLE in 2 mL MeOH). Subsequently, the organic solution was injected in an aqueous solution of PVA (1% w/v). The emulsion was left in magnetic stirring for 10 min at 250 rpm and then in shaker at 90 rpm, overnight, for evaporation of the solvents. Afterwards, the nanoparticles formed were recovered by centrifugation. An initial centrifugation at 17,000 rpm for 20 min at 10 °C was performed. The resulting supernatant (S1) was recovered and stored in a dark-coloured container. The nanoparticle sediment was re-suspended in deionized H_2O and centrifuged under the same conditions (17,000 rpm, 20 min and 10 °C) and the supernatant (S2) was recovered and stored. The NPs obtained were re-dispersed in doubly distilled (dd) H_2O (1 mL) and stored at 4 °C. Unloaded (blank) NPs were prepared using the same procedure without the addition of the OLE.

2.2.5. 1,1-Diphenyl-2-picryl-hydrazyl (DPPH) Radical Scavenging Assay

The DPPH method was used to determine antioxidant activity of olive leaves extract. Briefly, a solution of DPPH in methanol (0.1 M) was prepared and added (0.1 mL) to samples of different concentration OLE solution in methanol (3.9 mL, 0.03–0.4 mg/mL) and allowed to react in the dark, at room temperature. After 20 min, the absorbance values (Abs_{sample}) were measured at 515 nm against a blank sample (Abs_{blank}). The remaining free radical DPPH in percent was calculated using Equation (1):

$$\%RemDPPH = \frac{Abs_{sample}}{Abs_{blank}} \times 100 \tag{1}$$

In order to calculate the IC_{50} value, a graph of the remaining DPPH (% RemDPPH) against the sample concentration (C_{sample}) was plotted.

2.2.6. Total Phenolic Content

The total phenolic content of the OLE was determined by using the Folin-Ciocalteu method with some modifications. 100 µL of OLE or standard solution of Gallic acid (50, 100, 150, 250, 500 ppm) in MeOH were added to 500 µL of a Folin-Ciocalteu solution, followed by 1.5 mL of sodium carbonate solution. The reagents were mixed and incubated for 30 min in the dark at room temperature. Afterwards, the absorbance was measured at 765 nm in triplicate. The average data was interpolated in a gallic acid calibration curve and the total phenolic content was expressed as mg Gallic Acid Equivalents (GAE)/g of dry extract.

2.3. Nanoparticles (NPs) Characterization

2.3.1. Determination of Particle Size, Pdi and ζ-Potential

Mean particle size, polydispersity index (Pdi) and ζ-potential of loaded and blank nanoparticles were determined via Dynamic Light Scattering (DLS) technique, using a Zetasizer Nano ZS (Malvern Instruments, Malvern, UK). The samples were prepared by dispersing 0.2 mL of nanoparticle suspension in dd. H_2O (4 mL) resulting in off-white opaque aqueous suspensions. All measurements were performed in triplicate, at $25 \pm 1\ °C$ and results were reported as mean $\pm$ standard deviation (SD).

2.3.2. Morphology

The surface morphology of the nanoparticles prepared was examined using Scanning Electron Microscopy (SEM). The analysis was performed on a NanoSEM 230 (FEI Company, Hillsboro, OR, USA) equipped with an Everhart-Thornley Detector (ETD) and a Through Lens Detector (TLD). In order to secure conductivity of the surface for clear imaging, gold sputtering was applied with a nominal thickness of 7 nm using an EMS 550X Sputter Coater (Hatfield, PA, USA).

2.3.3. Encapsulation Efficiency Determination

Encapsulation efficiency (EE%) was determined indirectly using UV-Vis spectroscopy. For that purpose, the supernatants (S1, S2) from the centrifugation step of the preparation of loaded NPs were decanted and their UV-Vis spectrum was obtained at 287 nm. The concentration of OLE was calculated using the calibration curve shown in Figure 2.

The percent EE was then calculated using Equation (2):

$$EE\% = \frac{\text{Tatal amount of OLE(mg)} - \text{Free amount of OLE in superna tan ts(mg)}}{\text{Total initial amount of OLE(mg)}} \times 100 \qquad (2)$$

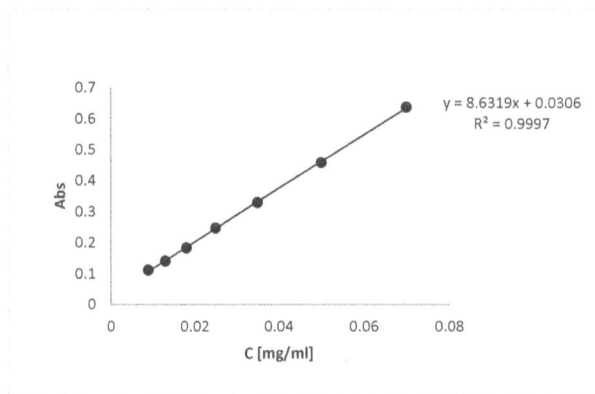

Figure 2. Calibration curve of OLE for the determination of EE% and in vitro release profile.

2.3.4. Thermal Properties

Differential scanning calorimetry (DSC) analysis was conducted on samples of OLE, PLA and OLE-loaded NPs using a Mettler DSC 1 STARe System® (Mettler Toledo, Columbus, OH, USA). The specimens were heated from 30 to 170 °C, with a heating rate of 10 °C/min, under nitrogen flow (20 mL/min). The mass fraction crystallinity of the PLA (pure PLA, blank NPs) was calculated by Equation (3):

$$x_c = \frac{\Delta H}{\Delta H_0} \times 100 \tag{3}$$

where, ΔH is the heat of fusion of the sample (J/g) and ΔH_0 is the heat of fusion of 100% crystalline polymer (J/g). ΔH_0 is considered equal to 93.1 J/g [35].

2.3.5. FT-IR Spectroscopy

FT-IR spectra of the OLE, the blank NPs and the OLE-NPs were obtained on a JASCO 4200 (JASCO Inc., Easton, MD, USA) using the ATR technique in the scanning range of 650–4000 cm^{-1}.

2.3.6. In Vitro Release Study

Preliminary in vitro release of OLE from the polymeric NPs was investigated using UV-vis spectroscopy, following a slightly modified literature procedure [38]. Experiments were carried out by suspending 12 mg of loaded nanoparticles into 4.2 mL of phosphate buffer (pH 5.6). The temperature was set at 37 ± 0.5 °C and the magnetic stirrer at 120 rpm. At appropriate intervals, the suspension was centrifuged at 12,000 rpm for 15 min. The supernatants were removed after every centrifugation and the precipitated nanoparticles were re-suspended in 4.2 mL of fresh buffer and were then put back in the magnetic stirring. The amount of OLE released in supernatants was inferred from the calibration curve used for the EE% calculation, in triplicate.

2.3.7. Incorporation of OLE-NPs in Cosmetic Formulation and Stability Studies

The pure extract and OLE-loaded NPs were incorporated in an o/w base cream and stability tests were performed: for a 3-month period, samples were stored at different temperatures (5, 25, 40 °C and freeze-thaw cycles 5–45 °C) and were examined at regular intervals. The tested parameters of the stability studies were: viscosity, pH, organoleptic characteristics, emulsions phases and grid. The main characteristics of the o/w base cream used for this study were: light beige-yellow cream of characteristic scent, pH: 5.47, viscosity (25 °C): 20450cSt.

3. Results and Discussion

3.1. Antioxidant Activity of Olive Leaves Extract (OLE), PLA and OLE-NPs

Taking the multifactorial character of oxidative stress into account, we decided to evaluate the in vitro antioxidant activity of OLE, using two different antioxidant assays: (a) the radical scavenging ability of OLE was tested against the 1,1-diphenyl-2-picryl-hydrazyl (DPPH) stable free radical; and (b) the ability of OLE, OLE-NPs and PLA to scavenge hydrogen peroxide (H_2O_2), a very important reactive oxygen species the production of which is increased during skin aging, was tested using the luminol chemiluminescence method. Moreover, the total phenolic content of the OLE was determined. Quercetin, a potent antioxidant flavonoid which is used in many cosmetic formulations was used as the reference compound. The results are presented in Table 1.

The results show that the OLE prepared in this study is a potent DPPH radical and H_2O_2 scavenger, although less effective than quercetin, therefore it constitutes a promising additive for cosmetic applications. PLA does not show important antioxidant activity (IC_{50} 36.45 mg/mL), whereas the OLE-NPs present a significantly higher antioxidant activity than PLA (IC_{50} 4.37 mg/mL).

Table 1. Antioxidant activity of olive leaves extract (OLE), poly(lactic acid) (PLA) and OLE-loaded nanoparticles (OLE-NPs). Quercetin was used as a reference antioxidant.

	DPPH Radical Scavenging Ability IC$_{50}$ (mg/mL)	Total Phenolic Content GAE (mg$_{gallic\ acid}$/g$_{of\ dry\ extract}$)	H$_2$O$_2$ Scavenging Ability IC$_{50}$ (mg/mL)
OLE	0.283	391.7	0.254 ± 0.007
PLA	n.t. *	n.t.	36.45 ± 2.03
OLE-NPs	n.t.	n.t.	4.37 ± 0.12
Quercetin	0.073	n.t.	0.049 ± 0.003

* n.t. = not tested.

3.2. Phytochemical Profile of Olive Leaves Extract

The polyphenolic profile of olive leaves' extract obtained from "Megaritiki" cultivar was determined using HPLC. A typical chromatogram of the olive leaves' extract is given in Figure 3. Oleuropein, vanillin and rutin were identified by comparison of the UV-VIS spectra of the peaks separated by HPLC (Figure 3). Table 2 shows the retention times, the calibration equations with the corresponding coefficients of determination, the variation coefficients obtained in the consecutive analysis of 10 samples of each compound and the concentration of oleuropein, vanillin and rutin in OLE.

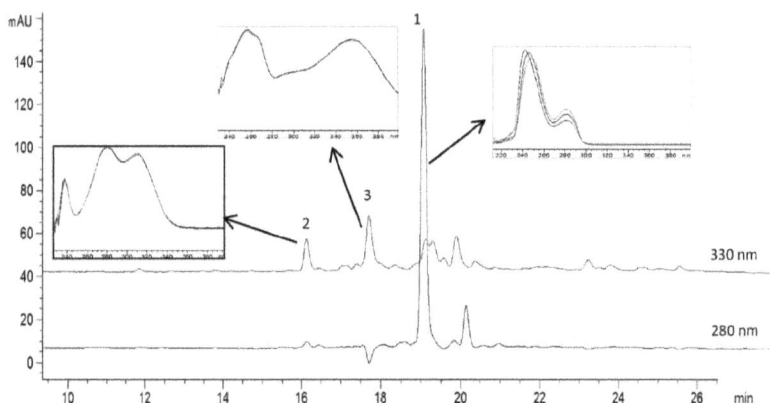

Figure 3. HPLC chromatogram of olive leaves extract (OLE). The peaks that were identified are: 1 oleuropein, 2 vanillin and 3 rutin. The UV-VIS spectra corresponding to the main polyphenols components are shown above the chromatogram.

Table 2. High-performance liquid chromatography (HPLC) of olive leaves extract (OLE): validation parameters and quantification of the identified phenolic compounds.

Phenolic Compound	Retention Time (min)	Variation Coefficient (%) for Retention Time (n = 10)	Calibration Equation	Variation Coefficient (%) for Concentration (n = 10)	C (mg/mL)	% in OLE
Oleuropein	18.4	0.46	y = 5730.3x − 98.3 R^2 = 0.9962	0.80	0.347 ± 0.035	69.5
Vanillin	15.0	0.19	y = 1755.5x + 3.51 R^2 = 1	0.15	0.005 ± 0.001	1.06
Rutin	17.1	0.44	y = 824.9x − 1.53 R^2 = 1	0.31	0.020 ± 0.005	4.03

The quantitative determination of oleuropein, vanillin and rutin in OLE was achieved with a retention time of 18.4, 15.0 and 17.1 min, respectively. The sensitivity of the method was evaluated by determining the limits of detection (LODs) (signal-to-noise ratio (s/n) = 3) and the limits of quantification (LOQs) (s/n = 10). High coefficients of determination were obtained for all three standards (R^2 = 0.9962, 1, 1 for oleuropein, vanillin and rutin, respectively) indicating good linearity response of the method proposed with LODs/LOQs (μg/mL) equal to: 44/135, 0.06/0.15 and 66/187 for oleuropein, vanillin and rutin, respectively.

The main phytochemical identified was the secoiridoid oleuropein (69.5%), as expected, because olive leaves are the richest source of this compound. Oleuropein content in OLEs can vary depending on plant maturation, cultivar type and harvest time. For example, Mourtzinos et al. found 90.2% oleuropein in the olive leaves extract obtained following exactly the same extraction procedure but another cultivar ("Kalamon") harvested in the Thermopylae region (Central Greece) [15]. Small amounts of the flavonoid rutin and vanillin (4% and 1%, respectively) were also present in the studied extract. Rutin has been reported to be present in olive leaves extract obtained from the same Greek cultivar [39] whereas vanillin is a common phenolic compound in other Greek cultivars but, to our knowledge, has not been reported from the OLE extract from "Megaritiki" cultivar.

3.3. Nanoparticles (NPs) Characterization and Encapsulation Efficiency (EE%)

Particle size and polydispersity are the most important characteristics of nanocarrier systems. They determine the targeting ability of NPs and toxicity, while they greatly influence the drug loading, drug release and the stability of NPs [31,40]. In the present study, PLA NPs prepared in different batches showed mean particle size in the range of 166.8–291.2 nm and polydispersity indices between 0.08–0.26, revealing a homogenous nanoparticle population (Table 3).

The morphology of discrete spherical polymeric nanoparticles was also verified by SEM indicating the effectiveness of the herein applied procedure to prepare OLE-loaded PLA nanospheres (Figure 4).

Table 3. Characterization of indicative batches of blank PLA nanoparticles (blank-NPs) and PLA nanoparticles loaded with oil leaves extract (OLE-loaded NPs): particle size, polydispersity index (Pdi), ζ-potential, encapsulation efficiency (EE).

	Size (nm)	Pdi	ζ-Potential (mV)	EE%
OLE-loaded NPs	246.3 ± 5.3	0.21 ± 0.01	−27.5 ± 0.12	49.2
Blank-NPs	220.6 ± 4.0	0.08 ± 0.00	−19.3 ± 0.74	-

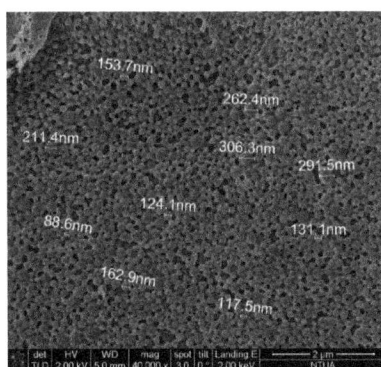

Figure 4. Scanning Electron Microscopy (SEM) image of PLA nanoparticles loaded with oil leaves extract (OLE-loaded NPs).

Zeta potential is also an important parameter in the characterization of NPs, since it measures the surface charge and gives information about suspension stability under defined conditions [24,31,41].

As can be observed in Table 3, the NPs prepared present negative ζ-potential values (-27.5 mV), which is indicative of a stable suspension without the tendency of aggregation. This value deviates from that of unloaded NPs (-19.3 mV), and this can be explained by the extract present on the surface of the NPs, as it is also shown in the FTIR-ATR spectra discussed below. Regarding the encapsulation efficiency of the extract, the loaded NPs showed a value of 49.2%. For comparison reasons, it can be cited at this point that higher EE value (82%) was reached by our group when using the same PLA grade as a carrier and a pure natural antioxidant (aureusidin) [24]. Obviously, the encapsulation of extracts, which are mixtures of compounds, presents a challenge regarding high EE values.

No quantification of residual methanol was performed in this study, as the main goal was to ensure the effective encapsulation of OLE extract to PLA nanoparticles, characterize the NPs and develop the encapsulation procedure. In the case that a commercial cosmetic product is going to be developed using these NPs, quantification of the residual methanol should definitely be performed in order to ensure that the product complies with international regulations.

3.4. Thermal Properties

DSC studies were performed in order to investigate the physical interactions between OLE and PLA in the formed nanoparticles. Different active substance/polymer combinations may coexist in the polymeric carriers, such as: (i) amorphous encapsulant in either an amorphous or a crystalline polymer and (ii) crystalline encapsulant in either an amorphous or a crystalline polymer [15,42–44]. Figure 5 shows the DSC thermograms of pure extract, pure PLA and loaded nanoparticles. The herein used PLA presented glass transition temperature (T_g) at 51.4 °C and double melting behaviour with a small endotherm at 130.6 °C and a stronger one on at 144.3 °C. The mass fraction crystallinity was calculated at 34%. The extract (OLE) exhibited a broad endotherm in the range of 92–121 °C, which, however, disappeared in the DSC curve of the loaded particles. The latter may indicate the homogenous dispersion or dissolution of OLE in the polymeric matrix, as it was also found in the case of embelin-loaded polycaprolactone samples [45]. Similarly, the endotherm of PLA polymer became much smoother appearing at slightly lower temperature (138 °C), demonstrating the prevention of polymer crystallization during the nanoparticles formation and the prevalence of matrix amorphous state. Finally, in the case of loaded NPs, an exothermic peak appeared at ca. 150 °C following polymer melting, which may be attributed to morphological changes and/or degradation occurred to the encapsulated extract.

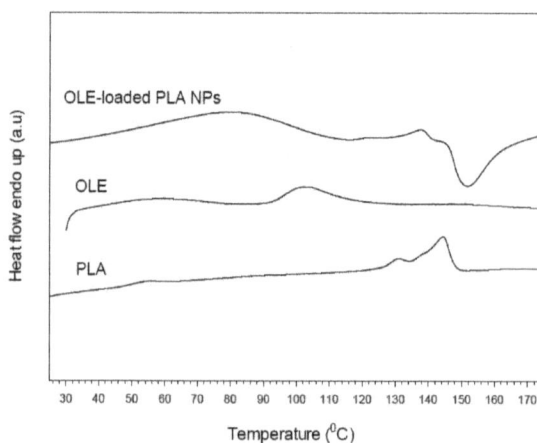

Figure 5. Differential scanning calorimetry (DSC) thermograms of pure poly(lactic acid) (PLA), olive leaves extract (OLE), and PLA nanoparticles loaded with oil leaves extract (OLE-loaded NPs).

3.5. FT-IR Spectroscopy

In order to obtain a better insight of the interaction between the encapsulated extract and PLA in the prepared NPs, the FT-IR (ATR) spectra of the free OLE, the polymer and the loaded NPs were obtained (Figure 6). The FT-IR spectrum of the pure extract is characterized by two absorption peaks at 1698.98 and 1629.11 cm^{-1}, owed to the C=O stretching of the carbonyl groups of oleuropein, rutin and vanillin or other flavonoids which are present in the extract. The band at 3299.51 cm^{-1} is attributed to O-H stretching whereas the strong absorptions at 1069.83 cm^{-1} and 1037.32 cm^{-1} should be attributed to the C-O stretching of the ester groups present in the aforementioned phytochemicals of the extract.

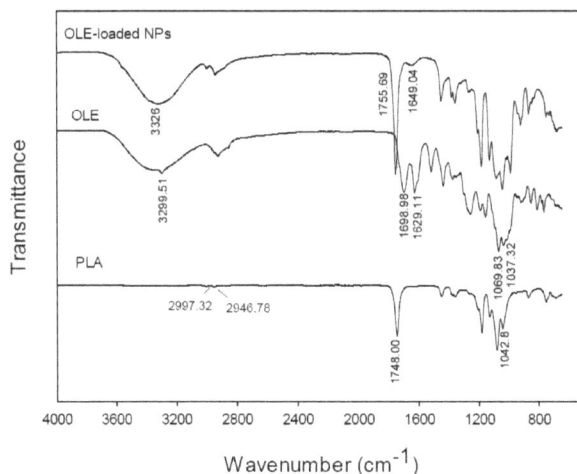

Figure 6. FT-IR (ATR) spectra of pure poly(lactic acid) (PLA), olive leaves extract (OLE), and PLA nanoparticles loaded with olive leaves extract (OLE-loaded NPs).

In the FT-IR spectrum of PLA, the most characteristic peaks appear at 2997.99 and 2950.82 cm^{-1} owing to C-H stretching from the main chain of PLA, 1746.01 cm^{-1} characteristic of C=O stretching from the carbonyl groups of the repeated ester units and 1081.61 cm^{-1} attributed to the C-C(=O)-O stretching from the ester units.

The spectrum of the OLE-loaded NPs shows mainly the absorptions owed to the PLA polymeric matrix, which in most cases are overlapping with those of the encapsulated OLE [23]. However, two significant observations can be made: (a) in the spectrum of OLE-NPs there is a strong broad band at 3326 cm^{-1} and a weak absorption peak at 1649.04 cm^{-1}, which can be attributed to the O-H stretching vibration of oleuropein as well as the other phytochemicals of the extract which are absorbed on the surface of the loaded NPs and are shifted in comparison to the spectrum of the pure extract (3299.51 and 1698.98, 1629.11 cm^{-1}, respectively); and (b) the peak owed to the C=O stretching of the carbonyl groups of PLA is shifted from 1746.01 cm^{-1} in the spectrum of pure PLA to 1755.69 cm^{-1} in the spectrum of OLE-NPs. It can be postulated that the shift in the wavenumbers is owed to the interactions of the phytochemicals of the encapsulated extract with the PLA matrix.

3.6. In Vitro Release Study

Preliminary in vitro release experiments were conducted in pH 5.6 at 37 ± 0.5 °C. This pH value was selected as it is the pH of healthy skin [46]. The release profile is depicted in Figure 7a,b. At t = 2 h a burst effect was observed in which a cumulative amount of 15.7% of OLE was released (Figure 7a). After that, it is obvious that OLE "escaped" at a constant rate from the NPs reaching almost 100% cumulative release after 168 h (7 days) (Figure 7b).

(a)

(b)

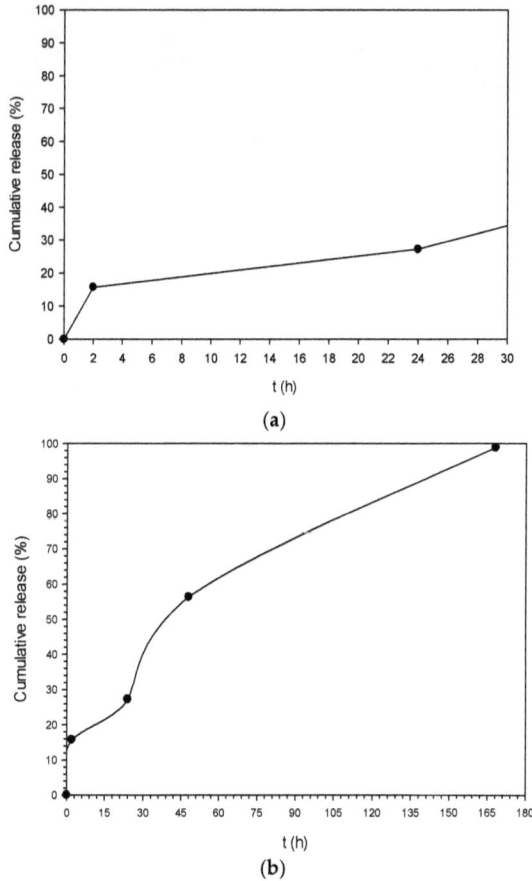

Figure 7. In vitro release profile of PLA nanoparticles loaded with oil leaves extract (OLE-loaded NPs) (pH 5.6, T = 37 °C). (**a**) 0–24 h; (**b**) 0–168 h.

3.7. Stability Studies

The results from the stability studies of the formulation incorporating the OLE-NPs prepared are shown in Tables 4 and 5. There were no significant differences between samples referring to scent, rheology and emulsion phases. The samples with OLE showed changes in the colour and pH, indications of reactions that could lead to instability. The browning which occurred was most probably caused by the oxidation of the extracts' polyphenols [10,19]. The results suggest that the formulation containing OLE-NPs is preferable since they do not affect the stability and appearance of the cosmetic emulsion.

Table 4. Results of the pH measurements during the stability studies.

pH Results		Freeze Cycles				Storage at 5 °C	Storage at 25 °C	Storage at 40 °C		
Sample	Initial Results	Day 7	Day 15	Day 21	Day 29	Month 3	Month 3	Month 1	Month 2	Month 3
o/w Base Cream	5.47	5.49	5.5	5.52	5.48	5.6	5.49	5.47	5.37	5.48
Base Cream with OLE-NPs	5.49	5.59	5.54	5.56	5.52	5.62	5.59	5.48	5.35	5.43
Base Cream with OLE	5.45	5.5	5.5	5.46	5.42	5.55	5.5	5.41	5.3	5.26

Table 5. Results of the viscosity measurements during the stability studies.

Viscosity Results [cSt]		Freeze Cycles				Storage at 5 °C	Storage at 25 °C	Storage at 40 °C		
Sample	Initial Results	Day 7	Day 15	Day 21	Day 29	Month 3	Month 3	Month 1	Month 2	Month 3
o/w Base Cream	20,450	47,600	48,532	38,501	39,231	30,598	33,032	40,922	39,163	34,870
Base Cream with OLE-NPs	20,219	46,813	47,408	38,612	39,688	30,703	32,760	41,224	37,817	35,268
Base Cream with OLE	17,319	45,314	45,347	38,614	40,302	29,623	32,814	39,602	39,084	34,286

4. Conclusions

The results of the current work demonstrated that the encapsulation of olive leaves extract in PLA NPs leads to nanoparticles-nanospheres with satisfactory characteristics, as initially observed in SEM images. The mean size of the particles formed was 246.3 ± 5.3 nm with satisfactory ζ-potential, polydispersity index and encapsulation efficiency. Moreover, based on the DSC and FT-IR studies, the olive leaves extract appeared to be protected inside the PLA matrix. The loaded NPs were successfully incorporated in a cosmetic emulsion without affecting its stability and appearance. Therefore, the encapsulation of sensitive polyphenolic extracts in biodegradable PLA nanoparticles provides the means to develop cosmetic formulations with advantageous characteristics.

Acknowledgments: The authors wish to cordially thank Professor Apostolos Kyritsis and Ph.D. student Stefanos Koutsoumpis for obtaining the SEM images.

Author Contributions: Anastasia Detsi and Stamatina Vouyiouka conceived and designed the experiments. Maritina Kesente, Eleni Kavetsou and Marina Roussaki performed the experiments and analyzed the data, under the supervision of Anastasia Detsi. Slim Blidi and Sofia Loupassaki performed the antioxidant activity experiments and analyzed the data. Sofia Chanioti and Paraskevi Siamandoura performed the HPLC analyses. Chrisoula Stamatogianni and Eleni Phillipou designed the stability studies and supervised Maritina Kesente while conducting the study. Maritina Kesente and Eleni Kavetsou wrote the paper with the suggestions/corrections of Anastasia Detsi, Stamatina Vouyiouka and Constantine Papaspyrides.

Conflicts of Interest: The authors declare no conflict of interest.

References

1. Afaq, F.; Mukhtar, H. Botanical antioxidants in the prevention of photocarcinogenesis and photoaging. *Exp. Dermatol.* **2006**, *15*, 678–684. [CrossRef] [PubMed]
2. Dtojiljkovic, D.; Pavlovic, D.; Arsic, I. Oxidative stress, skin aging and antioxidant therapy. *Sci. J. Fac. Med.* **2014**, *31*, 207–217.
3. Misaki, H. Role of antioxidants in the skin: Anti-aging effects. *J. Dermatol. Sci.* **2010**, *58*, 85–89. [CrossRef] [PubMed]
4. Miyachi, Y. Photoaging form an oxidative standpoint. *J. Dermatol. Sci.* **1995**, *9*, 79–86. [CrossRef]
5. Nishigori, C.; Hattori, Y.; Arima, Y.; Miyachi, Y. Photoaging and oxidative stress. *Exp. Dermatol.* **2003**, *12*, 18–21. [CrossRef] [PubMed]
6. Pandel, R.; Poljsak, B.; Godic, A.; Dahmane, R. Skin photoaging and the role of antioxidants in its prevention. *ISRN Dermatol.* **2013**, *2013*. [CrossRef] [PubMed]
7. Peres, P.S.; Terra, V.A.; Guarnier, F.A.; Cecchini, R.; Cecchini, A.L. Photoaging and chronological aging profile: Understanding oxidation of the skin. *J. Photochem. Photobiol. B* **2011**, *103*, 93–97. [CrossRef] [PubMed]
8. Ratz-Lyko, A.; Arct, J.; Pytkowska, K. Methods for evaluation of cosmetic antioxidant capacity. *Skin Res. Technol.* **2012**, *18*, 421–430. [CrossRef] [PubMed]
9. Zillich, O.V.; Schweiggert-Weisz, U.; Eisner, P.; Kerscher, M. Polyphenols as active ingredients for cosmetic products. *Int. J. Cosmet. Sci.* **2015**, *37*, 455–464. [CrossRef] [PubMed]
10. Ali, A.; Akhtar, N.; Mumtaz, A.M.; Khan, M.S.; Iqbal, F.M.; Zaidi, S.S. In vivo skin irritation potential of a cream containing Moringa oleifera leaf extract. *Afr. J. Pharm. Pharmacol.* **2013**, *7*, 289–293. [CrossRef]
11. Almeida, I.F.; Valentao, P.; Andradr, P.B.; Seabra, R.M.; Pereira, T.M.; Amaral, M.H.; Costa, P.C.; Bahia, M.F. In vivo skin irritation potential of a potential of a Castanea sativa (Chestnut) leaf extract, a putative natural antioxidant for topical application. *Basic Clin. Pharmacol. Toxicol.* **2008**, *103*, 461–467. [CrossRef] [PubMed]

12. Carvalho, I.T.; Estevinho, B.N.; Santos, L. Application of microencapsulated essential oils in personal healthcare products—A review. *Int. J. Cosmet. Sci.* **2016**, *38*, 109–119. [CrossRef] [PubMed]
13. Bouaziz, M.; Sayadi, S. Isolation and evaluation of antioxidants from leaves of Tunisian cultivar olive tree. *Eur. J. Lipid Sci. Technol.* **2005**, *107*, 497–504. [CrossRef]
14. Lee, O.; Lee, B.; Lee, J.; Lee, H.; Son, J.; Park, C.; Shetty, K.; Kim, Y. Assessment of phenolics-enriched extract and fractions of olive leaves and their antioxidant activities. *Bioresour. Technol.* **2009**, *100*, 6107–6113. [CrossRef] [PubMed]
15. Mourtzinos, I.; Salta, F.; Yannakopoulou, K.; Chiou, A.; Karathanos, V.T. Encapsulation of olive leaf extract in β-Cyclodextrin. *J. Agric. Food Chem.* **2007**, *55*, 8088–8094. [CrossRef] [PubMed]
16. Khan, Y.; Panchal, S.; Vyas, N.; Butani, A.; Kumar, V. Olea europaea: A phyto-pharmacological Review. *Pharmacogn. Rev.* **2007**, *1*, 112–116.
17. Xinos, N.; Papaefstathiou, G.; Psychis, M.; Argyropoulou, A.; Aligiannis, N.; Skaltsounis, A. Development of a green extraction procedure with super/subcritical fluid to produce extracts enriched in oleuropein from olive leaves. *J. Supercrit. Fluids* **2012**, *67*, 89–93. [CrossRef]
18. Manna, C.; Migliardi, V.; Golino, P.; Scognamiglio, A.; Galleti, P.; Chiariello, M.; Zappia, V. Oleuropein prevents oxidative myocardial injury induced by ischemia and reperfusion. *J. Nutr. Biochem.* **2004**, *15*, 461–466. [CrossRef] [PubMed]
19. Munin, A.; Edwards-Levy, F. Encapsulation of natural polyphenolic compounds; a review. *Pharmaceuticals* **2011**, *3*, 793–829. [CrossRef] [PubMed]
20. Ammala, A. Biodegradable polymers as encapsulation materials for cosmetics and personal care markets. *Int. J. Cosmet. Sci.* **2013**, *35*, 113–124. [CrossRef] [PubMed]
21. Duclairoir, C.; Orecchioni, A.M.; Depraetere, P.; Nakache, E. α-Tocopherol encapsulation and in vitro release from wheat gliadin nanoparticles. *J. Microencapsul.* **2002**, *19*, 53–60. [CrossRef] [PubMed]
22. Failloux, N.; Baron, M.H.; Abdul-Malak, N.; Perrier, E. Contribution of encapsulation on the biodisponibility of retinol. *Int. J. Cosmet. Sci.* **2004**, *26*, 71–77. [CrossRef] [PubMed]
23. Kumari, A.; Yadav, S.; Pakade, Y.; Singh, B.; Yadah, S. Development of biodegradable nanoparticles for delivery of quercetin. *Colloids Surf. B. Biointerfaces* **2010**, *80*, 184–192. [CrossRef] [PubMed]
24. Roussaki, M.; Gaitanarou, A.; Diamanti, P.Ch.; Vouyiouka, S.; Papaspyrides, C.; Kefalas, P.; Detsi, A. Encapsulation of the natural antioxidant aureusidin in biodegradable PLA nanoparticles. *Polym. Degrad. Stab.* **2014**, *108*, 182–187. [CrossRef]
25. Sanna, V.; Lubinu, G.; Madau, P.; Pala, N.; Nurra, S.; Mariani, A.; Sechi, M. Polymeric nanoparticles encapsulating white tea extract for nutraceutical application. *J. Agric. Food Chem.* **2015**, *63*, 2026–2032. [CrossRef] [PubMed]
26. Vettor, M.; Perugini, P.; Scalia, S.; Conti, B.; Genta, I.; Modena, T.; Pavanetto, F. Poly(D,L-lacticide) nanoencapsulation to reduce photoinactivation of a sunscreen agent. *Int. J. Cosmet. Sci.* **2008**, *30*, 219–227. [CrossRef] [PubMed]
27. Rancan, F.; Blum-Peytavi, U.; Vogt, A. Utilization of biodegradable polymeric materials as delivery agents in dermatology. *Clin. Cosmet. Investig. Dermatol.* **2014**, *7*, 23–34. [CrossRef] [PubMed]
28. Casanova, F.; Santos, L. Encapsulation of cosmetic active ingredients for topical application—A review. *J. Microencapsul.* **2016**, *33*, 1–17. [CrossRef] [PubMed]
29. Rancan, F.; Papakostas, D.; Hadam, S.; Hackbarth, S.; Delair, T.; Primard, C.; Verrier, B.; Sterry, W.; Blume-Peytavi, U.; Vogt, A. Investigation of polylactic acid (PLA) nanoparticles as drug delivery systems for local dermatotherapy. *Pharm. Res.* **2009**, *26*, 2027–2036. [CrossRef] [PubMed]
30. Lane, M.E. Nanoparticles and the skin—Applications and limitations. *J. Microencapsul.* **2011**, *28*, 709–716. [CrossRef] [PubMed]
31. Mohanraj, V.J.; Chen, Y. Nanoparticles—A review. *Trop. J. Pharm. Res.* **2006**, *5*, 561–573. [CrossRef]
32. Morganti, P. Use and potential of nanotechnology in cosmetic dermatology. *Clin. Cosmet. Investig. Dermatol.* **2010**, *3*, 5–13. [CrossRef] [PubMed]
33. Grabnar, P.A.; Kristl, J. The manufacturing techniques of drug-loaded polymeric nanoparticles from preformed polymers. *J. Microencapsul.* **2011**, *28*, 323–335. [CrossRef] [PubMed]
34. Mohamed, F.; Van der Walle, C.F. Engineering biodegradable polyester particles with specific drug targeting and drug release properties. *J. Pharm. Sci.* **2008**, *279*, 41–53. [CrossRef] [PubMed]

35. Vouyiouka, S.; Theodoulou, P.; Symeonidou, A.; Papaspyrides, C.D.; Pfaendner, P. Solid state polymerization of poly(lactic acid): Some fundamental parameters. *Polym. Degrad. Stab.* **2013**, *98*, 2473–2481. [CrossRef]

36. Chanioti, S.; Siamandoura, P.; Tzia, C. Evaluation of extracts prepared from olive oil by-products using microwave-assisted enzymatic extraction: Effect of encapsulation on the stability of final products. *Waste Biomass Valoriz.* **2016**, *7*, 831–842. [CrossRef]

37. Parejo, I.; Codina, C.; Petrakis, C.; Kefalas, P. Evaluation of scavenging activity assessed by Co(II)/EDTA-induced luminol chemiluminescence and DPPH (2,2-diphenyl-1-picrylhydrazyl) free radical assay. *J. Pharmacol. Toxicol. Methods* **2000**, *44*, 507–512. [CrossRef]

38. Mu, L.; Feng, S.S. A novel controlled release formulation for the anticancer drug paclitaxel (Taxol): PLGA nanoparticles containing vitamin E TPGS. *J. Control. Release* **2003**, *86*, 33–48. [CrossRef]

39. Kiritsakis, K.; Kontominas, M.G.; Kontogiorgis, C.; Hadjipavlou-Litina, D.; Moustakas, A.; Kiritsakis, A. Composition and antioxidant activity of olive leaf extracts from Greek olive cultivars. *J. Am. Oil Chem. Soc.* **2010**, *87*, 369–376. [CrossRef]

40. Wiechers, J.; Musee, N. Engineered inorganic nanoparticles and cosmetics: Facts, issues, knowledge gaps and challenges. *J. Biomed. Nanotechnol.* **2010**, *6*, 408–431. [CrossRef] [PubMed]

41. Soppimath, K.; Aminabhavi, T.M.; Kulkarni, A.; Rudzinski, W. Biodegradable polymeric nanoparticles as drug delivery devices. *J. Control. Release* **2001**, *70*, 1–20. [CrossRef]

42. Izumikawa, S.; Yoshioka, S.; Aso, Y.; Takeda, Y. Preparation of poly(L-lactide) microspheres of different crystalline morphology and effect of crystalline morphology on drug release rate. *J. Control. Release* **1991**, *15*, 133–140. [CrossRef]

43. Kalogeropoulos, N.; Yannakopoulou, K.; Gioxari, A.; Chiou, A.; Makris, D. Polyphenol characterization and encapsulation in β-cyclodextrin of flavonoid-rich *Hypericum perforatum* (St John's wort) extract. *LWT-Food Sci. Technol.* **2010**, *43*, 882–889. [CrossRef]

44. Musumeci, T.; Ventura, C.A.; Giannone, I.; Ruozi, B.; Montenegro, L.; Pignatello, R.; Puglisi, G. PLA/PLGA nanoparticles for sustained release of docetaxel. *Int. J. Pharm.* **2006**, *325*, 172–179. [CrossRef] [PubMed]

45. Cortez Tornello, P.; Feresin, G.; Tapia, A.; Veiga, I.G.; Moraes, Â.M.; Abraham, G.A.; Cuadrado, T.R. Dispersion and release of embelin from electrospun biodegradable, polymeric, membranes. *Polym. J.* **2012**, *44*, 1105–1111. [CrossRef]

46. Lambers, H.; Piessens, S.; Bloem, A.; Pronk, H.; Finkel, P. Natural skin surface pH is on average below 5, which is beneficial for its resident flora. *Int. J. Cosmet. Sci.* **2006**, *28*, 359–370. [CrossRef] [PubMed]

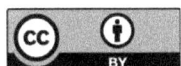

bioengineering

MDPI

Article

Encapsulation of Oregano (*Origanum onites* L.) Essential Oil in *β*-Cyclodextrin (*β*-CD): Synthesis and Characterization of the Inclusion Complexes

Margarita Kotronia [1,2], Eleni Kavetsou [1], Sofia Loupassaki [2], Stefanos Kikionis [3], Stamatina Vouyiouka [4] and Anastasia Detsi [1,*]

[1] Laboratory of Organic Chemistry, School of Chemical Engineering, National Technical University of Athens, Zografou Campus, 15780 Athens, Greece; margarita.kotronia@gmail.com (M.K.); eleni29@hotmail.com (E.K.)

[2] Department of Food Quality and Chemistry of Natural Products, Mediterranean Agronomic Institute of Chania (Centre International de Hautes Etudes Agronomiques Mediterraneennes), 73100 Chania, Crete, Greece; sofia@maich.gr

[3] Department of Pharmacognosy and Chemistry of Natural Products, Faculty of Pharmacy, National and Kapodistrian University of Athens, Panepistimiopolis Zografou, Athens 15771, Greece; skikionis@pharm.uoa.gr

[4] Laboratory of Polymer Technology, School of Chemical Engineering, National Technical University of Athens, Zografou Campus, 15780 Athens, Greece; mvuyiuka@central.ntua.gr

* Correspondence: adetsi@chemeng.ntua.gr ; Tel.: +30-210-772-4126

Academic Editor: Gary Chinga Carrasco
Received: 28 July 2017; Accepted: 4 September 2017; Published: 9 September 2017

Abstract: The aim of the present work was to study the encapsulation of *Origanum onites* L. essential oil (oregano EO) in β-cyclodextrin (β-CD) inclusion complexes (ICs), using the co-precipitation method. The formed β-CD–oregano EO ICs were characterized by diverse methods, such as Dynamic Light Scattering (DLS), FT-IR spectroscopy, Differential Scanning Calorimetry (DSC), Thermogravimetric Analysis (TGA), Nuclear Magnetic Resonance (NMR) spectroscopy and Scanning Electron Microscopy (SEM). UV-Vis spectroscopy was used for the determination of the inclusion efficacy and the study of the encapsulated oregano EO release profile. The interactions between host (β-CD) and guest (oregano EO) in the formed ICs were proven by the FT-IR, DSC, TG and NMR analyses. The ICs, which derived from different batches, presented nanoscale size (531.8 ± 7.7 nm and 450.3 ± 11.5 nm, respectively), good size dispersion (0.308 ± 0.062 and 0.484 ± 0.029, respectively) and satisfactory stability in suspension (ζ-potential = -21.5 ± 1.2 mV and -30.7 ± 1.8 mV). Inclusion efficiency reached up to 26%, whereas the oregano EO release from the ICs followed a continuous delivery profile for up to 11 days, based on *in vitro* experiments. The formed ICs can find diverse applications, such as in the preparation of films for active packaging of food products, in personal care products for the improvement of their properties (e.g., antioxidant, antimicrobial, etc.), as well as in insect repellent products.

Keywords: oregano essential oil; encapsulation; inclusion complexes; β-cyclodextrin; release

---

1. Introduction

Oregano is an aromatic plant which is commonly found growing wild in the countries of the Mediterranean basin [1,2]. In fact, although the name "Oregano" is used for several plants of different families and genera, the majority of the most well-known oregano plants, which have been traditionally used in cookery as food flavorings, as well as in the preservation of food products, belongs to the *Origanum* genus of the Lamiaceae or Labiatae family [1–3]. Although the *Origanum onites* L. plant and its essential oil (EO) are known and have been used for centuries, in the last decades the *Origanum onites* L.

EO has attracted the attention and the interest of the researchers and the industry, gaining extensive popularity and, consequently, proliferating its fields of application [3]. This occurred due to the growing social awareness and demand for safer, healthier and minimally processed products that present a more close-to-natural image, as well as respect product quality and environment [1].

The *Origanum onites* L. EO has been reported to present remarkable biological properties. Particularly, it has been shown to exhibit powerful antimicrobial, antimycotic, antioxidant, anti-inflammatory and insecticidal activity, which result from its phenolic content and mainly from its major component, carvacrol [1–3], having also been suggested to present a significant potential in preventing neurodegenerative disorders [1,2]. Furthermore, having been granted "Generally Recognized as Safe (GRAS)" status (ESO, GRAS—182.20) [1], the *Origanum onites* L. EO can be used in products without further approval. Consequently, it fulfils the requirements of promoting well-being and being environmentally friendly, meeting the consumers' expectations and demands [1–3]. Therefore, these quality characteristics render it as a valuable natural resource with great potential for industrial use, finding numerous applications among others in the food and pharmaceutical industry [1–3]. Certainly, the introduction and implementation of new technologies, which render the treatment of EOs and their use in several products more feasible and easier [1], have contributed to the increasing use and applications of the *Origanum onites* L. EO.

However, the EO's hydrophobic nature, volatility and high sensitivity in the presence of light, oxygen and heat, limit its use [4–7]. Concurrently, if it is going to be embedded into a complex product matrix, it is quite possible that its sensitivity could cause considerable problems to the product, concerning the organoleptic profile, physical stability and chemical integrity [5–8]. Hence, encapsulation of EOs in biodegradable nano-delivery systems seems to be a promising, viable and efficient approach for overcoming these problems. Specifically, nano-delivery systems would permit its targeted and controlled release, as well as the increase of its aqueous solubility and stability against evaporation and exposure to light, oxygen, or heat, maintaining its quality, maintaining or even improving its properties and protecting products from undesired alterations [8–11]. Consequently, encapsulation could also be an answer to consumers' demands for production of functional products with higher nutritional value, fewer synthetic additives and better organoleptic features [12].

Cyclodextrins (CDs) are cyclic, water-soluble oligosaccharides, which are produced from the enzymatic conversion, degradation and cyclization of starch and other related α-1,4-glucans, by CD glycosyltransferase and partly by α-amylases. They are composed of several D-glucose units linked by α-D-(1→4) linkages, exhibiting a three-dimensional structure, which is considered as a truncated cone. The most common of these ring-shaped molecules are α-CD, β-CD and γ-CD, which consist of six, seven and eight D-glucose units, respectively. Their depth is the same, irrespective of the glucose unit number, whereas their diameter, which is determined by the number of the glucose units, is different [5–7,11–16].

CDs have been extensively applied in various sectors as encapsulants of several organic substances, such as flavors, essential oils and spices, as well as individual compounds, such as carvacrol, thymol, menthol, ethylene and vanillin, as they present an inner hydrophobic cavity and a peripheral hydrophilic zone. Moreover, they are nontoxic, biodegradable polymers, not absorbed in the upper gastrointestinal tract, but completely metabolized by the gut microflora [5–7,11–16].

In particular, because of their hydrophobic cavity and hydrophilic external surface, CDs present the ability to interact with hydrophobic bioactive compounds and molecules (guest molecules), encapsulating them in their cavity. As a result, non-covalent CD—bioactive agent molecular complexes, which are also known as host—guest inclusion complexes (ICs), are formed. These complexes are mainly driven by hydrophobic or Van der Waals interactions, while their formation constitutes a dynamic equilibrium, allowing the guest molecule to diffuse reversibly from the CD cavity. Therefore, CDs constitute favorable and suitable molecules for the encapsulation of poorly soluble, temperature sensitive, or chemically labile bioactive agents, in order to protect them against diverse environmental conditions, to improve their physical and chemical stability, to retain or even enhance their biological properties, as well as to improve or extend their physical and chemical properties [5–7,11–16].

To our knowledge, a significantly large part of the current literature is focused on the encapsulation of the main oregano EO component, carvacrol [5,15,17–19], whereas little systematic research has been conducted to evaluate the encapsulation of oregano EO, with most of the studies dealing with encapsulation matrices other than β-CD [1,2,6,17,20–23] or using other methods like spray-drying [24]. In the current study, a detailed research on the encapsulation of the oregano EO in β-CD was conducted, using the co-precipitation method. The formed ICs were characterized using diverse analytical techniques, and the main parameters that affect the encapsulation procedure were investigated. In addition, the release profile of the encapsulated oregano EO in media of different temperatures and pH values was determined.

2. Materials and Methods

2.1. Materials

Oregano (*Origanum onites* L.) essential oil (EO) of food-grade quality was kindly supplied by the Laboratory of Nutritional Physiology and Feeding, of the Animal Sciences and Aquaculture Faculty, of the Agricultural University of Athens (A.U.A., Athens, Greece). β-Cyclodextrin (β-CD) of >99% purity was purchased from Fluka (Gillingham, England), while ethanol of analytical reagent grade was purchased from Merck Millipore (Billerica, MA, USA). Ethyl acetate of ACS grade was purchased from Chem-Lab (Zedelgem, Belgium). For the preparation of solutions double deionized water was used. The aforementioned materials were used without further purification.

2.2. Preparation of β-CD—Oregano EO Inclusion Complexes (ICs)

The co-precipitation method of Sun et al. [15], slightly modified, was used to prepare the β-CD—oregano EO ICs. Briefly, β-CD was dissolved in defined volumes of ethanol and double deionized water mixture (1:2 v/v), in order for each time a concentration of 100 mg of β-CD per 1 mL of solvents' total volume to be achieved. In a typical experiment, β-CD (500 mg) was dissolved in ethanol-double deionized water solution (5 mL). The solution was magnetically stirred at $55 \pm 2\,^{\circ}C$, until the complete dissolution of β-CD. Subsequently, oregano EO (125 mg) was added dropwise in the β-CD solution, in order for a EO/β-CD ratio of 20:80 w/w to be obtained. The formed emulsion was continuously stirred at room temperature, until the β-CD–oregano EO ICs were formed. The elimination of the oily phase from the emulsion indicated the formation of the ICs. The final dispersion was kept in the refrigerator for approximately 1 h, after which the β-CD–oregano EO ICs were recovered by vacuum filtration, using a Hirsch filter funnel (pore size 3). The recovered ICs were washed twice with ethanol, in order for the unencapsulated oregano EO or the oregano EO absorbed on the surface of β-CD to be removed, and they were dried in vacuo for 3 h at 40 °C. Finally, 445 mg of dried ICs were obtained and stored in airtight glass containers, under refrigeration, for further analysis and characterization.

2.3. Characterization of the β-CD—Oregano EO ICs

2.3.1. Dynamic Light Scattering (DLS)

Size, size distribution (PDI) and zeta-potential (ζ-potential) determinations were performed by Dynamic Light Scattering (DLS) method, using the Zetasizer Nano ZS device (Malvern Instruments, Malvern, UK). The samples for the DLS measurements were adequately diluted aqueous solutions of the final dried β-CD—oregano EO ICs (pH 6), prepared by dispersing 1 mg of ICs in 4 mL of double deionized water and the solution being left in stirring for 48 hours at room temperature. For both size and ζ-potential measurements, folded capillary cells DTS1070 were used, while for each sample the measurements for the size, PDI and ζ-potential were carried out at 25 ± 1 °C and in triplicate. The results were reported as mean ± standard deviation (SD).

2.3.2. Fourier Transform Infrared Spectroscopy (FT-IR (ATR) Spectroscopy)

The ICs' formation, as well as the interactions between the oregano EO and the β-CD, were confirmed and determined by Fourier Transform Infrared spectroscopy (FT-IR spectroscopy), using a JASCO FT/IR-4200 spectrometer (Japan Spectroscopic Company, Tokyo, Japan). The IR analyses were conducted in the final dried β-CD–oregano EO ICs, while for each sample, the IR analysis was carried out in the scanning range of 650–4000 cm^{-1}.

2.3.3. Differential Scanning Calorimetry (DSC)

The thermal characteristics of the ICs were studied with the Differential Scanning Calorimetry (DSC) method, using the DSC 1 STAR^e System device (Mettler Toledo, Columbus, OH, USA). DSC analyses were conducted in the final dried β-CD—oregano EO ICs, as well as in β-CD and pure oregano EO. The samples were heated from 25 °C to 400 °C, respectively, with a heating rate of 10 °C/min under nitrogen gas flow (20 mL/min).

2.3.4. Thermogravimetric Analysis (TGA)

Thermogravimetric (TG) analyses were also conducted in the final dried β-CD–oregano EO ICs, β-CD and oregano EO. The TG analyses were performed in the TGA/DSC 1 STAR^e System Thermobalance (Mettler Toledo, Columbus, OH, USA), with the samples being heated from 25 °C to 600 °C, at a heating rate of 10 °C/min under nitrogen gas flow (10 mL/min).

2.3.5. Nuclear Magnetic Resonance Spectroscopy (NMR Spectroscopy)

The ^{1}H-NMR spectra of the final dried β-CD – oregano EO ICs and β-CD were recorded on a Varian 300 MHz spectrometer (Varian, Palo Alto, CA, USA).The used solvent for the preparation of the solutions was deuterium oxide (D_2O). The coupling constants (J) are expressed in hertz (Hz) and the chemical shifts (δ) are reported in parts per million (ppm) relative to the solvent.

2.3.6. Scanning Electron Microscopy (SEM)

The SEM analyses were conducted in the final dried β-CD–oregano EO ICs, using a PhenomWorld desktop scanning electron microscope (Phenom-World, Eindhoven, The Netherlands) with tungsten filament (10 kV) and a charge reduction sample holder. The size of 100 particles from each SEM image was measured, using the embedded image analysis software (Phenom Pro Suite/ParticleMetric), and the average particle size was determined.

2.4. Inclusion Efficiency of the β-CD—Oregano EO ICs

The inclusion efficiency (IE) represents the percentage of oregano EO encapsulated in the formed β-CD—oregano EO ICs, relative to the total initial amount of oregano EO used:

$$(\%IE) = 100 \times \frac{mass\ of\ the\ encapsulated\ oregan\ EO\ (mg)}{initial\ oregano\ EO\ mass\ to\ be\ encapsulated\ (mg)} \tag{1}$$

The % IE of oregano EO in the β-CD–oregano EO ICs was determined directly, using Ultraviolet-Visible Spectroscopy (UV-Vis Spectroscopy), by quantification of the encapsulated oregano EO. The UV-Vis analyses were conducted in the final dried ICs, being performed on a JASCO double beam V-770 UV-Vis/NIR spectrophotometer (Japan Spectroscopic Company, Tokyo, Japan). For the UV-Vis analyses, 10 mg of ICs were dispersed in 10 mL of ethyl acetate, with the solution being left in stirring for 48 h at room temperature. Subsequently, the solution was filtered in vacuo and from this resulting solution, proper volumes were obtained for the performance of the analysis. The IE was quantified by measuring the absorption of the major oregano EO component, carvacrol, at 275 nm. From this absorption the mass of the encapsulated oregano EO in the ethyl acetate–oregano EO solution was calculated and used in Equation 1, in order for the IE to be determined. Furthermore, a calibration curve of the absorbance versus the concentration of the oregano EO, constructed by standard ethyl acetate–oregano EO solutions of known concentrations, was used for the quantitative determinations of oregano EO. For each sample, the UV-Vis analysis was carried out in triplicate.

2.5. In Vitro Release Studies of the Oregano EO from the β-CD—Oregano EO ICs

In vitro release experiments were performed, in order for the oregano EO release profile from the formed β-CD—oregano EO ICs to be evaluated. The release profile of the oregano EO was studied under specified conditions, in media of different temperatures and pH values. Particularly, three release experiments were conducted: (a) using deionized water as medium, at 37 °C and under neutral pH conditions, 7.4, (b) using deionized water as medium, at 50 °C and under neutral pH conditions, 7.4, as well as (c) using phosphate buffer solution as medium, at 37 °C and under slightly acidic pH conditions, 5.5. For each experiment, 100 mg of β-CD—oregano EO ICs were dispersed into 25 mL of medium and the entire system was kept at the specified temperature and pH values, being under continuous magnetic stirring (450 rpm) for approximately 10 days. At regular predetermined time intervals, 2 mL samples from the solution were taken and were analyzed by UV-Vis spectroscopy, so that the amount of the released oregano EO as a function of time to be calculated, by measuring the absorbance at 275 nm. The quantification of the released oregano EO was performed by a calibration curve. Each time a 2 mL sample was withdrawn, 2 mL of fresh medium were added at the solutions. For each experiment, two replicates were performed.

3. Results and Discussion

3.1. Characterization of the β-CD—Oregano EO ICs

3.1.1. Size, Size Distribution and Zeta-Potential (ζ-Potential)

The size, size distribution and ζ-potential of the produced ICs determine to a great extent their ability to be used in certain applications. They constitute the most important parameters in the characterization of the produced ICs. The size of the ICs affects their nature and attributes, such as their surface characteristics, their physicochemical stability, the bioactive agent's loading and targeted delivery, as well as the bioactive agent's release profile [25–29]. Nevertheless, the type of application determines the range of the values that the size of the ICs should obtain; hence, there is no optimal size. For this reason, most of the times polydispersity index (PDI), which represents the size distribution of the produced ICs, presents greater interest. The PDI is a measure of the uniformity of the ICs' sizes, constituting a significant indicator concerning the uniformity of the attributes that the ICs present (i.e., ICs of uniform sizes bring similarly loads of the bioactive agent, which leads to a uniform release of it.). As far as the ζ-potential is concerned, it constitutes an indicator of the ICs' stability in suspension [30]. As the absolute value of the ζ-potential increases, the greater the repulsive forces between them, reducing their tendency to aggregate; therefore, the more stable the ICs become.

In the present study the obtained size, PDI and ζ-potential values for the formed β-CD–oregano EO ICs, which were derived from different batches, are presented in Table 1. As can be observed, the size and PDI values of the formed β-CD–oregano EO ICs were reproducible, presenting no significant variations. Specifically, the formed ICs exhibited a mean diameter in the range of 450.3 ± 11.5 nm–531.8 ± 7.7 nm, while their PDI values ranged from 0.308 ± 0.062 to 0.484 ± 0.029, indicating moderately uniform size dispersion. This moderate homogeneity of the ICs populations was also being perceived through their size distribution graphs (Figure S1), in which two groups of β-CD—oregano EO ICs, regarding the size, could be observed. The obtained size and PDI values could be attributed to the strong tendency of the β-CD ICs to agglomerate, as a consequence of their self-assembly in aqueous solutions [7]. This phenomenon is attributed to the absence of strong repulsive forces between the particles, as a result of the lack of significant net charge on the β-CD ICs' surface [7]. Generally, the agglomeration does not occur uniformly, potentially creating more variability in ICs' size [7], something that explains the obtained PDI values. Nevertheless, the obtained size values were much smaller than that found by Hill L. E. et al. (2013) [7] concerning β-CD ICs with different EOs. Furthermore, the obtained absolute ζ-potential values for the formed β-CD–oregano EO ICs were high enough to indicate the formation of stable ICs, which present a low tendency to aggregate. Particularly, the obtained ζ-potential values ranged from -21.5 ± 1.2 mV to -30.7 ± 1.8 mV, values which render the dispersion quite stable.

Table 1. Size, polydispersity index (PDI) and ζ-potential average values of the formed β-CD—oregano EO ICs.

	Size (nm)	Polydispersity Index (PDI)	ζ-potential (mV)
ICs (1)	531.8 ± 7.7	0.308 ± 0.062	-21.5 ± 1.2
ICs (2)	450.3 ± 11.5	0.484 ± 0.029	-30.7 ± 1.8

3.1.2. FT-IR Analysis

FT-IR Spectroscopy is a commonly used method for the examination of ICs' structure, through the determination of the interactions between the guest molecules and the carrier material [31–33]. The obtained FT-IR spectra are presented in Figure S2.

In the FT-IR spectrum of oregano EO (Figure S2a) the most characteristic absorptions that could be observed are present at 2961.16 cm^{-1}, 1579.41 cm^{-1}, 1428.03 cm^{-1}, 1251.58 cm^{-1} and 938.19 cm^{-1}. Specifically, the peak at 2961.16 cm^{-1} is owed to the aromatic C-H stretching vibration, while the peaks at 1579.41 cm^{-1} and 1428.03 cm^{-1} can be attributed to the C-C stretch of the aromatic ring of carvacrol, the main oregano EO component. The characteristic absorption of the C-O stretching vibration appears at 1251.58 cm^{-1}, while the absorption of the ring C-H bending vibration gives a characteristic peak at 938.19 cm^{-1}.

As far as the FT-IR spectrum of β-CD (Figure S2b) is concerned, the most characteristic peaks appear at 3292.35 cm^{-1} owed to the -OH stretching vibration, at 2924.63 cm^{-1} attributed to the C-H stretching vibration, at 1643.67 cm^{-1} due to the asymmetric C-H stretching of -CH$_2$, as well as at 1414.33 cm^{-1} owing to the O-H bending vibration. Additionally, the absorption at 1020.75 cm^{-1} is attributed to the C-O stretching vibration of the secondary alcohol groups that are present in the β-CD molecule.

The FT-IR spectrum of the β-CD–oregano EO ICs (Figure S2c) significantly differs from the respective ones of oregano EO and β-CD. In this particular spectrum, the most characteristic absorptions appear at 2965.14 cm^{-1}, 2917.71 cm^{-1}, 1644.88 cm^{-1}, 1436.03 cm^{-1} and 885.58 cm^{-1}. Particularly, the peak at 2965.14 cm^{-1} can be attributed to the C-H stretching vibration of carvacrol, the major component of oregano EO, while the peak at 2917.71 cm^{-1} is attributed to the C-H stretching vibration of β-CD. The peak at 1644.88 cm^{-1} results from the shift of the characteristic peak that appears at 1643.67 cm^{-1} in the IR spectrum of β-CD, and consequently, is owed to the asymmetric C-H stretching of the –CH$_2$. Similarly, the peak at 1436.03 cm^{-1} could possibly result from the shift of the characteristic peak that appears at 1414.33 cm^{-1} in the IR spectrum of β-CD, being attributed to the O-H bending vibration. The peak at 885.58 cm^{-1} most probably constitutes a combined result of the overlap and shift of the peak at 1020.75 cm^{-1} of the β-CD IR spectrum and the peak at 938.19 cm^{-1} of the oregano EO IR spectrum, which, along with the characteristic absorption at 1436.03 cm^{-1}, prove the encapsulation of the oregano EO in the β-CD ICs, by indicating the presence of host-guest interaction.

3.1.3. Thermal Analysis by Differential Scanning Calorimetry (DSC) and Thermogravimetric Analysis (TGA)

Thermal analysis was conducted in order to confirm the formation of the ICs. Figure 1 presents the DSC curves under nitrogen flow of the three samples: β-CD, pure oregano EO, and β-CD—oregano EO ICs. Starting with the oregano EO, it is liquid at room temperature; therefore, it exhibited an endothermic peak at 228.2 °C that corresponds to the boiling point. The relevant thermal transition was also seen in its TGA graph (Figure 2), where the oregano EO weight loss starts at roughly 80 °C, reaching a maximum rate at 207.4 °C, with a residue at 8%. As far as the β-CD DSC curve is concerned, the observed endothermic peak at 130.9 °C can be attributed to water evaporation from the β-CD cavity, as it was suggested in the work of Karathanos et al. [34] and Gomes et al. [35] for the β-CD endotherm peaks at 175 °C and 165 °C, respectively. For the same reason of water elimination, ca. 10% weight loss is observed in the β-CD TGA graph (Figure 2) in the temperature range of 60 °C–120 °C. On the other hand, in the DSC of the β-CD—oregano EO ICs, the endothermic peak of the oregano EO disappeared and the curve was found slightly different compared to the respective one of the β-CD, indicating the ICs formation. This is in agreement with the work of Seo et al. [36], where the endothermic peak of eugenol boiling point also disappeared in the DSC curve of the relevant β-CD ICs.

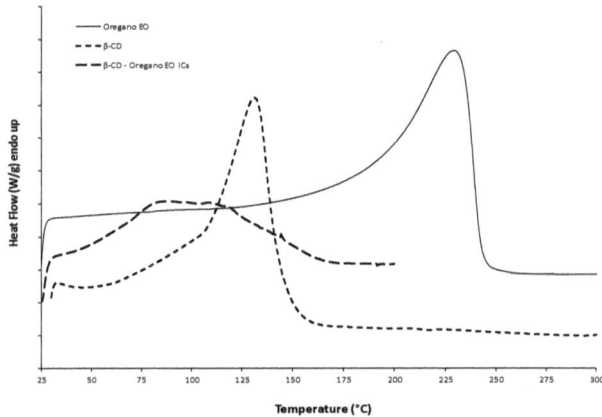

Figure 1. The DSC curves of the oregano EO, β-CD and β-CD—oregano EO ICs.

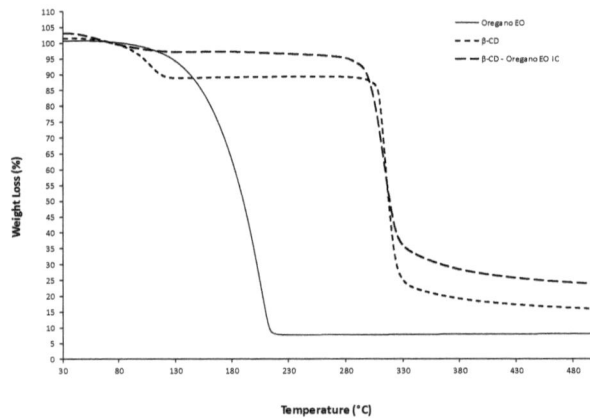

Figure 2. The TGA graphs of the oregano EO, β-CD and β-CD—oregano EO ICs.

The TGA results (Figure 2) also confirmed the ICs' formation. The TGA graph of the β-CD—oregano EO ICs follows a similar pattern to the TGA graph of the β-CD, with slightly higher weight residue (27% and 18%, respectively) and maximum degradation temperature at ca. 320 °C. In particular, in the β-CD–oregano EO ICs TGA graph, the first step of weight loss in the range of 60–120 °C was not so distinctly observed as it was in the β-CD TGA graph, something that could be attributed to the partial displacement of the water molecules in the β-CD cavity by the encapsulated oregano EO. Additionally, in the range of 80–220 °C, where the oregano EO loss occurs, no significant weight loss is observed, something that suggests the protection of the oregano EO by being inside the β-CD cavity.

3.1.4. Nuclear Magnetic Resonance (NMR) Analysis

NMR can provide useful evidence to support the formation of the ICs and help structure characterization [14,37,38]. The NMR analysis of β-CD and β-CD—oregano EO ICs was performed at 300 MHz in D_2O. The structure of β-CD showing the numbering of β-glucose monomer is shown in Figure 3.

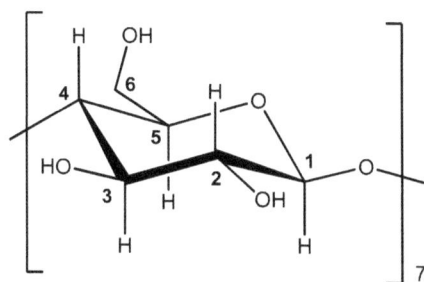

Figure 3. Structure of β-CD showing the numbering of β-glucose monomer.

The ICs' formation can lead to changes of the chemical shifts of H-3 and H-5, which are located in the interior of the β-CD cavity, and possibly the chemical shift of H-6, which is located near the cavity (Figure 3). These changes can provide information concerning the inclusion mode and binding affinity between β-CD and guest molecule. The ^{1}H-NMR spectra of β-CD and β-CD–oregano EO ICs are shown in Figure S3. The Δδ values of selected NMR signals of β-CD before and after the formation of the ICs are presented in Table 2.

Table 2. Chemical shift changes of ^{1}H-NMR signals of β-CD and β-CD–oregano EO ICs.

Proton	Chemical Shifts (δ_1) of β-CD Protons (ppm)	Chemical Shifts (δ_2) of β-CD Protons in β-CD—oregano EO ICs (ppm)	Δδ = $\delta_2 - \delta_1$ (ppm)
H-1	5.089	5.082	−0.007
H-2	3.675	3.670	−0.005
H-3	3.991	3.961	−0.030
H-4	3.610	3.610	0
H-5	3.875	3.836	−0.039
H-6	3.905	3.882	−0.023

The H-3 and H-5 β-CD proton signals showed an upfield shift (Δδ = −0.030 ppm and −0.039 ppm, respectively) after the formation of the IC with oregano EO (Table 2). This is in accordance with the work of Locci et al. [38], who studied the inclusion of carvacrol in β-CD. A Δδ = −0.023 ppm for H-6 was also observed, whereas for the rest of the β-CD protons no noteworthy changes in their chemical shift values were detected. The significant differences in chemical shifts observed for H-3 and H-5 corroborate that an IC between the oregano EO constituents and β-CD is formed. The shift of the signal of H-5 allows also for the multiplicity of the signal (doublet) to be revealed in the spectrum of the ICs.

The observed shielding of H-3 and H-5 in the ICs can be attributed to the hydrophobic interactions with the guest molecules (oregano EO constituents), which are located inside the β-CD cavity. The downfield shift of the signal of H-6 is also indicative of an interaction between the oregano EO constituents, potentially trapped on the outer β-CD surface, with these protons which rest near the cavity of β-CD. This assumption is supported by the appearance of signals at the aromatic region (6.7–7 ppm) and the region 1–2.2 ppm, which can be attributed to some of the oregano EO constituents located on the surface of β-CD.

3.1.5. Morphology

Evidence concerning the morphological characteristics of the formed β-CD—oregano EO ICs was obtained using SEM. Figure 4 presents the SEM images of the ICs at (a) ×2000, (b) ×2500, (c) ×5000 and (d) ×10,000 magnification.

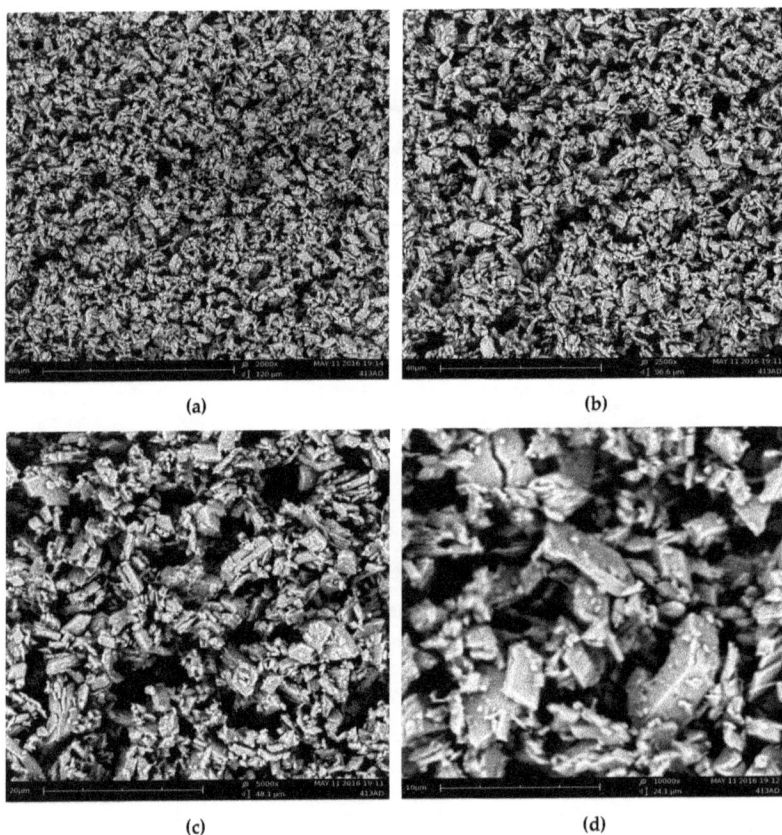

Figure 4. SEM images of the formed β-CD—oregano EO ICs at (a) × 2000, (b) × 2500, (c) × 5000 and (d) × 10000 magnification.

As can be observed, the β-CD–oregano EO ICs present a non-spherical morphology which resembles that of prisms, having parallel and rather smooth sides. Moreover, the images reveal that the β-CD – oregano EO ICs form agglomerates of different sizes, with the larger particles possibly attracting the smaller ones, while a size analysis of the particles through the obtained SEM images revealed an average particle size of 2.2 μm (Figure 5). Similar observations have been previously reported by Ikuta et al. [39], Dima et al. [40] and Rakmai et al. [31].

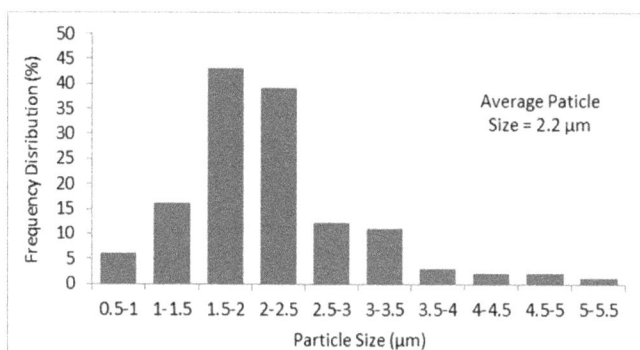

Figure 5. Size distribution bar chart of the particles, resulted from the analysis of the SEM images.

3.2. Inclusion Efficiency of the β-CD—Oregano EO ICs

Determination of the inclusion efficiency (IE) of the β-CD–oregano EO ICs is of great importance, as it provides a direct estimation concerning the effectiveness of the oregano EO encapsulation, as well as evidence concerning the available oregano EO quantity in the ICs, which along with its release profile affect directly the way that the ICs are going to be used in several applications.

The obtained IEs for the formed β-CD–oregano EO ICs that derived from different batches, as determined through Equation (1), are presented in Table 3. The IEs were significantly lower than the ones reported in the literature for the main oregano EO component, carvacrol [31,41]. This was expected as the EOs constitute complex mixtures of different compounds that present high affinities for CD molecules, competing against each other for IC formation with the β-CD [7,31]. Nevertheless, the obtained IEs were reproducible and, interestingly, much higher than the range of the theoretical maximum loading for β-CD with other EOs (8%–12%) [42], suggesting an efficient encapsulation of the oregano EO in β-CD. Moreover, the obtained IEs were in accordance with those of Parris N. et al. (2005) [20], who studied the encapsulation of EOs, including that of oregano, in zein nanospherical particles.

Table 3. Inclusion efficiency (IE) of the formed β-CD–oregano EO ICs.

	β-CD—Oregano EO ICs (*Exp. 1*)	β-CD—Oregano EO ICs (*Exp. 2*)
Initial Oregano EO Mass (mg)	124.60	124.70
Encapsulated Oregano EO Mass (mg)	28.16	31.84
IE (%)	22.60	25.53

3.3. In Vitro Release Studies of the Oregano EO from the β-CD—Oregano EO ICs

The study of the oregano EO release profile from the formed β-CD–oregano EO ICs was performed in order for the effectiveness of the oregano EO encapsulation, concerning the retention, as well as the controlled and targeted release of the encapsulated oregano EO, to be estimated. Concurrently, the release profile under various conditions provides crucial information concerning the range of applications that the ICs could be used.

The release profiles of the ICs are depicted in Figures 6–8. As it can be observed in Figure 6a, at 37 °C and pH 7.4, the release profile is characterized by two different phases; an initial relatively rapid release phase (0 h–1 h and 45 min) ("burst effect") (Figure 6b), during which a 29.6% of oregano EO was released, followed by a slower, more constant release phase (after 1 h and 45 min) ("lag time"), during which an additional 21.5% of oregano EO was released. Normally, the initial rapid release is attributed to the fraction of oregano EO which was adsorbed on the surface of the ICs, having as a result this fraction to diffuse rapidly into the medium, while at the second phase, the sustained release of oregano EO is attributed to the diffusion of the encapsulated oregano EO within the ICs cavity. After 11 days, a cumulative release of 51.2% was reached.

As far as the release profiles at 50 °C and pH 7.4 (Figure 7a), as well as at 37 °C and pH 5.5 (Figure 8a), are concerned, a similar pattern to that described above (37 °C, pH 7.4) is followed. In particular, at 50 °C and pH 7.4, a cumulative amount of 51.7% of oregano EO was released after 11 days, out of which 34.7% was released during the "burst effect" (0 h–1 h and 45 min) (Figure 7b) and 17% during the "lag time" (after 1 h and 45 min). On the other hand, at 37 °C and pH 5.5, 35.5% of the oregano EO was released within 1 h and 45 min at a fast rate (Figure 8b), while the rest 12.6% was constantly released at a slower rate for the next 10 days, after which no more oregano EO was released.

Although the oregano EO release was slightly higher at the first 1 h and 45 min of the experiments as the temperature was increased from 37 °C to 50 °C and the pH was decreased from 7.4 to 5.5 (Figures 6b, 7b and 8b), the release rate profiles of the formed β-CD—oregano EO ICs are very similar to each other, indicating that the changes in the temperature and pH did not significantly affect the oregano EO release. Interestingly, in all conducted experiments continuous release of the loaded oregano EO for up to 11 days was observed.

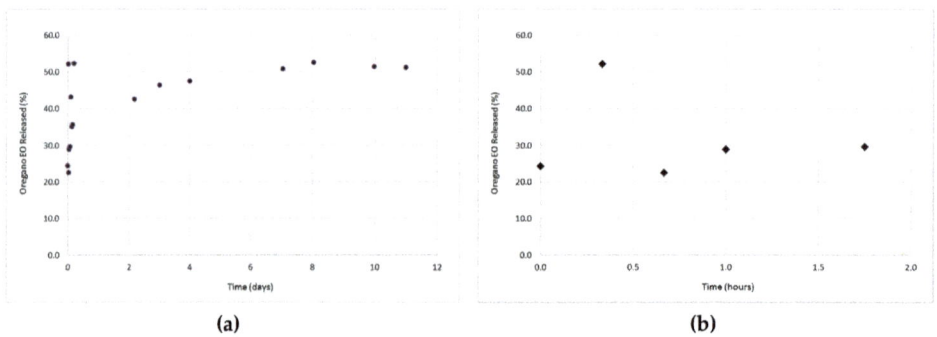

(a)   (b)

Figure 6. The release profile of the encapsulated oregano EO at 37 °C and pH 7.4, during 11 days (a), as well as at the first 1 h and 45 min of the experiment (b).

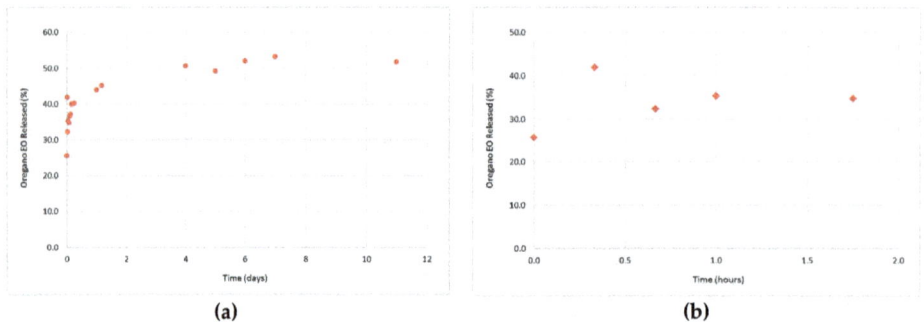

(a)   (b)

Figure 7. Release profile of the encapsulated oregano EO at 50 °C and pH 7.4, during 11 days (a), as well as at the first 1 h and 45 min of the experiment (b).

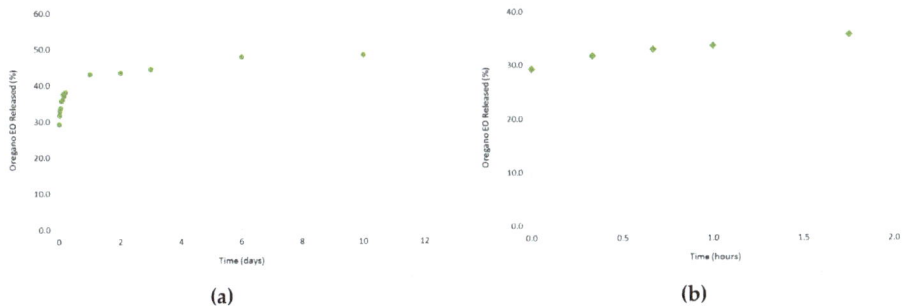

Figure 8. Release profile of the encapsulated oregano EO at 37 °C and pH 5.5, during 11 days (**a**), as well as at the first 1 h and 45 min of the experiment (**b**).

4. Conclusions

In the present study, the encapsulation of oregano EO into β-CD ICs was achieved. The formed β-CD–oregano EO ICs, derived from different batches, presented satisfactory characteristics concerning their size (531.8 ± 7.7 nm and 450.3 ± 11.5 nm, respectively), stability (−21.5 ± 1.2 mV and −30.7 ± 1.8 mV) and morphology, according to the obtained DLS and SEM results. The successful formation of the ICs and encapsulation of oregano EO was confirmed by FT-IR spectroscopy, NMR spectroscopy, DSC and TG analyses. The obtained results corroborate the presence of host (β-CD)–guest (oregano EO) interactions and the location of the oregano EO within the β-CD cavity, being protected inside the β-CD molecules. Moreover, the obtained inclusion efficiency was satisfactory, reaching up to 26%, while the oregano EO release profile was found to follow a continuous pattern. Hence, encapsulation of the oregano EO in β-CD could be an efficient approach to overcome the problem of its high sensitivity, as well as to enhance its bioavailability, providing the means to develop products with advantageous characteristics. The encapsulated EO can be used in diverse applications in the food, cosmetic and agriculture sectors, such as in the preparation of antimicrobial films for active packaging of food products [15,17], in personal care products for the improvement of their properties (e.g., antioxidant, antimicrobial, *etc.*) [43], as well as in insect repellent products for a safer and more environmentally friendly protection of cultivations and crops [44,45].

Supplementary Materials: The following are available online at www.mdpi.com/2306-5354/4/3/74/s1, Figure S1: The size distribution of the β-CD-oregano EO ICs (2); Figure S2: The IR spectra of the oregano EO (a), β-CD (b) and β-CD-oregano EO ICs (c); Figure S3: The 1H NMR spectra (300 MHz, D2O) of β-CD (a), β-CD-oregano EO ICs (expanded region 3–5.5 ppm) (b) and β-CD-oregano EO ICs (c).

Acknowledgments: Eleni Kavetsou gratefully acknowledges financial support from the Research Committee of the National Technical University of Athens (scholarship for postgraduate studies).

Author Contributions: Anastasia Detsi and Stamatina Vouyiouka conceived and designed the experiments. Margarita Kotronia and Eleni Kavetsou performed the experiments and analyzed the data, under the supervision of Anastasia Detsi. Margarita Kotronia, Eleni Kavetsou and Sofia Loupassaki wrote the paper with the suggestions/corrections of Anastasia Detsi and Stamatina Vouyiouka. Stefanos Kikionis obtained and analyzed the SEM data.

Conflicts of Interest: The authors declare no conflict of interest.

References

1. Almeida, A.P.; Rodríguez-Rojo, S.; Serra, A.T.; Vila-Real, H.; Simplicio, A.L.; Delgadilho, I.; Beirão da Costa, S.; Beirão da Costa, L.; Nogueira, I.D.; Duarte, C.M.M. Microencapsulation of oregano essential oil in starch-based materials using supercritical fluid technology. *Innov. Food Sci. Emerg. Technol.* **2013**, *20*, 140–145. [CrossRef]

2. Beirão da Costa, S.; Duarte, C.; Bourbon, A.I.; Pinheiro, A.C.; Serra, A.T.; Moldão Martins, M.; Nunes Januário, M.I.; Vicente, A.A.; Delgadillo, I.; Duarte, C.; et al. Effect of the matrix system in the delivery and in vitro bioactivity of microencapsulated Oregano essential oil. *J. Food Eng.* **2012**, *110*, 190–199. [CrossRef]

3. Stefanaki, A.; Cook, C.M.; Lanaras, T.; Kokkini, S. The Oregano plants of Chios Island (Greece): Essential oils of *Origanum onites* L. growing wild in different habitats. *Ind. Crops Prod.* **2016**, *82*, 107–113. [CrossRef]

4. Burt, S. Essential oils: Their antibacterial properties and potential applications in foods—A review. *Int. J. Food Microbiol.* **2004**, *94*, 223–253. [CrossRef] [PubMed]

5. Lavoine, N.; Givord, C.; Tabary, N.; Desloges, I.; Martel, B.; Bras, J. Elaboration of a new antibacterial bio-nano-material for food-packaging by synergistic action of cyclodextrin and microfibrillated cellulose. *Innov. Food Sci. Emerg. Technol.* **2014**, *26*, 330–340. [CrossRef]

6. Kfoury, M.; Auezova, L.; Greige-Gerges, H.; Fourmentin, S. Promising applications of cyclodextrins in food: Improvement of essential oils retention, controlled release and antiradical activity. *Carbohydr. Polym.* **2015**, *131*, 264–272. [CrossRef] [PubMed]

7. Hill, L.E.; Gomes, C.; Taylor, T.M. Characterization of beta-cyclodextrin inclusion complexes containing essential oils (*trans*-cinnamaldehyde, eugenol, cinnamon bark, and clove bud extracts) for antimicrobial delivery applications. *LWT Food Sci. Technol.* **2013**, *51*, 86–93. [CrossRef]

8. Donsì, F.; Annunziata, M.; Sessa, M.; Ferrari, G. Nanoencapsulation of essential oils to enhance their antimicrobial activity in foods. *LWT Food Sci. Technol.* **2011**, *44*, 1908–1914. [CrossRef]

9. Ezhilarasi, P.N.; Karthik, P.; Chhanwal, N.; Anandharamakrishnan, C. Nanoencapsulation Techniques for Food Bioactive Components: A Review. *Food Bioprocess Technol.* **2013**, *6*, 628–647. [CrossRef]

10. Fathi, M.; Mozafari, M.R.; Mohebbi, M. Nanoencapsulation of food ingredients using lipid based delivery systems. *Trends Food Sci. Technol.* **2012**, *23*, 13–27. [CrossRef]

11. Marques, C.H.M. A review on cyclodextrin encapsulation of essential oils and volatiles. *Flavour Fragr. J.* **2010**, *25*, 313–326. [CrossRef]

12. Fathi, M.; Martín, A.; McClements, D.J. Nanoencapsulation of Food Ingredients using Carbohydrate Based Delivery Systems. *Trends Food Sci. Technol.* **2014**, *39*, 18–39. [CrossRef]

13. Costa, P.; Medronho, B.; Gonçalves, S.; Romano, A. Cyclodextrins enhance the antioxidant activity of essential oils from three Lamiaceae species. *Ind. Crops Prod.* **2015**, *70*, 341–346. [CrossRef]

14. Song, L.X.; Wang, H.M.; Xu, P.; Yang, Y.; Zhang, Z.Q. Experimental and Theoretical Studies on the Inclusion Complexation of Syringic Acid with α-, β-, γ- and Heptakis(2,6-di-O-methyl)-β- cyclodextrin. *Chem. Pharmaceut. Bull.* **2008**, *56*, 468–474. [CrossRef]

15. Sun, X.; Sui, S.; Ference, C.; Zhang, Y.; Sun, S.; Zhou, N.; Zhu, W.; Zhou, K. Antimicrobial and Mechanical Properties of β-Cyclodextrin Inclusion with Essential Oils in Chitosan Films. *J. Agricult. Food Chem.* **2014**, *62*, 8914–8918. [CrossRef] [PubMed]

16. Voncina, B.; Vivod, V. Cyclodextrins in Textile Finishing. In *Eco-Friendly Textile Dyeing and Finishing*; Günay, M., Ed.; INTECH Open Access Publisher: Rijeka, Croatia, 2013; pp. 53–76.

17. Guarda, A.; Rubilar, J.F.; Miltz, J.; Galotto, M.J. The antimicrobial activity of microencapsulated thymol and carvacrol. *Int. J. Food Microbiol.* **2011**, *146*, 144–150. [CrossRef] [PubMed]

18. Chang, Y.; McLandsborough, L.; McClements, D.J. Physicochemical Properties and Antimicrobial Efficacy of Carvacrol Nanoemulsions Formed by Spontaneous Emulsification. *J. Agricult. Food Chem.* **2013**, *61*, 8906–8913. [CrossRef] [PubMed]

19. Wu, Y.; Luo, Y.; Wang, Q. Antioxidant and antimicrobial properties of essential oils encapsulated in zein nanoparticles prepared by liquid-liquid dispersion method. *LWT Food Sci. Technol.* **2012**, *48*, 283–290. [CrossRef]

20. Parris, N.; Cooke, P.H.; Hicks, K.B. Encapsulation of Essential Oils in Zein Nanospherical Particles. *J. Agric. Food Chem.* **2005**, *53*, 4788–4792. [CrossRef] [PubMed]

21. Beirão-da-Costa, S.; Duarte, C.; Bourbon, A.I.; Pinheiro, A.C.; Januário, M.I.N.; Vicente, A.A.; Beirão-da-Costa, M.L.; Delgadillo, I. Inulin potential for encapsulation and controlled delivery of Oregano essential oil. *Food Hydrocoll.* **2013**, *33*, 199–206. [CrossRef]

22. Hosseini, S.F.; Zandi, M.; Rezaei, M.; Farahmandghavi, F. Two-step method for encapsulation of oregano essential oil in chitosan nanoparticles: Preparation, characterization and in vitro release study. *Carbohydr. Polym.* **2013**, *95*, 50–56. [CrossRef] [PubMed]

23. Bhargava, K.; Conti, D.S.; Da Rocha, S.R.P.; Zhang, Y. Application of an oregano oil nanoemulsion to the control of foodborne bacteria on fresh lettuce. *Food Microbiol.* **2015**, *47*, 69–73. [CrossRef] [PubMed]

24. Arana-Sánchez, A.; Estarrón-Espinosa, M.; Obledo-Vázquez, E.N.; Padilla-Camberos, E.; Silva-Vázquez, R.; Lugo-Cervantes, E. Antimicrobial and antioxidant activities of Mexican oregano essential oils (Lippia graveolens HBK) with different composition when microencapsulated in β-cyclodextrin. *Lett. Appl. Microbiol.* **2010**, *50*, 585–590. [CrossRef] [PubMed]

25. Judefeind, A.; de Villiers, M.M. Drug Loading into and In Vitro Release from Nanosized Drug Delivery Systems. In *Nanotechnology in Drug Delivery*; De Villiers, M.M., Aramwit, P., Kwon, G.S., Eds.; Springer: New York, NY, USA, 2009; Volume X, pp. 129–162.

26. Kohane, D.S. Microparticles and Nanoparticles for Drug Delivery. *Biotechnol. Bioeng.* **2007**, *96*, 203–209. [CrossRef] [PubMed]

27. Wendorf, J.R.; Singh, M.; O'Hagan, D.T. Nanoparticles and Microparticles as Vaccine Adjuvants. In *Nanoparticulates as Drug Carriers*; Torchilin, V.P., Ed.; Imperial College Press: London, UK, 2006; pp. 675–696.

28. Mohanraj, V.J.; Chen, Y. Nanoparticles—A Review. *Trop. J. Pharm. Res.* **2006**, *5*, 561–573. [CrossRef]

29. Wiechers, J.W.; Musee, N. Engineered inorganic nanoparticles and cosmetics: Facts, issues, knowledge gaps and challenges. *J. Biomed. Nanotechnol.* **2010**, *6*, 408–431. [CrossRef] [PubMed]

30. Roussaki, M.; Gaitanarou, A.; Diamanti, P.C.; Vouyiouka, S.; Papaspyrides, C.; Kefalas, P.; Detsi, A. Encapsulation of the natural antioxidant aureusidin in biodegradable PLA nanoparticles. *Polym. Degrad. Stab.* **2014**, *108*, 182–187. [CrossRef]

31. Rakmaia, J.; Cheirsilp, B.; Torrado-Agrasar, A.; Simal-Gándara, J.; Mejuto, J.C. Encapsulation of yarrow essential oil in hydroxypropyl-beta-cyclodextrin: Physiochemical characterization and evaluation of bio-efficacies. *CyTA J. Food* **2017**, 1–9. [CrossRef]

32. Sancho, M.I.; Andujar, S.; Porasso, R.D.; Enriz, R.D. Theoretical and Experimental Study of Inclusion Complexes of β-Cyclodextrins with Chalcone and 2′,4′-Dihydroxychalcone. *J. Phys. Chem. B* **2016**, *120*, 3000–3011. [CrossRef] [PubMed]

33. Cannava, C.; Crupi, V.; Guardo, M.; Majolino, D.; Stancanelli, R.; Tommasini, S.; Ventura, C.A.; Venuti, V. Phase solubility and FTIR-ATR studies of idebenone/sulfobutyl ether b-cyclodextrin inclusion complex. *J. Incl. Phenom. Macrocycl. Chem.* **2013**, *75*, 255–262. [CrossRef]

34. Karathanos, V.; Mourtzinos, I.; Yannakopoulou, K.; Andrikopoulos, N. Study of the solubility, antioxidant activity and structure of inclusion complex of vanillin with β-cyclodextrin. *Food Chem.* **2007**, *101*, 652–658. [CrossRef]

35. Gomes, C.; Moreira, R.; Castell-Perez, E. Microencapsulated antimicrobial compounds as a means to enhance electron beam irradiation treatment for inactivation of pathogens on fresh spinach leaves. *J. Food Sci.* **2011**, *76*, 479–488. [CrossRef] [PubMed]

36. Seo, E.; Min, S.; Choi, M. Release characteristics of freeze-dried eugenol encapsulated with β-cyclodextrin by molecular inclusion method. *J Microencapsul.* **2010**, *27*, 496–505. [CrossRef] [PubMed]

37. Pessine, F.B.T.; Calderini, A.; Alexandrino, G.L. Review: Cyclodextrin Inclusion Complexes Probed by NMR Techniques. In *Magnetic Resonance Spectroscopy*; Kim, D.H., Ed.; InTech: Rijeka, Croatia, 2012; pp. 238–264.

38. Locci, E.; Lai, S.; Piras, A.; Marongiu, B.; Lai, A. ^{13}C-CPMAS and ^{1}H-NMR Study of the Inclusion Complexes of β-Cyclodextrin with Carvacrol, Thymol, and Eugenol Prepared in Supercritical Carbon Dioxide. *Chem. Biodivers.* **2004**, *1*, 1354–1366. [CrossRef] [PubMed]

39. Ikuta, N.; Sugiyama, H.; Shimosegawa, H.; Nakane, R.; Ishida, Y.; Uekaji, Y.; Nakata, D.; Pallauf, K.; Rimbach, G.; Terao, K.; et al. Analysis of the Enhanced Stability of R(+)-Alpha Lipoic Acid by the Complex Formation with Cyclodextrins. *Int. J. Molecul. Sci.* **2013**, *14*, 3639–3655. [CrossRef] [PubMed]

40. Dima, C.; Cotarlet, M.; Tiberius, B.; Bahrim, G.; Alexe, P.; Dima, S. Encapsulation of Coriander Essential Oil in Beta-Cyclodextrin: Antioxidant and Antimicrobial Properties Evaluation. *Rom. Biotechnol. Lett.* **2014**, *19*, 9128–9140.

41. Kamimura, J.A.; Santos, E.H.; Hill, L.E.; Gomes, C.L. Antimicrobial and antioxidant activities of carvacrol microencapsulated in hydroxypropyl-beta-cyclodextrin. *LWT Food Sci. Technol.* **2014**, *57*, 701–709. [CrossRef]

42. Pagington, J.S. β-cyclodextrin and its uses in the flavour industry. In *Developments in Food Flavors*; Birch, G.G., Linley, M.G., Eds.; Elsevier Applied Science: London, UK, 1986; pp. 131–150.

43. Carvalho, I.T.; Estevinho, B.N.; Santos, L. Application of microencapsulated essential oils in cosmetic and personal healthcare products—A review. *Int. J. Cosmet. Sci.* **2016**, *38*, 109–119. [CrossRef] [PubMed]
44. Pavela, R.; Benelli, G. Essential oils as ecofriendly biopesticides? Challenges and constraints. *Trends Plant Sci.* **2016**, *21*, 1000–1007. [CrossRef] [PubMed]
45. Bakry, A.M.; Abbas, S.; Ali, B.; Majeed, H.; Abouelwafa, M.Y.; Mousa, A.; Liang, L. Microencapsulation of oils: A comprehensive review of benefits, techniques, and applications. *Comprehens. Rev. Food Sci. Food Safet.* **2016**, *15*, 143–182. [CrossRef]

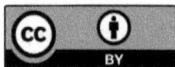

bioengineering

MDPI

Review

Recent Advances in 3D Printing of Aliphatic Polyesters

Ioana Chiulan [1,*], Adriana Nicoleta Frone [1,*], Călin Brandabur [2] and Denis Mihaela Panaitescu [1]

[1]   Polymer Department, National Institute for R&D in Chemistry and Petrochemistry ICECHIM,
      202 Splaiul Independentei, 060021 Bucharest, Romania; panaitescu@icechim.ro
[2]   Symme3D and LTHD Corporation SRL, 300425 Timisoara, Romania; calin.brandabur@symme3d.com
*   Correspondence: ioana.chiulan@icechim-rezultate.ro (I.C.); ciucu_adriana@yahoo.com (A.N.F.);
      Tel.: +40-724-523-149 (I.C.)

Academic Editor: Gary Chinga Carrasco
Received: 3 November 2017; Accepted: 22 December 2017; Published: 24 December 2017

Abstract: 3D printing represents a valuable alternative to traditional processing methods, clearly demonstrated by the promising results obtained in the manufacture of various products, such as scaffolds for regenerative medicine, artificial tissues and organs, electronics, components for the automotive industry, art objects and so on. This revolutionary technique showed unique capabilities for fabricating complex structures, with precisely controlled physical characteristics, facile tunable mechanical properties, biological functionality and easily customizable architecture. In this paper, we provide an overview of the main 3D-printing technologies currently employed in the case of poly (lactic acid) (PLA) and polyhydroxyalkanoates (PHA), two of the most important classes of thermoplastic aliphatic polyesters. Moreover, a short presentation of the main 3D-printing methods is briefly discussed. Both PLA and PHA, in the form of filaments or powder, proved to be suitable for the fabrication of artificial tissue or scaffolds for bone regeneration. The processability of PLA and PHB blends and composites fabricated through different 3D-printing techniques, their final characteristics and targeted applications in bioengineering are thoroughly reviewed.

Keywords: 3D printing; aliphatic polyesters; scaffolds; tissue engineering; polylactic acid; polyhydroxyalkanoates

---

1. Introduction

The diversity and complexity of materials expands continuously with a speed that is beyond of any expectations. Traditional manufacturing cannot meet all the requirements of the new products, especially when they are of small dimension and with high shape complexity. 3D printing, usually called "additive manufacturing", is a useful tool for scalable fabrication of high complexity devices, or materials with multiple functions such as smart materials or customized products. It is very important in the process of prototyping and may also lead to the improvement of manufacturing by increasing the speed of production and lowering product cost. The first 3D printer was invented in 1987 and since then, this technology has grown rapidly because it brings multiple advantages over traditional production methods: (i) very complex structures can be created without added costs; (ii) the pieces are fabricated directly in assembled forms and the number of the components is consistently smaller compared to the same piece obtained by classical methods; and (iii) small series of personalized products can be obtained by this technique [1–3]. The interest for this technology is highlighted by the vibrant growth of the sales reported by 3D printer producers, who claim an increase of 17.4% in worldwide revenues, in 2016, as compared with previous years [4]. A substantial amount of research predicts the proliferation of this industry and a potential increase of the products and services from $6 billion in 2016 to $21 billion worldwide by 2021 [4].

3D-printing technology is attractive for many applications: (i) in the research field for prototyping or for a limited production of prototypes; (ii) in medicine to create 3D biomedical structures using digital models obtained with different medical imaging techniques (computer tomography, magnetic resonance imaging, ultrasound); (iii) in industry for prototyping and manufacture of spare parts for automotive, airplanes, etc. 3D-printing development is speeding up annually due to the reduction of the production cycles, waste, limited use of cutting fluids, and it becomes more accessible for small companies etc. [5]. Thus, 3D printing is often used to develop medical devices [6], flexible electronics [7,8], various pieces for automotive or robotics [9], art objects [2,3], precise replica of archeological objects [10] etc. Dental implants and porous scaffolds for tissue engineering, with increased surface roughness and improved mechanical performance and biocompatibility, used for bone fixation [11,12] are among the most studied medical devices.

The additive manufacturing methods are suitable for multiple types of materials, such as thermoplastics (acrylonitrile-butadiene-styrene (ABS), poly (lactic acid) (PLA), polyamide 6 (PA6), high-impact polystyrene, etc.), resins, metals (Al, steel, Au, Ag, Ti, alloys), gypsum-based powders, ceramics, waxed materials, biomaterials, paper, food. Polymers are by far the most used materials for 3D printing [13]. Likewise, aliphatic polyesters are among the most used biopolymers in the biomedical field due to their non-toxic, biodegradable and biocompatible character [14].

This mini-review deals with the use of aliphatic polyesters in 3D printing for medical applications, with a deeper attention on materials and methods suitable to construct scaffolds for tissue engineering. The industrial applications of 3D printing of aliphatic polyesters are quickly reviewed. The motivation behind this work resides from the recent scientific reports that highlight the ability of additive manufacturing to overcome the limitations of traditional methods such as molding, electrospinning, solvent casting, gas foaming, leaching etc. in the fabrication of medical products. Through 3D-printing techniques it is now possible to obtain superior control of the pore size, to manufacture scaffolds with complex architecture, and to implement biological functions in order to mimic the natural tissue [15,16]. A short presentation of the main 3D-printing methods will be followed by an overview of two most important classes of thermoplastic aliphatic polyesters, poly(lactic acid) and polyhydroxyalkanoates (PHA), their blends and composites that were processed by these methods. Finally, a discussion of the future perspectives and research approaches is included.

2. Short Overview of the Main 3D-Printing Techniques

Broadly, the main 3D-printing techniques commercially available are: (i) selective layer/laser sintering (SLS); (ii) fused filament fabrication (FFF), also known as fused deposition modeling (FDM, trademark of Stratasys) or molten polymer deposition; (iii) stereolithography; (iv) digital light processing; (v) polyjet / inkjet 3D printing and (vi) electronic beam melting [3,16]. Only SLS and FDM have been used for the 3D printing of aliphatic polyesters (Figure 1).

2.1. Selective Laser Sintering

In SLS technique, the 3D-designed model is transferred to the printer, where an infrared laser beam fuses the polymeric powder, especially polyamides and thermoplastic polyurethanes (TPU), as well as metal and ceramic powders, into thin layers, one layer at a time [17]. After the completion of a layer, a new layer of powder is applied to it and then subjected to another round of heating action and sintering. The process is repeated and the completed object is removed from the printer, brushed and sandblasted in order to remove any trace of powder [18]. Depending on the application and material used, the printed object can be further polished and/or dyed. This technique is characterized by a high resolution, is suitable for functional polymers and does not require a support material or structures, so the printed structures can be used without further cleaning steps [19]. Polyamide 12 (PA12) or its powdered blends with PA6 were successfully printed through SLS and represents around 90% of the total industrial consumption [20]. Other materials processed to a much lesser extent through SLS are polyamide 11, PLA and polyether ether ketone.

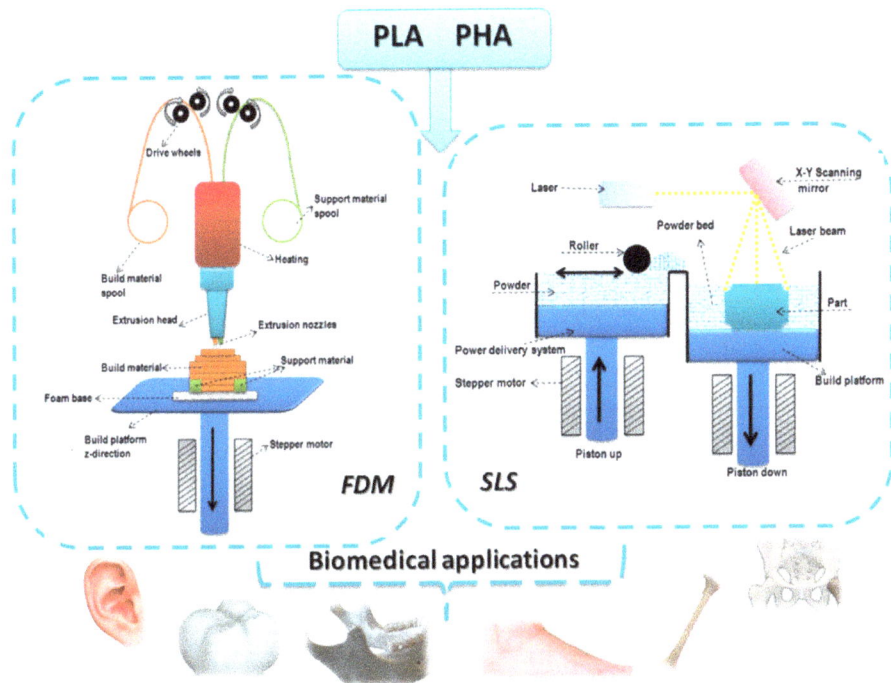

Figure 1. 3D-printing techniques employed for PLA and PHA.

2.2. Fused Deposition Modeling

Through this technique, filaments made of thermoplastic materials are extruded in thin threads and deposited layer by layer in the desired 3D structure and adhere to each other by physical interactions. The layer underneath hardens as it cools and binds with the new layer that is added on the top, remaining a fully solidified structure throughout the process. FDM is already used to produce commercial plastics and, in general, is the most used among all the techniques; this is partially because of the low price of the printer and the facile manipulation, which makes it possible even for home use. Thermoplastic polymers currently processed with FDM are ABS and PLA. Other polymers were also found suitable for this technique: acrylonitrile-styrene-acrylate, PA12, polycarbonate, polyethylene terephtalate, TPU and thermoplastic elastomers. The roughness of the 3D-printed structures is an important issue in the case of FDM, since it affects not only the appearance but also the mechanical resistance of the products. A polishing device connected to the 3D printer [21], the use of the vaporized acetone to melt uniformly the surface of 3D-printed prostheses made of ABS [22] and filling the grooves with the material dissolved by the solvent stored in a pen-style device [23] were among the solutions proposed to remove the layer grooves. FDM technology also allows the printing of cells suspension into a scaffold support. A schematic illustration of a tissue-engineered structure obtained by FDM bioprinter is presented in Figure 2.

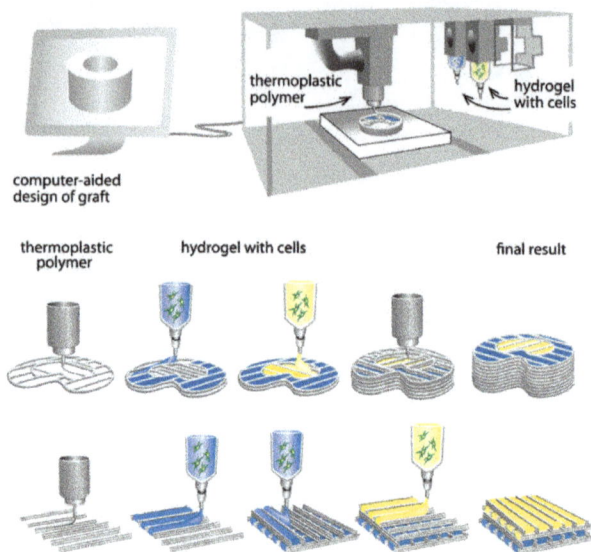

Figure 2. FDM schematic of the bioprinting of tissue and organs.

3. Aliphatic Polyesters for Additive Manufacturing

Well selected and up-to-date information on the additive manufacturing of various polymers were recently reported [13]. Considering the huge importance of aliphatic polyesters for biomedical applications, this review gives thorough information on the use of 3D-printing techniques in the case of PLA and PHA, correlated with the properties of the manufactured products and their applications in bioengineering.

3.1. Poly(Lactic Acid)

PLA is up to now the most used bioplastic for 3D printing by FDM, intended to be used in regenerative medicine, mostly as scaffolds for tissue engineering. PLA is thermoplastic aliphatic polyester (Figure 3a) prepared from fossil fuels or derived from renewable resources such as cornstarch or sugarcanes, rendering it accessible and inexpensive. PLA properties are strongly influenced by even small amounts of enantiomeric impurities. Pure poly(L-lactic acid) (PLLA) or poly(D-lactic acid) are semicrystalline polymers with a glass transition temperature (T_g) around 57 °C and a melting temperature of about 175 °C while PLA with a content of 50–93% L-lactic acid is completely amorphous [24]. Generally, amorphous grades have better processability and wider processing window than the crystalline grades [25] but much lower mechanical properties (Table 1). T_g value is important for amorphous PLA because it determines the maximum usage temperature in most applications while both T_g and T_m vales are important in the case of crystalline PLA applications. Some thermal and mechanical characteristics of PLA are given in Table 1.

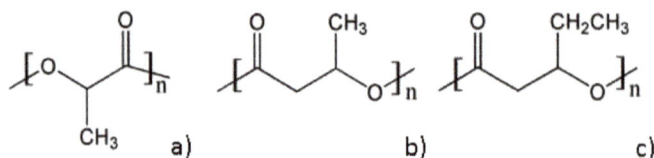

Figure 3. Chemical structures of PLA (**a**), PHB (**b**) and PHV (**c**).

PLA is the most studied aliphatic polyester for biomedical and packaging applications, due to its biocompatibility, biodegradability, clarity, high mechanical strength and modulus, and facile processability through extrusion, injection molding or casting [14]. Moreover, its lower coefficient of thermal expansion and non-adherent properties to the printed surface makes PLA a suitable material for 3D printing. In addition, it is already approved by the Food and Drug Administration (FDA) and European Medicines Agency (EMA), which makes it suitable for rapid transfer from production to clinical trials and fabrication of medical devices, pharmaceutics or various consumer products [26]. This material was intensively studied for applications such as sutures, scaffolds, extracellular matrix, dental implants, drug delivery systems, cell carriers, bioresorbable screws for bones fractures, bioabsorbable meniscus repair and stents, hernia meshes, to name just a few [27].

Table 1. Mechanical and thermal properties of PLA.

Properties	T_g, °C	T_m, °C	Tensile Strength, MPa	Young's Modulus, GPa	References
PLA (Bio-flex®F 6510) solution casting from chloroform	57.5	156.3	15.2	1.17	[28]
PLA (Nature Works™ 4032D) solution casting from DMF	-	-	32.8	2.5	[29]
PLA (Nature Works™ 4031D) extrusion	-	-	40.9	2.9	[30]
PLA film extrusion grade (Nature Works™)	55.3	151.3	40.0	1.4	[31]
PLA (Nature Works™ 4032D) Melt compounding	60.0	167.0	40.0	2.7	[32]

DMF—dimethylformamide

To date, the most common technique for 3D printing of PLA is fused deposition modeling [12,33–51]. Printing parameters such as build orientation, layer thickness, raster angle, raster width, air gap, infill density and pattern, feed rate and others directly influence the quality and the mechanical properties of the FDM printed parts [35]. Considering the importance of mechanical performance for the printed parts, the majority of current studies are focused on the influence of printing parameters on the mechanical properties of the resulted parts [33–35]. Therefore, many recent studies highlighted the mechanical and biocompatibility characteristics of PLA or its composites after 3D printing [36–40].

3.1.1. 3D Printing of PLA through Fused Deposition Modeling

A detailed study comparing the mechanical response of 3D-printed PLA blocks versus that of injection-molded PLA was provided by Song et al. [33]. PLA filament (commercial, diameter 1.75 mm) was deposited in a single direction using FDM method. Specimens cut from the printed blocks were measured along different material directions. 3D printing had a limited influence upon material elasticity; both axial and transverse stiffness being similar to that of injection-molded PLA while the inelastic response of the 3D-printed material was ductile and orthotropic. It was observed that the fracture response of the 3D-printed product was tougher when loaded in the extrusion direction than in the transverse direction. Moreover, the unidirectional 3D-printed material showed an increased toughness as compared to injection-molded PLA, due to its layered and filamentous nature. By controlling the process parameters (extruder temperature, extrusion speed, and deposition speed during 3D printing) the porosity of the material can be controlled.

Other authors used a custom 3D-printing profile for printing the specimen entirely in a single raster orientation in order to evaluate the connection between printing orientation and the material anisotropy [34]. It was found that the 45° raster orientation resulted in a slight improvement of the ultimate tensile strength and fatigue endurance limit as compared to the specimens printed at 0° and 90° raster orientation angles. Still, the mechanical properties of printed specimens were similar to those of PLA filament.

In addition to mechanical properties, 3D-printing process parameters have also great influence on the shape-memory properties of the printed parts, as reported by Wu et al. [26]. Authors used orthogonal experimental design method in order to evaluate the influence of four FDM parameters (layer thickness, raster angle, deformation temperature and recovery temperature) on the shape-recovery ratio and maximum shape-recovery rate of 3D-printed PLA. Authors concluded that the shape-memory effect of 3D-printed PLA parts depended more on recovery temperature and less on the deformation temperature and 3D-printing parameters. These findings could be of great interest for biomedical applications (self-expanding vascular stents, the elimination of thrombus) as well as the selection of parameters for 4D printing.

The possibility to replace conventional processing technique with additive manufacturing is considered by most to be unrealistic and the reasons for this opinion come from some drawbacks of the latter, such as the impossibility of manufacturing very large objects, the limitation to a small range of materials and the cost of high-performance 3D printers. This cost is subsequently reflected by the price of the final product. In order to evaluate the cost of the 3D procedure and the possibility to reduce it, Chacón et al. tried to find a connection between printing parameters and the FDM manufacturing cost [35]. Thus, PLA samples were obtained from a filament with a diameter of 1.75 mm using a low cost desktop 3D printer. Build orientation, layer thickness and feed rate parameters were analyzed and it was found that printing time decreases as layer thickness and feed rate increase. Thus, the manufacturing cost is directly related to the layer thickness and feed rate parameters.

It has been shown previously that it is possible to control the mechanical properties of PLA printed parts using an optimal selection of FDM parameters but other properties are also of great importance when referring, for example, to biomedical applications. In this respect, recent studies focused on the evaluation of PLA printed parts for reconstructive surgery and tissue engineering [36–39]. In a paper by Wurm et al. [39] FDM was successfully employed for the fabrication of PLA discs and the influence of processing technique upon biocompatibility of printed parts was assessed. In vitro tests, using human fetal osteoblasts showed no cytotoxic effects of PLA discs. Since FDM proved no negative influence on the biocompatibility of PLA, this 3D-printing technique could be further used in the reconstructive surgery for the production of individual shaped scaffolds or other implants. The filaments were printed at a nozzle temperature of 225 °C, which led to an enhanced degree of crystallinity of 22% and, finally, to a modulus of elasticity of 3.2 GPa that fits the requirements for maxillofacial implants [39].

PLA membranes, with a thickness of 100 μm and pores diameter of 200 μm, were also fabricated by direct 3D-printing method, using a PLA chloroform solution, of 5%, well dissolved by heating at 45 °C, for 24 h [40]. The PLA membranes were further seeded with human osteoprogenitors and endothelial progenitor cells and then assembled one above the other, to form a layer-by-layer (LBL) structure. After evaluating the properties of LBL constructs in vitro, in 2D – 3D, the authors stated that LBL approach could be suitable for bone tissue engineering in order to promote cells proliferation and a homogenous distribution into the scaffold.

The surface roughness of the 3D structure is very important, since cell attachment and proliferation are mainly influenced by the surface tension, roughness and stiffness of the substrate [41]. In order to enhance the roughness of the surface, Wang et al. used cold atmospheric plasma (CAP) to treat a 3D-printed PLA scaffold fabricated using a FDM printer [12]. They obtained an increase of roughness from 1.20 nm to 27.60 nm upon exposure to CAP for 5 min as compared to the untreated PLA scaffold. A significant increase of the hydrophilicity, revealed by a decrease of the contact angle from 70° to 24°, was obtained after the CAP treatment, which was proven to be a facile route to positively impact the proliferation of the osteoblasts on the PLA scaffold.

Another research study proposed a design process for FDM 3D printing of a prosthetic foot made from PLA which can significantly reduce the prosthetic weight, design and manufacturing cycle [42]. Through this process the initial model was optimized using topology optimization methods. The optimized model was printed directly from a 3D desktop printer. The authors obtained a reduction of the prosthetic feet weight by 62% compared to the initial model and a more accurate 3D-printed product (Figure 4). The proposed method facilitates the manufacturing process and reduces the fabrication time, by skipping the transfer to computer-aided design software. This research can contribute to the improvement of the quality of life of patients who need foot-customized prostheses.

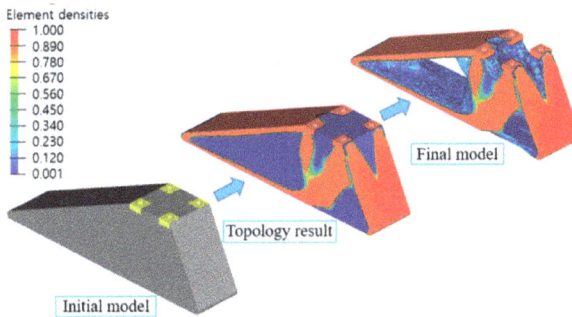

Figure 4. Topology optimization process of designed prosthetic foot. Reproduced with permission from [42].

Flores et al. also emphasized the cost effectiveness, easy manufacturing and high accuracy of the 3D-printing technology. They successfully obtained auricular prosthesis, fully customizable, which replicate in an astonishing degree the skin color and texture of the patient. However, further maintenance and potential replacement of this 3D ear prosthesis may convince the patient to agree with other alternative options [43].

3.1.2. 3D Printing of PLA Composites through Fused Deposition Modeling

PLA has relatively low glass transition temperature (55–60 °C), low toughness and weak heat resistance, which limits its application. Scaffolds made only of PLA do not mimic sufficiently the native bone architecture and they do not ensure properly the cell colonization or mechanical properties. For some uses, PLA needs to be mixed with other polymers or fillers in order to create materials with improved thermal and mechanical properties, or higher biocompatibility for biomedical purposes.

Good improvement of properties was achieved by adding 15 wt.% of nano-hydroxyapatite (HA) to PLA [47,48]. The composite was extruded in filaments and then 3D printed at a nozzle temperature of 220 °C [47]. Long-term creep test revealed a superior hardness of the 3D-printed composite as compared with PLA scaffold and consequently an increase in creep resistance. However, both samples displayed identical delamination destruction, due to limitations of the 3D-printing technique that cannot ensure completely sinterization between the layers. This causes the air to be trapped between layers, which lead to creation of voids. As expected, in vivo tests made on mice showed no inflammatory reaction even after 2 months and a slow biodegradation rate. Corcione et al. used filaments made of PLA and HA in different concentrations to obtain a molar tooth (Figure 5); this was successfully printed using FDM [48].

No noticeable difference was observed for both composites in terms of morphology, thermal behavior and crystallinity. A good dispersion of the filler was observed, but some expectable agglomerations of the nanoparticles took place, both at 5 and 15 wt.% HA. Similar values of the glass transition temperature and crystallization degree were obtained for PLA and PLA/HA samples. The addition of 15% HA influenced the rheological behavior by a significant increase of viscosity and the mechanical properties by the increase with almost 4% of the average compressive modulus as compared with the PLA sample.

Zhuang et al. used 3D printing to obtain plastic items with anisotropic heat and resistance distribution, which allows storing a simple message as color information in the printed objects. These were obtained from conductive graphene doped poly(lactic acid) (G-PLA) [50]. The authors used a method of programmed mixed printing to manufacture PLA composites with anisotropic properties. They stated that the method could be applied to other polymeric materials for a wide range of applications including biomedical ones.

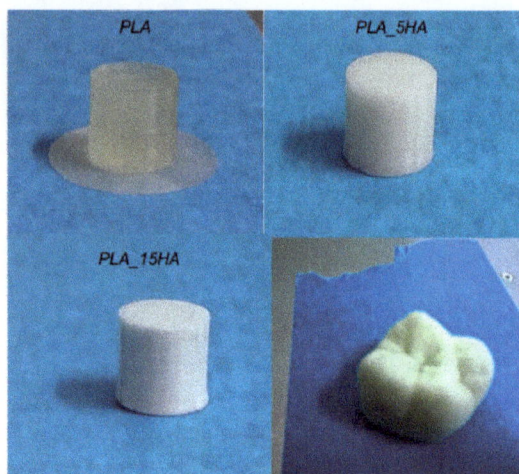

Figure 5. PLA/HA nanocomposites by FDM 3D printer. Reproduced with permission from [48].

For some medical applications, the rigidity and brittleness of the PLA are undesirable and the addition of elastomers is the easiest solution to overcome this drawback. TPU are among the most used polymers in 3D printing. They are also attractive for some biomedical applications due to their biocompatibility, high elongation at break and good abrasion resistance. As shown before, the use of different fillers impart to PLA exceptional mechanical strength, electrical conductivity, and enhanced thermal stability. Among them, composites with carbon fibers and graphene oxide (GO) proved to be also suitable for 3D-printing process. The addition of GO and TPU may have a cumulative effect of increased flexibility and mechanical strength. Chen et al. studied both the influence of the GO concentration and printing orientation on the mechanical properties of a TPU/PLA (7/3) blend [51]. Compression modulus tests have shown an increasing trend with the increase of GO content from 0.5 to 5 wt.% for both printing orientations, but the highest values were found for the specimens having the same printing orientation and height direction. The addition of only 0.5 wt.% GO determined an increase of the tensile modulus by 75% as compared with TPU/PLA sample, further addition of nanofiller determining a reduction of properties. This was explained by the percolation effect, which appeared below 2 wt.% GO content. All TPU/PLA/GO scaffolds supported fibroblast cells growth and proliferation, with the optimum effect at 0.5 wt.%.

3.1.3. 3D Printing of PLA and PLA Composites through SLS

An important requirement for the powders intended for SLS is the sintering behavior, which is greatly influenced by the thermal properties, melt viscosity, melt surface tension, and powder surface energy [13]. Semicrystalline polymers such as PLA exhibit a large change in both viscosity and density within a narrow temperature range upon melting and crystallization, which affects their processing through SLS method. Therefore, the consolidation of semicrystalline powders is conducted by local heating to temperatures slightly above melting temperature [13].

Thus, a porous scaffold was sintered from PLLA using a modified commercial Sinterstation® 2000 system (3D Systems, Valencia, CA, USA), adapted for the use of small amount of raw material [52]. The PLLA was in the form of microsphere of 5–30 μm in diameter, obtained by oil-in-water emulsion solvent evaporation technique. The SLS was conducted at 15 watts, the PLLA powder bed was preheated at 60 °C and the scan spacing was 0.15 mm. The control of the 3D scaffold porosity was difficult, since PLLA microspheres were partially melted and entangled, as revealed by SEM images [52].

The same equipment was further used to manufacture scaffolds made of PLLA and carbonated hydroxyapatite (CHAp) nanospheres, intended for bone tissue reconstruction [52–55]. Both PLLA microspheres and the PLLA/CHAp nanocomposite with 10 wt.% CHAp were prepared by emulsion method. The good dispersion and embedment of the CHAp nanoparticles in the PLLA matrix conducted to the increase of nanocomposite hardness, as revealed by the nanoindentation test. The SLS processing parameters (laser power, scan spacing, part bed temperature, roller speed, scan speed) were optimized in order to obtain adequate porosity, good compression properties, osteoconductivity and biodegradability of the PLLA and PLLA/CHAp scaffolds. The addition of the CHAp was found to influence the thermal behavior, by lowering the glass transition temperature and cold crystallization temperature and increasing to a lesser extent the melting temperature of PLLA. CHAp addition favored the powder deposition but reduced the fusion degree compared with pure PLLA powder. The porosity was mostly influenced by the part bed temperature, being enlarged in the case of nanocomposite [53–55].

Duan et al. reported the fabrication of PLLA/CHAp nanocomposite scaffolds with controllable architecture and pore size for bone tissue engineering starting from PLLA microspheres and PLLA/CHAp nanocomposite microspheres through SLS method [56]. Both raw CHAp microspheres and nanocomposite microspheres were made "in house" using a nanoemulsion method in the first case and double emulsion solvent evaporation method in the second case. More than that, in order to ensure a firm foundation and to facilitate handling of the sintered scaffold a solid base was incorporated into the scaffold design. The sintered PLLA/CHAp nanocomposite scaffolds exhibited a lower porosity value ($66.8 \pm 2.5\%$) as compared with the control PLLA scaffolds ($69.5 \pm 1.3\%$). The mechanical response (the compressive strength and modulus) of 3D scaffolds under dry conditions was higher than the one obtained under wet conditions (immersion in phosphate-buffered saline at 37 °C). In terms of biological evaluation, the PLLA/CHAp nanocomposite scaffolds exhibited a similar level of cell response compared with control PLLA scaffolds. After 7 days culture, the human osteoblastic cells were found to be well attached and spread over the strut surface and interacted favorably with all scaffolds [56].

3.1.4. Other Directions in 3D Printing of PLA Based Materials

PLA may also fit the requirements for electronic devices and other fields by chemical modification or by the addition of different fillers and polymers [44]. The presence of ionic liquids (IL) in a PLA 3D-printed structure provides unique features to PLA-based electronics; IL were recently added in the process of additive manufacturing of PLA filaments by Dichtl et al. [45]. The mixture was prepared by simply adding IL (5 and 10 wt.%) into a PLA chloroform solution, stirring for 12 h and then casting on a teflon plate. A significant enhancement of the PLA conductivity was noticed after the addition of trihexyl tetradecyl phosphonium decanoate, but further mechanical investigations are required to certify that this mixture is suitable for different applications. Prashantha and Roger studied the mechanical and electrical properties of 3D-printed specimens made from commercially available PLA filaments filled with 10 wt.% graphene [46]. The porosity distribution of the structure and the adhesion between layers were characterized through X-ray computed tomography. The results suggested that a shorter deposition time is favorable to obtain better interactions between the fused filaments and the maximum concentration for a suitable graphene dispersion is 10 wt.%. The increase of the electrical resistivity of the 3D-printed specimens, compared with the same composite before FDM processing, was explained by the alignment of the graphene nanoplatelets in the same direction with the deposited filaments. The reinforcing effect of graphene was highlighted by the increase of the storage modulus with more than 20% and tensile strength with 27%, with respect to PLA, as revealed by the DMA and static mechanical analysis [46].

PLA reinforced with 15 wt.% short carbon fibers (length about 60 mm) was manufactured by 3D printing based on fused filament fabrication and tested for mechanical and morphological properties [49]. The PLA composite showed a higher increase in stiffness in the direction of printing.

This behavior was explained by the morphological results, which revealed that the short carbon fibers were mostly aligned with the length of the 3D-printing filament, and remained aligned with the direction of printing within the PLA composite.

Wood pulp fibers (WPF) are valuable reinforcements for many polymers but the application of FDM technology for 3D printing of biocomposites with WPF is a difficult process [57]. The issues are related to the low thermal degradation temperature of the fibers, the small size of the nozzle used in FDM process and the poor dispersion of the fibers in the hydrophobic matrix, which causes fibers accumulation in the nozzle. A full enzymatic treatment was used to modify the surface of thermomechanical pulp (TMP) fibers [57]; TMP fibers modified via laccase-assisted grafting of octyl gallate (OG) showed improved interfacial adhesion with PLA and a remarkable impact on the mechanical properties of PLA-TMP fibers composites. Moreover, filaments obtained from PLA reinforced with OG-treated fibers showed a good behavior during the 3D printing [57].

3D printing of a recycled PLA composite has proved to be a viable solution to the environmental issues, since the remanufactured 3D structure showed even better mechanical properties than the original one. Tian et al. have managed to recover a PLA/carbon fiber composite in a 100% rate for the carbon fiber and 73% for PLA matrix. They reused the material for the fabrication of new filaments, with a carbon fiber content of 10 wt.%, that were further processed by 3D printing [58]. No increase of the tensile strength was observed for the remanufactured composites as compared with the original composite, but other representative characteristics were improved, such as flexural strength, which increased with around 25%. The aging process of the PLA matrix was impossible to be avoided due to repeated thermal cycles, but the mechanical performances were maintained by the addition of pure PLA in the 3D printing of the recycled composite.

3.2. Polyhydroxyalkanoates

The polyesters of aliphatic hydroxyacids, PHA, are natural polymers with some of their properties similar to those of conventional plastic materials but, in addition, they show biodegradability and biocompatibility. PHA are biosynthesized intracellularly as spherical inclusions by some bacterial strains in unbalanced growing conditions (low concentrations of nitrogen, phosphorus, oxygen or magnesium and an excess of carbon). Depending on the number of carbon atoms in the lateral chain, they may be brittle materials or elastomers. Both types are interesting materials for the biomedical field, especially for scaffolds and implants.

Short-chain-length PHA contain 3–5 carbon atoms and show high stiffness and brittleness in relation to their high crystallinity (50–80%) [24]. Poly(3-hydroxybutyrate) (PHB) (Figure 3b) and poly(3-hydroxybutyrate-co-3-hydroxyvalerate) (PHBV) are by far the most studied of PHA and are commercially available. PHB is biodegradable and biocompatible and can be processed with common plastic manufacturing equipment. However, its brittleness and small processing window limits its applications. PHBV, obtained by copolymerization with hydroxyvalerate (HV), is a more ductile material, with lower melting point and decreased strength and stiffness [24,59]. The properties of PHB or PHBV strongly depend on the processing conditions and composition (Table 2).

Table 2. Mechanical and thermal properties of some PHA.

Properties	T_g, °C	T_m, °C	Tensile Strength, MPa	Young's Modulus, GPa	Reference
PHB (Biocycle)—compression molding		164/174	43	3.5	[60]
PHB—solution casting from chloroform			28	2.1	[61]
PHBV 12 mol% HV (Metabolix Inc.)—solvent casting from DMF		140	17		[59]
PHBV 12 mol% HV (Metabolix Inc.)—solvent casting from DMF	~0	140/154	14	0.8	[62]

Cell attachment and viability tests were performed using various cultures and revealed a good biocompatibility of PHA to these cells. For example, CHL fibroblast cells showed good adhesion and proliferation on PHB scaffolds [60]. Moreover, polyhydroxyalkanoates degrade into non-toxic oligomers being suitable candidates for in vivo use in medical applications.

However, the reconstruction of some parts of the human body and organs using PHA is a very complex and difficult process because of the large differences between patients. The patient specific anatomical data should be considered for reconstruction and 3D printing is a promising technique to produce complex medical devices according to the computer aided design of the damage part or organ. Only few data were reported regarding the application of rapid prototyping techniques (RP) for the fabrication of PHA scaffolds [63–70]. Comparing to PLA, PHA cover a much broader range of properties and, therefore multiple possibilities of 3D printing.

3.2.1. PHA Filaments for Fused Deposition Modeling

PHA filaments can be used to obtain scaffolds by using FDM. Wu et al [63] obtained PHBV/palm fibers (PF) composite for 3D printers by melt mixing PHBV grafted with maleic anhydride (PHBV-g-MA) and silane treated PF. The filaments (diameter 1.75 ± 0.05 mm) were obtained from these composite materials by extrusion at 130–140 °C and 50 rpm [63]. The treatments ensured a better adhesion at polymer–filler interface and avoided the phase separation and fluctuation in the filaments diameter. The treated composites showed enhanced mechanical properties compared to that of PHBV matrix and untreated composites and higher biodegradation rate than that of PHBV when incubated in soil. Increased tensile strength and antibacterial activity were also reported for PHBV-g-MA/wood flower (WF) composites prepared with the same purpose, for 3D-printing filaments [64]. Thus, the tensile strength of PHBV-g-MA/WF composites was 6–18 MPa greater than that of untreated composites and increased with the increase of WF content [63]. Wu and Liao [65] have also prepared 3D-printing filaments from PHBV-g-MA composites with acid oxidized multi-walled carbon nanotubes (MWCNTs) using a similar method. Highly improved thermal stability, Young's modulus and antibacterial activity were obtained for only 1.0 wt.% MWCNTs in PHA-g-MA matrix [65]. However, no study on the behavior of these types of filaments in a real 3D-printing process was reported.

3.2.2. PHA Structures Obtained by Selective Laser Sintering

SLS Applied to Pure PHB

SLS technique is very attractive because porous structures with very controlled pore size may be built up without the need of any additives such as plasticizers. Preliminary RP tests with a polyhydroxyalkanoate were done by Oliveira et al. using SLS technique [66]. They worked with a polyhydroxybutyrate powder in pure form (without additives) and obtained structures of about 2.5 mm in thickness (up to 10 layers) with 1 mm holes by SLS (Figure 6).

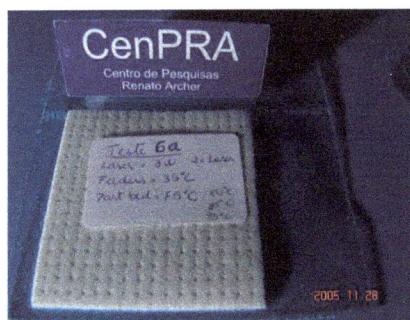

Figure 6. Sintered PHB using SLS containing pores of 1 mm in diameter [66].

They also reported the difficulties encountered with the application of SLS technique to PHB powder, such as excessive dust drag, curbing of the coating or release of vapors and the solutions adopted to solve these problems [66].

Pereira et al synthesized porous 3D cubes with orthogonal channels measuring 0.836 mm in diameter by SLS, starting from a poly(3-hydroxybutyrate) powder from PHB Industrial S/A (Brazil) [67]. A thin layer of powdered PHB was scanned by a CO_2 laser and sintered, the polymer layers being deposited one on the top of each other until the object reached the dimensions of the virtual model. The obtained objects showed geometrical and dimensional features closed to the model [67]. No significant change in crystallinity, glass transition, melting or crystallization temperatures of PHB were detected after SLS process, suggesting no thermal degradation [67]. Moreover, the possibility to recycle PHB through 3 rounds of SLS processes without any sign of degradation was also demonstrated.

SLS Applied to PHA Nanocomposites

One of the most studied applications of PHA based materials is in bone tissue engineering. PHA nanocomposites were designed to obtain 3D scaffolds that mimic the structure and function of an extracellular matrix (ECM) and support cells adhesion and proliferation [56,68–70]. Thus, bionanocomposites microspheres from PHBV and nano-sized osteoconductive inorganic fillers were obtained using a solid-in-oil-in-water emulsion/solvent evaporation method [56]. Nano-sized calcium phosphate (Ca-P) was prepared for this purpose and dispersed in a PHBV-chloroform solution by ultrasonication to form a solid-in-oil nano-suspension which was added to an aqueous solution containing 1% of poly(vinyl alcohol) and maintained at room temperature until total evaporation of the solvent, resulting Ca-P/PHBV nanocomposite microspheres. Tetragonal scaffolds with porosity around 60% were obtained from these nanocomposite microspheres using selective laser sintering. These 3D scaffolds show many advantages related to (i) the nanodimension of the inorganic filler which may provide a better cell response and osteoconductivity, (ii) the nanocomposite microspheres that ensure better dispersion of the nanofiller and (iii) the SLS technique which resulted in a controlled microstructure with totally interconnected pores [56]. Moreover, improved cell proliferation was obtained for Ca-P/PHBV nanocomposite compared to pure PHBV scaffolds.

Porous scaffolds with complex shapes and architecture (Figure 7) were constructed by SLS using Ca–P/PHBV nanocomposite [69]. Moreover, Ca–P/PHBV scaffold representing a human proximal femoral condyle (40% scale-down) was produced by SLS technique. The surface modification of Ca–P/PHBV nanocomposite scaffolds by physically entrapping gelatin and subsequent immobilization of heparin improved the wettability and provided affinity to the growth factor recombinant human bone morphogenetic protein-2 [68]. This osteoconductive nanocomposite with controlled architecture also showed sustained release behavior of osteogenic growth factor and had a great potential for bone tissue engineering [68].

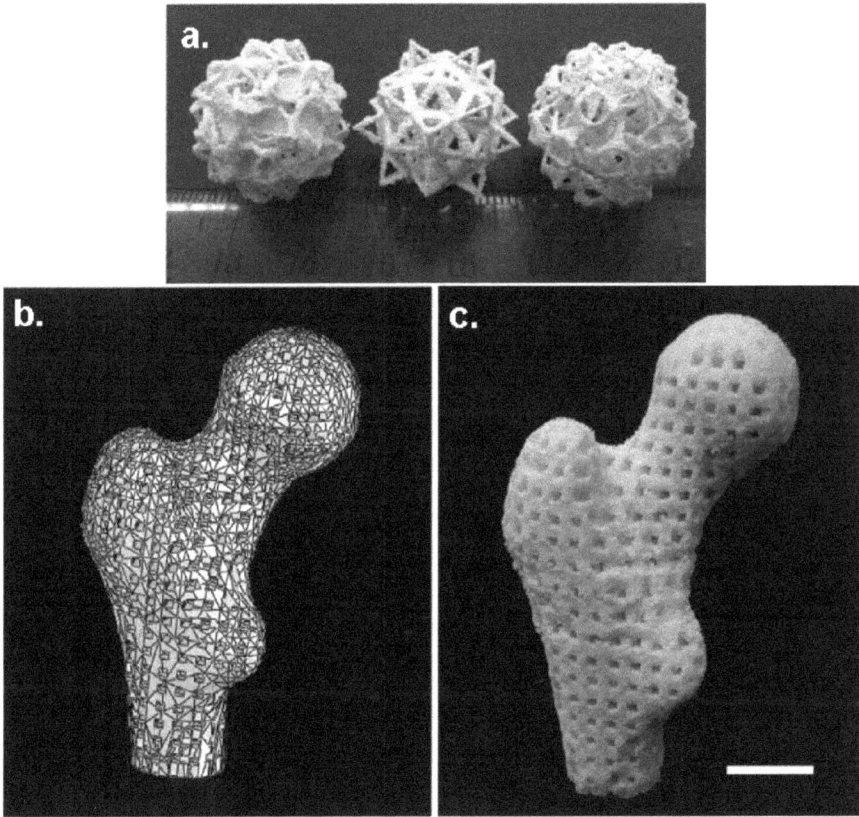

Figure 7. (**a**) Sintered Ca–P/PHBV nanocomposite porous structures based on the following models: salamanders, elevated icosidodecahedron and snarl (from left to right) (**b**) three-dimensional model of a human proximal femoral condyle reconstructed from CT images and then processed into porous scaffold using cubic cells; (**c**) sintered Ca–P/PHBV nanocomposite proximal femoral condyle scaffold. Scale bar, 1 cm. Reproduced with permission from [68].

The technique of preparation of Ca-P/PHBV nanocomposite coupled with SLS also offers the possibility of incorporating biomolecules in the nanocomposite microspheres [69]. The advantage of incorporating biomolecules in nanocomposite microspheres is related to the preservation of their biological activity and controlled release. For this purpose, a model protein, bovine serum albumin (BSA), was encapsulated into Ca-P/PHBV nanocomposite microspheres and Ca-P/PHBV/BSA 3D scaffolds with good dimensional accuracy were produced by SLS [69]. It is worth mentioning that the bioactivity of BSA was maintained during SLS processing. In vitro BSA release test showed an initial high activity followed by a slow release of BSA and a slight degradation of the PHBV matrix after 28 days in vitro test [69].

The influence of the SLS process parameters (laser power, scan spacing, layer thickness) on the quality of Ca–P/PHBV nanocomposite scaffolds was also studied [70]. The quality of the scaffolds was quantified by their structure and handling stability, their dimensional accuracy and their compressive properties and the optimized SLS parameters were determined [70].

The most important results regarding the application of 3D-printing techniques to PLA and PHA-based materials are summarized in Table 3.

Table 3. Summary of 3D-printed PLA-based materials.

Technique	Material	Results	Application	Reference
FDM	PLA	Controllable porosity and pore size by controlling the extrusion and 3D-printing parameters	quantifying anisotropic responses of PLA parts	[33]
FDM	PLA	The 3D-printed samples supports the growth of human fetal osteoblast	Bone reconstruction	[39]
FDM	PLA	The 3D-printed model with optimized design displayed a reduction with 62% of the weight as compared to the initial model	Prosthetic foot	[42]
FDM	PLA	Accurate anatomic aspect, reduced amount of raw material, inexpensive final product	Artificial ear	[43]
FDM	PLA, PLA/ionic liquid (IL)	The addition of IL led to enhanced conductivity	Electronic devices	[45]
FDM	PLA/HA	Good dispersion of the HA in the PLA matrix; increased viscosity and compressive modulus for the composites with 15 wt.% HA	Molar tooth	[48]
FDM	PLA, PLA/graphene	Enhanced electrical resistivity and mechanical strength	Electronics	[46]
FDM	PLA	The increased surface roughness and hydrophilicity conducted to cells attachment and proliferation	Bone regeneration	[12]
FDM	TPU/PLA/GO	0.5 wt.% GO led to the highest tensile modulus and cell proliferation	Tissue engineering scaffolds	[51]
FDM	PHA, PHA-g-MA, PHA/palm fibers, PHA-g-MA/ wood flower	Silane treatment of the palm fibers enhanced the adhesion with the polymer matrix; increased mechanical properties and higher degradation rate of the treated composites as compared to pure PHA and untreated composites; Increased tensile strength and antibacterial activity for PHA-g-MA/ wood flower		[63,64]
SLS	PHB	Fidel replication of the 3D-printed structure with the design model; no thermal degradation of the PHB observed after 3D printing	Tissue engineering	[66,67]
SLS	PHBV/Ca-P	The addition of the inorganic filler led to improved cell proliferation; the SLS process didn't influenced the bioactivity of the incorporated model protein	Bone tissue	[56,68,69]

4. Future Perspectives

The use of additive manufacturing methods for the production of artificial organs, tissues or bone implants is an effervescent research area with a promising future. The new era of artificial tissues and organs started twenty years ago with the production of the first 3D FDM printer and since then significant advancements have been made. However, only a few materials have been transferred to mass production and explored with 3D printing and even less of them were found suitable for medical applications. Aliphatic polyesters and, especially, PLA and PHA are suitable materials for in vivo applications due to their biocompatibility, biodegradability, good mechanical strength and processability. The continuous development of new or more specialized biomaterials is often correlated with the progress in the 3D-printing technology enhancing its potential and forcing its rapid development. There are still some challenges in the introduction of 3D-printing technologies as industrial manufacturing tools competing with injection molding and other well-established techniques. They are related to both material and equipment limits, such as reaching high accuracy of the porosity and morphology of the 3D-printed structure according to design specifications, improving the adhesion between layers, fitting the properties and their spatial distribution are some of these challenges. However, the implementation of 3D printing in biomedicine for building prosthetics, tissue grafts and other surgical implants is much more rapid than in other fields. The actual bioprinting technology is suited for the production of artificial organs or implants containing living cells, which requires a sterile environment, but avoiding contamination while handling and keeping the cells alive until they are placed into the patient are still challenges. Likewise, tuning the mechanical and biological properties of artificial tissues and organs is still a challenge and new biocompatible materials are needed to replicate parts of the human body. In addition, it is important for these future materials to be easily combined and manufactured in order to obtain adjustable properties (strength,

Bioengineering **2018**, *5*, 2

elasticity, color) for each individual, in respect to its age, gender or race. Besides the aliphatic polyesters presented in this mini-review, some elastomers such as TPU or silicones, which can be processed through different 3D-printing technologies, deserve more attention.

Acknowledgments: This work was partially supported by a grant of Ministry of Research and Innovation, CNCS–UEFISCDI, project number PN-III-P4-ID-PCE-2016-0431, within PNCDI III, Contract no. 148/2017, (CELL-3D) and partially by a grant of the Romanian National Authority for Scientific Research and Innovation, CCCDI-UEFISCDI, project number 107 BM.

Author Contributions: Ioana Chiulan, Adriana Nicoleta Frone and Denis Mihaela Panaitescu have equally revised current literature. Calin Brandabur provided the schematic illustration of the FDM bioprinting technique and the technical information about 3D printing.

Conflicts of Interest: The authors declare no conflict of interest.

References

1. Wüst, S.; Müller, R.; Hofmann, S. Controlled positioning of cells in biomaterials—Approaches towards 3D tissue printing. *J. Funct. Biomater.* **2011**, *2*, 119–154. [CrossRef] [PubMed]
2. Balletti, C.; Ballarin, M.; Guerra, F. 3D printing: State of the art and future perspectives. *J. Cult. Herit.* **2017**, *26*, 172–182. [CrossRef]
3. Lee, J.-Y.; An, J.; Chua, C.K. Fundamentals and applications of 3D printing for novel materials. *Appl. Mater. Today* **2017**, *7*, 120–133. [CrossRef]
4. Wohlers, T. *Wohlers Report 2016*; WOHLERS Associates: Fort Collins, CO, USA, 2016.
5. Kamei, K.-I.; Mashimo, Y.; Koyama, Y.; Fockenberg, C.; Nakashima, M.; Nakajima, M.; Li, J.; Chen, Y. 3D printing of soft lithography mold for rapid production of polydimethylsiloxane-based microfluidic devices for cell stimulation with concentration gradients. *Biomed. Microdevices* **2015**, *17*, 36. [CrossRef] [PubMed]
6. Shahali, H.; Jaggessar, A.; Yarlagadda, P.K.D.V. Recent advances in manufacturing and surface modification of titanium orthopaedic applications. *Procedia Eng.* **2017**, *174*, 1067–1076. [CrossRef]
7. Patel, D.K.; Sakhaei, A.H.; Layani, M.; Zhang, B.; Ge, Q.; Magdassi, S. Highly stretchable and UV curable elastomers for digital light processing based 3D printing. *Adv. Mater.* **2017**, *29*, 1606000. [CrossRef] [PubMed]
8. Muth, J.T.; Vogt, D.M.; Truby, R.L.; Mengüç, Y.; Kolesky, D.B.; Wood, R.J.; Lewis, J.A. Embedded 3D printing of strain sensors within highly stretchable elastomers. *Adv. Mater.* **2014**, *26*, 6307–6312. [CrossRef] [PubMed]
9. Bâlc, N.; Vilău, C. Design for additive manufacturing, to produce assembled products, by SLS. *MATEC Web Conf.* **2017**, *121*, 04002. [CrossRef]
10. Additive Manufacturing in Archeology. Available online: http://3dprintingcenter.net/2017/06/16/additive-manufacturing-in-archeology/ (accessed on 3 November 2017).
11. David, O.T.; Szuhanek, C.; Tuce, R.A.; David, A.P.; Leretter, M. Polylactic acid 3D printed drill guide for dental implants using CBCT. *Rev. Chim.-Bucharest* **2017**, *68*, 341–342.
12. Wang, M.; Favi, P.; Cheng, X.; Golshan, N.H.; Ziemer, K.S.; Keidar, M.; Webster, T.J. Cold atmospheric plasma (CAP) surface nanomodified 3D printed polylactic acid (PLA) scaffolds for bone regeneration. *Acta Biomater.* **2016**, *46*, 256–265. [CrossRef] [PubMed]
13. Ligon, S.C.; Liska, R.; Stampfl, J.; Gurr, M.; Mülhaupt, R. Polymers for 3D Printing and Customized Additive Manufacturing. *Chem. Rev.* **2017**, *117*, 10212–10290. [CrossRef] [PubMed]
14. Panaitescu, D.M.; Frone, A.N.; Chiulan, I. Nanostructured biocomposites from aliphatic polyesters and bacterial cellulose. *Ind. Crops Prod.* **2016**, *93*, 251–266. [CrossRef]
15. Mondschein, R.J.; Kanitkar, A.; Williams, C.B.; Verbridge, S.S.; Long, T.E. Polymer structure-property requirements for stereolithographic 3D printing of soft tissue engineering scaffolds. *Biomaterials* **2017**, *140*, 170–188. [CrossRef] [PubMed]
16. Wu, G.-H.; Hsu, S. Polymeric-based 3D printing for tissue engineering. *J. Med. Biol. Eng.* **2015**, *35*, 285–292. [CrossRef] [PubMed]
17. Kruth, J.P.; Wang, X.; Laoui, T.; Froyen, L. Lasers and materials in selective laser sintering. *Assem. Autom.* **2003**, *23*, 357–371. [CrossRef]
18. 3D Printing Material: Alumide. Available online: https://www.sculpteo.com/en/materials/alumide-material/ (accessed on 3 November 2017).

19. Türk, D.-A.; Kussmaul, R.; Zogg, M.; Klahn, C.; Leutenecker-Twelsiek, B.; Meboldt, M. Composites part production with additive manufacturing technologies. *Procedia CIRP* **2017**, *66*, 306–311. [CrossRef]

20. Schmid, M.; Amado, A.; Wegener, K. Polymer powders for selective laser sintering (sls). *AIP Conf. Proc.* **2015**, *1664*, 160009.

21. Dieste, J.A.; Fernández, A.; Roba, D.; Gonzalvo, B.; Lucas, P. Automatic grinding and polishing using spherical robot. *Procedia Eng.* **2013**, *63*, 938–946. [CrossRef]

22. He, Y.; Xue, G.; Fu, J. Fabrication of low cost soft tissue prostheses with the desktop 3D printer. *Sci. Rep.-UK* **2014**, *4*, 6973. [CrossRef] [PubMed]

23. Takagishi, K.; Umezu, S. Development of the improving process for the 3D printed structure. *Sci. Rep.-UK* **2017**, *7*, 39852. [CrossRef] [PubMed]

24. Panaitescu, D.; Frone, A.N.; Chiulan, I. Green Composites with Cellulose Nanoreinforcements. In *Handbook of Composites from Renewable Materials*; Thakur, V.K., Thakur, M.K., Kessler, M.R., Eds.; Scrivener Publishing LLC: Beverly, MA, USA, 2017; Volume 7, pp. 299–338.

25. Farah, S.; Anderson, D.G.; Langer, R. Physical and mechanical properties of PLA, and their functions in widespread applications—A comprehensive review. *Adv. Drug Deliv. Rev.* **2016**, *107*, 367–392. [CrossRef] [PubMed]

26. Wu, W.; Ye, W.; Wu, Z.; Geng, P.; Wang, Y.; Zhao, J. Influence of layer thickness, raster angle, deformation temperature and recovery temperature on the shape-memory effect of 3D-printed polylactic acid samples. *Materials* **2017**, *10*, 970. [CrossRef] [PubMed]

27. Tyler, B.; Gullotti, D.; Mangraviti, A.; Utsuki, T.; Brem, H. Polylactic acid (pla) controlled delivery carriers for biomedical applications. *Adv. Drug Deliv. Rev.* **2016**, *107*, 163–175. [CrossRef] [PubMed]

28. Abdulkhani, A.; Hosseinzadeh, J.; Ashori, A.; Dadashi, S.; Takzare, Z. Preparation and characterization of modified cellulose nanofibers reinforced polylactic acid nano composite. *Polym. Test.* **2014**, *35*, 73–79. [CrossRef]

29. Gu, J.; Catchmark, J.M. Polylactic acid composites incorporating casein functionalized cellulose nanowhiskers. *J. Biol. Eng.* **2013**, *7*, 31. [CrossRef] [PubMed]

30. Oksman, K.; Mathew, A.P.; Bondeson, D.; Kvien, I. Manufacturing process of cellulose whiskers/polylactic acid nanocomposites. *Compos. Sci. Technol.* **2006**, *66*, 2776–2784. [CrossRef]

31. Ambrosio-Martın, J.; Fabra, M.J.; Lopez-Rubio, A.; Lagaron, J.M. Melt polycondensation to improve the dispersion of bacterial cellulose into polylactide via melt compounding: Enhanced barrier and mechanical properties. *Cellulose* **2015**, *22*, 1201–1226. [CrossRef]

32. Frone, A.N.; Panaitescu, D.; Chiulan, I.; Nicolae, C.A.; Vuluga, Z.; Vitelaru, C.; Damian, C.M. The effect of cellulose nanofibers on the crystallinity and nanostructure of poly(lactic acid) composites. *J. Mater. Sci.* **2016**, *51*, 9771–9791. [CrossRef]

33. Song, Y.; Li, Y.; Song, W.; Yee, K.; Lee, K.Y.; Tagarielli, V.L. Measurements of the mechanical response of unidirectional 3D-printed pla. *Mater. Des.* **2017**, *123*, 154–164. [CrossRef]

34. Letcher, T.; Waytashek, M. Material property testing of 3D-printed specimen in PLA on an entry-level 3D printer. *Adv. Manuf.* **2014**, *2A*, IMECE2014-39379.

35. Chacón, J.M.; Caminero, M.A.; García-Plaza, E.; Núñez, P.J. Additive manufacturing of pla structures using fused deposition modelling: Effect of process parameters on mechanical properties and their optimal selection. *Mater. Des.* **2017**, *124*, 143–157. [CrossRef]

36. Guo, R.; Lu, S.; Page, J.M.; Merkel, A.R.; Basu, S.; Sterling, J.A.; Guelcher, S.A. Fabrication of 3D scaffolds with precisely controlled substrate modulus and pore size by templated-fused deposition modeling to direct osteogenic differentiation. *Adv. Healthc. Mater.* **2015**, *4*, 1826–1832. [CrossRef] [PubMed]

37. Pedro, F.C.; Cédryck, V.; Jeremy, B.; Mohit, C.; Manuela, E.G.; Rui, L.R.; Christina, T.; Dietmar, W.H. Biofabrication of customized bone grafts by combination of additive manufacturing and bioreactor knowhow. *Biofabrication* **2014**, *6*, 035006.

38. Almeida, C.R.; Serra, T.; Oliveira, M.I.; Planell, J.A.; Barbosa, M.A.; Navarro, M. Impact of 3-d printed pla- and chitosan-based scaffolds on human monocyte/macrophage responses: Unraveling the effect of 3-d structures on inflammation. *Acta Biomater.* **2014**, *10*, 613–622. [CrossRef] [PubMed]

39. Wurm, M.C.; Möst, T.; Bergauer, B.; Rietzel, D.; Neukam, F.W.; Cifuentes, S.C.; Wilmowsky, C.V. In-vitro evaluation of polylactic acid (PLA) manufactured by fused deposition modeling. *J. Biol. Eng.* **2017**, *11*, 29. [CrossRef] [PubMed]

Bioengineering **2018**, *5*, 2

40. Guduric, V.; Metz, C.; Siadous, R.; Bareille, R.; Levato, R.; Engel, E.; Fricain, J.-C.; Devillard, R.; Luzanin, O.; Catros, S. Layer-by-layer bioassembly of cellularized polylactic acid porous membranes for bone tissue engineering. *J. Mater. Sci. Mater. Med.* **2017**, *28*, 78. [CrossRef] [PubMed]

41. Chiulan, I.; Mihaela Panaitescu, D.; Nicoleta Frone, A.; Teodorescu, M.; Andi Nicolae, C.; Căşărică, A.; Tofan, V.; Sălăgeanu, A. Biocompatible polyhydroxyalkanoates/bacterial cellulose composites: Preparation, characterization, and in vitro evaluation. *J. Biomed. Mater. Res. A* **2016**, *104*, 2576–2584. [CrossRef] [PubMed]

42. Tao, Z.; Ahn, H.-J.; Lian, C.; Lee, K.-H.; Lee, C.-H. Design and optimization of prosthetic foot by using polylactic acid 3D printing. *J. Mech. Sci. Technol.* **2017**, *31*, 2393–2398. [CrossRef]

43. Flores, R.L.; Liss, H.; Raffaelli, S.; Humayun, A.; Khouri, K.S.; Coelho, P.G.; Witek, L. The technique for 3D printing patient-specific models for auricular reconstruction. *J. Cranio Maxill. Surg.* **2017**, *45*, 937–943. [CrossRef] [PubMed]

44. Nakatsuka, T. Polylactic acid-coated cable. *Fujikura Tech. Rev.* **2011**, *40*, 39–45.

45. Dichtl, C.; Sippel, P.; Krohns, S. Dielectric properties of 3D printed polylactic acid. *Adv. Mater. Sci. Eng.* **2017**, *2017*, 10. [CrossRef]

46. Prashantha, K.; Roger, F. Multifunctional properties of 3D printed poly(lactic acid)/graphene nanocomposites by fused deposition modeling. *J. Macromol. Sci. A* **2017**, *54*, 24–29. [CrossRef]

47. Niaza, K.V.; Senatov, F.S.; Stepashkin, A.; Anisimova, N.Y.; Kiselevsky, M.V. Long-term creep and impact strength of biocompatible 3D-printed PLA-based scaffolds. *Nano Hybrids Compos.* **2017**, *13*, 15–20. [CrossRef]

48. Esposito Corcione, C.; Gervaso, F.; Scalera, F.; Montagna, F.; Sannino, A.; Maffezzoli, A. The feasibility of printing polylactic acid–nanohydroxyapatite composites using a low-cost fused deposition modeling 3D printer. *J. Appl. Polym. Sci.* **2017**, *134*. [CrossRef]

49. Ferreira, R.T.L.; Amatte, I.C.; Dutra, T.A.; Bürger, D. Experimental characterization and micrography of 3D printed PLA and PLA reinforced with short carbon fibers. *Compos. B-Eng.* **2017**, *124*, 88–100. [CrossRef]

50. Zhuang, Y.; Song, W.; Ning, G.; Sun, X.; Sun, Z.; Xu, G.; Zhang, B.; Chen, Y.; Tao, S. 3D–printing of materials with anisotropic heat distribution using conductive polylactic acid composites. *Mater. Des.* **2017**, *126*, 135–140. [CrossRef]

51. Chen, Q.; Mangadlao, J.D.; Wallat, J.; De Leon, A.; Pokorski, J.K.; Advincula, R.C. 3D printing biocompatible polyurethane/poly(lactic acid)/graphene oxide nanocomposites: Anisotropic properties. *ACS Appl. Mater. Interfaces* **2017**, *9*, 4015–4023. [CrossRef] [PubMed]

52. Zhou, W.Y.; Lee, S.H.; Wang, M.; Cheung, W.L. Selective Laser Sintering of Tissue Engineering Scaffolds Using Poly(L-Lactide) Microspheres. *Key Eng. Mater.* **2007**, *334–335*, 1225–1228. [CrossRef]

53. Zhou, W.Y.; Lee, S.H.; Wang, M.; Cheung, W.L.; Ip, W.Y. Selective laser sintering of porous tissue engineering scaffolds from poly(L-lactide)/carbonated hydroxyapatite nanocomposite microspheres. *J. Mater. Sci.-Mater. Med.* **2008**, *19*, 2535–2540. [CrossRef] [PubMed]

54. Zhou, W.Y.; Duan, B.; Wang, M.; Cheung, W.L. Crystallization Kinetics of Poly(L-Lactide)/Carbonated Hydroxyapatite Nanocomposite Microspheres. *J. Appl. Polym. Sci.* **2009**, *113*, 4100–4115. [CrossRef]

55. Zhou, W.Y.; Wang, M.; Cheung, W.L.; Ip, W.Y. Selective Laser Sintering of Poly(L-Lactide)/Carbonated Hydroxyapatite Nanocomposite Porous Scaffolds for Bone Tissue Engineering. In *Tissue Engineering*; Eberli, D., Ed.; InTech: Vukovar, Croatia, 2010; pp. 179–204.

56. Duan, B.; Wang, M.; Zhou, W.Y.; Cheung, W.L.; Li, Z.Y.; Lu, W.W. Three-dimensional nanocomposite scaffolds fabricated via selective laser sintering for bone tissue engineering. *Acta Biomater.* **2010**, *6*, 4495–4505. [CrossRef] [PubMed]

57. Filgueira, D.; Holmen, S.; Melbø, J.K.; Moldes, D.; Echtermeyer, A.T.; Chinga-Carrasco, G. Enzymatic-assisted modification of TMP fibers for improving the interfacial adhesion with PLA for 3D printing. *ACS Sustain. Chem. Eng.* **2017**, *5*, 9338–9346. [CrossRef]

58. Tian, X.; Liu, T.; Wang, Q.; Dilmurat, A.; Li, D.; Ziegmann, G. Recycling and remanufacturing of 3D printed continuous carbon fiber reinforced PLA composites. *J Clean. Prod.* **2017**, *142*, 1609–1618. [CrossRef]

59. Ten, E.; Turtle, J.; Bahr, D.; Jiang, L.; Wolcott, M. Thermal and mechanical properties of poly(3-hydroxybutyrate-co-3-hydroxyvalerate)/cellulose nanowhiskers composites. *Polymer* **2010**, *51*, 2652–2660. [CrossRef]

60. Pinto, C.E.D.S.; Arizaga, G.G.C.; Wypych, F.; Ramos, L.P.; Satyanarayana, K.G. Studies of the effect of molding pressure and incorporation of sugarcane bagasse fibers on the structure andproperties of poly (hydroxy butyrate). *Compos. A-Appl. Sci. Manuf.* **2009**, *40*, 573–582. [CrossRef]

61. Cai, Z.; Ynag, G.; Kim, J. Biocompatible nanocomposites prepared by impregnating bacterial cellulose nanofibrils into poly(3-hydroxybutyrate). *Curr. Appl. Phys.* **2011**, *11*, 247–249.
62. Jiang, L.; Morelius, E.; Zhang, J.; Wolcott, M. Study of the poly(3-hydroxybutyrate-co-3-hydroxyvalerate)/ cellulose nanowhisker composites prepared by solution casting and melt processing. *J. Compos. Mater.* **2008**, *42*, 2629–2645. [CrossRef]
63. Wu, C.-S.; Liao, H.; Cai, Y.-X. Characterisation, biodegradability and application of palm fibre-reinforced polyhydroxyalkanoate composites. *Polym. Degrad. Stabil.* **2017**, *140*, 55–63. [CrossRef]
64. Wu, C.-S.; Liao, H. Fabrication, characterization, and application of polyester/wood flour composites. *J. Polym. Eng.* **2017**, *37*, 689–698. [CrossRef]
65. Wu, C.-S.; Liao, H. Interface design of environmentally friendly carbon nanotube-filled polyester composites: Fabrication, characterisation, functionality and application. *Express Polym. Lett.* **2017**, *11*, 187–198. [CrossRef]
66. Oliveira, M.F.; Maia, I.A.; Noritomi, P.Y.; Nargi, G.C.; Silva, J.V.L.; Ferreira, B.M.P.; Duek, E.A.R. Construção de Scaffolds para engenharia tecidual utilizando prototipagem rápida. *Matéria* **2007**, *12*, 373–382. [CrossRef]
67. Pereira, T.F.; Oliveira, M.F.; Maia, I.A.; Silva, J.V.L.; Costa, M.F.; Thire, R.M.S.M. 3D Printing of Poly(3-hydroxybutyrate) Porous Structures Using Selective Laser Sintering. *Macromol. Symp.* **2012**, *319*, 64–73. [CrossRef]
68. Duan, B.; Wang, M. Customized Ca–P/PHBV nanocomposite scaffolds for bone tissue engineering: design, fabrication, surface modification and sustained release of growth factor. *J. R. Soc. Interface* **2010**, *7*, S615–S629. [CrossRef] [PubMed]
69. Duan, B.; Wang, M. Encapsulation and release of biomolecules from Ca-P/PHBV nanocomposite microspheres and three-dimensional scaffolds fabricated by selective laser sintering. *Polym. Degrad. Stabil.* **2010**, *95*, 1655–1664. [CrossRef]
70. Duan, B.; Cheung, W.L.; Wang, M. Optimized fabrication of Ca–P/PHBV nanocomposite scaffolds via selective laser sintering for bone tissue engineering. *Biofabrication* **2011**, *3*, 015001. [CrossRef] [PubMed]

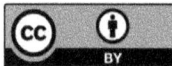

bioengineering

MDPI

Article

Modification of Bacterial Cellulose Biofilms with Xylan Polyelectrolytes

Sara M. Santos [1,*]**, José M. Carbajo** [1]**, Nuria Gómez** [1]**, Miguel Ladero** [2] **and Juan C. Villar** [1]

[1]   Laboratory of Cellulose and Paper, INIA, Forest Research Center, Ctra. De la Coruña km 7.5,
      28040 Madrid, Spain; chema@inia.es (J.M.C.); nuria@inia.es (N.G.); villar@inia.es (J.C.V.)
[2]   Department of Chemical Engineering and Materials, Universidad Complutense de Madrid,
      Avda. Complutense s/n, 28040 Madrid, Spain; mladero@quim.ucm.es
*   Correspondence: santos@inia.es; Tel.: +37-913-476-834

Academic Editor: Gary Chinga Carrasco
Received: 31 October 2017; Accepted: 23 November 2017; Published: 28 November 2017

Abstract: The effect of the addition of two [4-butyltrimethylammonium]-xylan chloride polyelectrolytes (BTMAXs) on bacterial cellulose (BC) was evaluated. The first strategy was to add the polyelectrolytes to the culture medium together with a cell suspension of the bacterium. After one week of cultivation, the films were collected and purified. The second approach consisted of obtaining a purified and homogenized BC, to which the polyelectrolytes were added subsequently. The films were characterized in terms of tear and burst indexes, optical properties, surface free energy, static contact angle, Gurley porosity, SEM, X-ray diffraction and AFM. Although there are small differences in mechanical and optical properties between the nanocomposites and control films, the films obtained by BC synthesis in the presence of BTMAXs were remarkably less opaque, rougher, and had a much lower specular gloss. The surface free energy depends on the BTMAXs addition method. The crystallinity of the composites is lower than that of the control material, with a higher reduction of this parameter in the composites obtained by adding the BTMAXs to the culture medium. In view of these results, it can be concluded that BC–BTMAX composites are a promising new material, for example, for paper restoration.

Keywords: bacterial cellulose; xylan polyelectrolytes; nanocomposites

1. Introduction

Bacterial cellulose (BC) is produced by certain bacterial species. BC consists of elementary fibrils of pure cellulose, free of lignin and hemicellulose, and it is considered a natural nanocellulose [1,2]. These elementary fibrils make up a flat, ribbon like microfibril, which are branched together in the BC films, providing high mechanical strength [3]. BC shows high crystallinity, high water absorption capacity, and high degree of polymerization [4]. These properties, along with its biocompatibility, make it an attractive candidate for a big range of applications in various fields, receiving much attention as potential materials associated with biomedical and biotechnology applications [2].

BC is an excellent matrix for the preparation of composites. The use of cellulosic materials in polymer composites has been growing over the past, due to advantages such as low density, renewability, and biodegradability [5]. BC may be used in high quality special applications of bio-based composites, because of the small fibril dimensions that enable direct contact between cellulose and polymers, allowing for a large contact surface, and thus, excellent adhesion. BC composites showed considerably improved properties, leading to additional applications in the medical and other industrial fields [6].

BC permits two ways of composites forming: by in situ BC modification, adding composite partners to the culture medium, or by processing BC previously synthesized [7]. In the literature, different compounds have been added to study their influence on yield, morphology, and crystalline constituents of BC, including agar [8], sodium alginate [9], carboxymethylcellulose [10,11], pectin [9], carbon nanotubes [12], polyacrylamide [13], xylan [14], xyloglucan [15], acetyl glucomannan [16], lignosulfonate [17], and microcrystalline cellulose [18].

It has been proven that xylans interact with cellulose, and are irreversibly absorbed onto cellulosic surfaces [19]. Adsorption of the pre-isolated xylans has been shown to improve pulp properties, such as tensile strength, beatability and resistance to hornification [20]. However, it is well known that only low amounts of xylan can be adsorbed in comparison with xylan derivatives [21]. Despite the use of xylans for cellulose fiber modification, these polymers can be transformed into new polymers with promising properties by chemical modification [22]. The cationic ammonium xylan derivatives are described to enhance the tensile modulus of pulp, compared to the untreated pulp [23]. Vega et al. [24] produced and characterized [4-butyltrimethylammonium]-xylan chloride polyelectrolytes. They observed, by using time-of-flight secondary ion mass spectrometry (ToF-SIMS), that BTMAXs were adsorbed onto the surface of cellulosic fibers of bleached pine kraft pulp. They concluded that a positive polyelectrolyte prepared from extracted xylan could be used as a modifying fiber surface agent. Therefore, certain improvements on BC properties are expected by including BTMAXs during its production.

In the present study, we have produced BC/xylan polyelectrolytes nanocomposites by incorporating xylan polyelectrolytes by two different approaches. In the first process, xylan polyelectrolytes were incorporated in BC hydrogels by adding them to the medium for *Gluconacetobacter sucrofermentans*. The second process was based on the penetration and adsorption of the xylan polyelectrolytes in a BC hydrogel that was previously produced and homogenized. The obtained BC composites were characterized in terms of tear and burst indexes, optical properties, static and dynamic contact angles, Gurley porosity, SEM, X-ray diffraction, and AFM.

2. Materials and Methods

2.1. Microorganism

Gluconacetobacter sucrofermentans CECT 7291 was obtained from the Spanish Type Culture Collection (CECT, Valencia, Spain). For maintenance, it was subcultured periodically in HS medium [25]. *G. sucrofermentans* was grown in HS solid medium placed in Petri dishes for 6 days, in order to obtain the suspension of bacterial cells to be utilized in further experiments. Five hundred milliliter Erlenmeyer flasks containing 100 mL of liquid HS medium were inoculated with biomass from these dishes, and cultivated in static conditions for 4 days. Subsequently, the pellicles formed were cut in small pieces (about 1 cm × 1 cm) in sterile conditions, and shaken with the liquid medium at 700 rpm for 30 min. The suspension obtained was filtered through gauze, centrifuged at 4000 rpm for 10 min, and after removing the supernatant, the pellet was washed with Ringer's solution (NaCl, 2.5 g/L; KCl, 0.105 g/L; $CaCl_2 \cdot 2H_2O$, 0.120 g/L; and $NaHCO_3$, 0.05 g/L). The solid phase was centrifuged again in the same conditions, and the final pellets were re-suspended in a small volume of Ringer's solution. The optical density of the suspension at a wavelength of 600 nm was adjusted to 0.59–0.64 (McFarland standards 3-4) diluting when needed with Ringer's solution. Of this final solution, 250 µL was used to inoculate 100 mL of medium.

2.2. Films Production and Purification

The objective is to obtain BC films modified with xylan derivatives by two different strategies, one based on the addition of the polymers to the culture medium during the synthesis of BC (s), and a second one adding the polymers to the BC already generated and homogenized (h).

Polymers, named PS5 and PS6, are two xylan derivatives modified with 4-[*N,N,N*-trimethylammonium]butyrate chloride (XTMAB), with different degrees of substitution (0.13 for PS5 and 0.58 for PS6). These polyelectrolytes were a kind gift from the research group of P. Fardim at

Åbo Akademi in Turku (Finland). According to Vega et al. [24], the molecular weight of the repeating unit of the polymer is 200 g/mol, and the saturation of cellulose with the polymer is reached with 70 μmol of functional groups per gram of pulp (BC in this case). In order to maximize xylan–BC interactions, xylan derivatives were added so as to reach the saturation point (27 mg of PS5/BC sheet and 6 mg of PS6/BC sheet).

Culture medium employed for BC production in both cases, (s) and (h), was a modified HS medium (fructose, 20 g/L; yeast extract, 5 g/L; corn steep liquor, 5 g/L; Na_2HPO_4, 2.7 g/L; and citric acid, 1.15 g/L). In all cases, 100 mL of liquid medium were added to 150 mm Petri dishes, inoculated with the suspension described above, and cultivated at 30 °C under static conditions. As it has been described previously [26], in one week under these conditions, BC films of approximately 0.25 g dry weight are obtained.

For BC composites generated during BC synthesis (s), polymers were added to the culture medium as inoculation was performed (BC_PS5$_s$; BC_PS6$_s$). Also, control films without polymer have been generated (BC_C$_s$). All sheets were collected after 7 days of culture, purified by boiling them for 1 h at 90 °C in 1% NaOH, and washing them afterwards, thoroughly with distilled water. They were dried by filtration on a Büchner funnel and air-dried afterwards.

For BC composites from the BC previously homogenized (h), BC films have been obtained in the same way as control ones. After washing them as described previously, they were gelled using a Panda Plus 2000 homogenizer (GEA Niro Soavi, Parma, Italy), treating them five consecutive times at a pressure of 600 bar, with a subsequent consistency adjustment at 1%. After that, xylan derivatives have been added, adjusting again the consistency at 0.5%. Appropriate amounts of gel were placed in Petri dishes and allowed to dry in order to obtain layers (BC_PS5$_h$; BC_PS6$_h$). Control layers (BC_C$_h$) were prepared in the same way, but avoiding addition of xylan derivatives.

2.3. X-ray Diffraction (XRD)

BC crystallinity was studied by XRD using a multipurpose PAN analytical diffractometer (PANalytical, Almelo, Netherlands), model X'PertMPD. This diffractometer is equipped with a copper X-ray tube and two goniometers with vertical configuration th-2th and Bragg–Brentano optic. One of the goniometers has a multipurpose sample support, which can hold large samples as heavy as 1 kg and measuring up to 10 cm × 10 cm × 10 cm. The supporting platform of the second goniometer is a sample spinner fitted with an automatic sampler with 21 positions. The diffractometer is used in phase analysis and, in this study, the angular range between $2\theta = 5°–40°$ was studied. The crystallinity indexes for the BC samples have been calculated in each case using the Equation (1) [27]:

$$Crystallinity~(\%) = \frac{I_{200} - I_{2\theta=18}}{I_{200}} \times 100 \tag{1}$$

2.4. Contact Angle Measurements and Surface Free Energy Determination

The samples' wettability was studied by means of contact angle measurements in air (α), using distilled water. This technique has been also used to obtain the samples surface free energy, since the contact angle measurement, using liquids whose surface tension is known, is an indirect method to analyze this parameter, being fast, simple, and based on easy-to-use equations. Several studies can be found in the open literature concerning the fundamentals of this method [28–30].

The measurements were performed in a DataPhysics Instrument OCA 15 plus, running on SCA 20/21 software (DataPhysics Instruments GmbH, Filderstand, Germany) and using the sessile drop method. A CCD camera takes the images of the initial resting drop immediately after the drop impacts on the paper surface. The corresponding contact angle is calculated after fitting the drop contour line numerically, using the Young–Laplace method. In this study, a 15 drop test was made for distilled water, applying a drop volume of 2 μL.

The surface free energy (γ) was calculated by the OWRK (Owens, Wendt, Rabel and Kaelble) method, which considers the interfacial tension as a function of the dispersive (γ_d) and polar (γ_p) interactions [30]. In this study, the probe liquids were *n*-hexane, ethylene glycol, 1,2-propanediol, formamide, and distilled water, using the 15 drop test, and 5 μL for each one.

The influence of surface topography in the contact angle has been rather reported by several authors, who recommended using the Wenzel´s roughness correction [31–33]. The Wenzel Equation (2) establishes that the relationship between the measured contact angle (α_m) and the corrected angle in an ideal flat surface (α_c) may be written as follows:

$$\cos \alpha_m = r \times \cos \alpha_c \qquad (2)$$

where *r* is the topographical correction factor Equation (3) obtained as:

$$r = 1 + \frac{Sdr}{100} \qquad (3)$$

where *Sdr* is the developed interfacial area ratio provided by atomic force microscopy (AFM). The Wenzel's correction was carried out for each contact angle measured in this study.

2.5. Scanning Electron Microscopy (SEM)

The morphology of the BC layers was studied by SEM microscopy using a JEOL JSM 6335F (JEOL, Peabody, MA, USA) at 1 kV (with maximum resolution of 5 nm) to avoid energetic degradation of the samples during SEM observation. Samples have been previously cryo-fractured after immersing them into liquid nitrogen, and metalized with gold during 3 min and stored for 16–18 h at 50° in a vacuum stove (20 mmHg) before proceeding with SEM observations. This latter treatment led to total dryness of the samples.

2.6. Atomic Force Microscopy (AFM)

The BC derivatives were characterized by means of AFM imaging using a Nanoscope IIIa Bruker microscope (Bruker, Billerica, MA, USA). The images were scanned in the AFM in tapping mode in air using 2 nm radio cantilevers (TESP-SS Bruker, Bruker, Billerica, MA, USA). The drive frequency of the cantilever was approximately 0.4–0.5 Hz. The images were 10 × 10 μm. Scan size 10 μm, tip velocity 8 μm/s, 256 lines, aspect ratio: 1:1, scan angle 0, Z range 1500 nm. Except for flattening, no image processing was conducted. The surface roughness was evaluated with the root mean square average of height deviation taken from the mean image data plane (Rq).

2.7. Mechanical and Optical Properties

The following mechanical properties were determined: basic weight (ISO 536:2012), burst strength (ISO 2759:2001), and tear strength (ISO 1974:2012). A Color Touch reflectometer (Datacolor®, Lawrenceville, NJ, USA) was used to assess the optical properties: ISO brightness (ISO 2470-1:2009), opacity (ISO 2471:2008), and yellowness index (SCAN-G 5:03). Yellowness is defined as the attribute by which an object color is judged to depart from a preferred white toward yellow.

The specular gloss was determined using an angle of incidence of 75° (ISO 8254-1:1999). To measure the air permeance of papers, a Gurley porosimeter was used (ISO 5636-5:2013).

3. Results and Discussion

3.1. X-ray Diffraction

X-ray diffraction was used to study the structure of the obtained materials (Figure 1). Each of them has two diffraction dominant peaks, one disposed between 14° and 15°, and the other between 22° and 24°. Each of the peaks presents the two crystalline phases, Iα and Iβ. According to Barud et al. [34],

Bioengineering **2017**, *4*, 93

who investigated membranes of BC, the first peak represents the projection of the planes (1 0 0) of fraction Iα and (1 1 0 and 0 1 0) of fraction Iβ, and the second peak represents the projection of the planes (1 1 0) Iα and (2 0 0) I Iβ.

The obtained diffractograms suggest that the addition of BTMAXs did not alter BC crystalline morphology in any case, which is consistent with the results obtained by Huang et al. [35]. A decrease in peak intensity can be observed around $2\theta = 17°$ in the samples from the generation with the BTMAXs in culture medium, compared with their control (Figure 1a). This behavior was also observed by Khan et al. [36]. This peak is also evident in the samples from the homogenized BC (Figure 1b), regardless of whether they have polyelectrolytes or not.

(a)   (b)

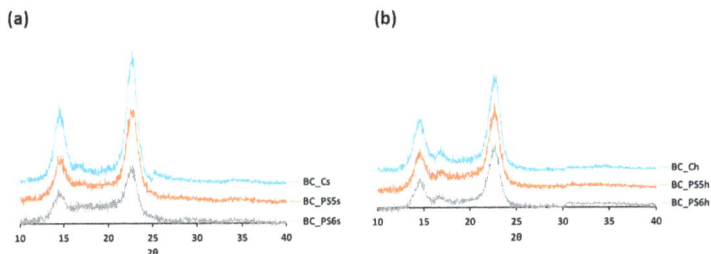

Figure 1. X-Ray diffraction patterns of (a) samples obtained from non-homogenized bacterial cellulose (BC), and (b) samples obtained from homogenized BC.

The crystallinity indexes of the materials are shown on Table 1. It can be observed that materials made only with BC are more crystalline than the materials with xylan polyelectrolytes, regardless of the method of production. The amorphous nature of BTMAXs could be the cause of decreased crystallinity, being these results in agreement with previous studies showing a reduction in crystallinity due to the presence of additives [36,37].

Table 1. Crystallinity index (%) of pure BC and composites made by adding [4-butyltrimethylammonium]-xylan chloride polyelectrolytes (BTMAXs) to the culture medium and to the homogenized BC.

	Crystallinity Index (%)
BC_C$_s$	82.61
BC_PS5$_s$	75.45
BC_PS6$_s$	72.86
BC_C$_h$	80.92
BC_PS5$_h$	74.48
BC_PS6$_h$	78.68

As it can be observed, when BTMAXs are added to the culture medium, the crystallinity decrement is more pronounced than if the addition of the polymer is done to the homogenized BC. The reason may be found by Huang et al. [35], who observed that hydroxypropylmethyl cellulose or carboxymethyl cellulose do not stick regularly on individual microfibrils, preventing the aggregation of microfibrils and ribbon formation during fermentation. Hirai et al. [11] concluded that the effect of polymer additives on the formation of microfibrils of BC depends on their degrees of polymerization or substitution, which can explain the differences in the crystallinity between PS5 and PS6.

When the addition of the polyelectrolytes is carried out after the homogenization of BC, the decrease in crystallinity is slight. This was also observed when chitosan (Ch) is included after the BC formation: the intermolecular hydrogen bonding interaction between the BC and Ch molecules promotes a slight decrease in the crystallinity index of the BC_C$_h$ composites, compared to pure BC [38].

Yano et al. [39] used two processes to prepare nanocomposites of BC filled with silica particles. In one of them, *G. xylinus* was incubated in medium containing silica particles, which disturbs the formation of ribbon-shaped fibrils and affects the preferential orientation of the (110) plane, modifying the crystallinity. In the other process, the BC hydrogel was immersed in different concentrations of silica solutions, allowing silica particles to diffuse into the BC hydrogel and lodge in the spaces between the ribbon-shaped fibrils, hardly affecting the crystallinity.

3.2. Contact Angle Measurements

The surface free energy and polar/dispersive components of samples are presented in Table 2. As it can be seen, both biofilm controls showed similar values of surface free energy and its components, as expected.

Table 2. Surface free energy of samples: polar and dispersive components and contact angle with water.

	Surface Free Energy-γ- (mN/m)	Dispersive Component-γ_d- (mN/m)	Polar Component-γ_p- (mN/m)	Polar Component/Surface Free Energy-γ_p/γ- (%)	Contact Angle with Water-α_w- (°)
BC_C$_s$	37.7	12.6	25.03	66.5	62.4
BC_PS5$_s$	24.9	18.2	6.67	26.8	88.6
BC_PS6$_s$	32.5	16.2	16.28	50.1	73.2
BC_C$_h$	35.2	14.2	21.00	59.7	65.4
BC_PS5$_h$	47.7	10.0	37.78	79.1	46.3
BC_PS6$_h$	42.0	11.8	30.22	71.9	54.0

The use of BTMAXs to obtain composites led to a change in the surface free energy and its components, but the behavior depends on the way of obtaining the biofilms.

When the BTMAXs were added to culture medium, the resulting γ values were smaller than the control one, whereas the γ values were increased when blending them with the homogenized BC. These data are in agreement with those by Lopes et al. [40], who suggested that hyaluronic acid (HA) added to the culture medium are retained inside the membrane. Therefore, during the BC synthesis, the free hydroxyl groups of the newly formed BC fibrils orientate toward the HA, becoming no longer available to occupy the surface, and lowering the surface hydrophilicity of the material.

On the contrary, when BTMAXs are mixed with the homogenized BC, there could be polar groups on the surface of the composite, from both the BC and the polyelectrolytes. This would increase their surface free energy. The more hydrophilic character of these surfaces is in accordance with Harnett et al. [41], who observed that low surface energy values correspond to surfaces with high hydrophobic character. This is in accordance with Vega et al. [24], who observed that the BTMAXs were evenly adsorbed onto the surface of pulp fibers, following Langmuir model.

The composites showed quite similar values of dispersive component (γ_d), ranging from 10.0 mN/m to 18.2 mN/m, whereas variability in the polar component (γ_p) was greater, from 6.7 mN/m to 37.8 mN/m. This polar component is related to the cellulose wettability with water. Thus, material with a high γ_p has greater affinity for water, resulting in low static contact angles [31,42,43]. Figure 2 shows the relationship between polar component and static contact angle with water (α_w). It can be observed that α_w decreased when the polar component of samples increased. The regression analysis between these two component reveals a significant correlation between both parameters at a 95% confidence level ($r = 0.99$), confirming that the static contact angle between water and material increases with decreasing γ_p. This finding may provide an important understanding about how to modify the BC to obtain hydrophobic surfaces.

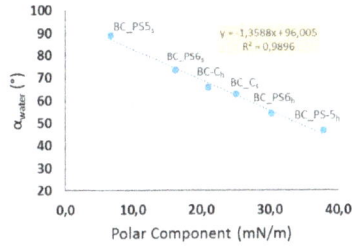

Figure 2. Relation between the polar component of surface free energy of the samples and their static contact angles obtained with water.

3.3. Scanning Electron Microscopy

The morphology of BC dried layers has been studied by SEM microscopy (Figure 3). This technique allows obtaining images of the surface and the cross sections of the samples, so evident qualitative differences between pure BC films and those of nanocomposites can be appreciated.

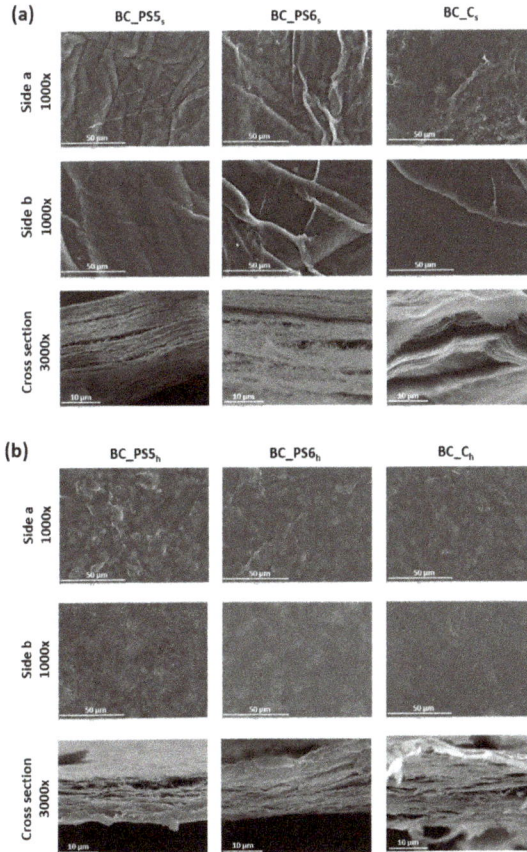

Figure 3. SEM images at different magnifications of samples. (**a**) Samples obtained from non-homogenized BC. (**b**) Samples obtained from homogenized BC.

SEM microscopic images of samples obtained from adding polyelectrolytes to the culture medium (Figure 3a) reveal that the surface of the films depends on their composition. The presence of BTMAX promotes a rougher surface, which supports the specular gloss results (Table 4).

When the BTMAXs were added to the BC previously homogenized (Figure 3b), the resulting gels were placed in Petri dishes, and allowed to air dry. This resulted in that the faces of the composites that were in contact with the Petri dishes (face b) are clearly smoother. This is confirmed by AFM data and images (Figure 4) and, as will be seen later, by greater gloss values (Table 4). In this case, SEM micrographs of the samples from gel (Figure 3b) allowed us to observe that there are no differences on the surfaces between the added BTMAXs. This is in accordance with data obtained from surface free energy (Table 2), as it was mentioned before.

It was also observed the morphology of cryo-fractured samples, corresponding to the cross sections. The structures of pure BC and nanocomposites were formed by a group of thin sheets, forming a pile. The fact that pure BC and nanocomposites have similar morphology at these scales, confirm that the blending of the BTMAX with BC took place on the nano scale. SEM micrographs corresponding to the transversal sections of the sheets reveal that the process in which the BTMAXs are added to the homogenized BC promotes a more compact structure, if compared to other studied samples.

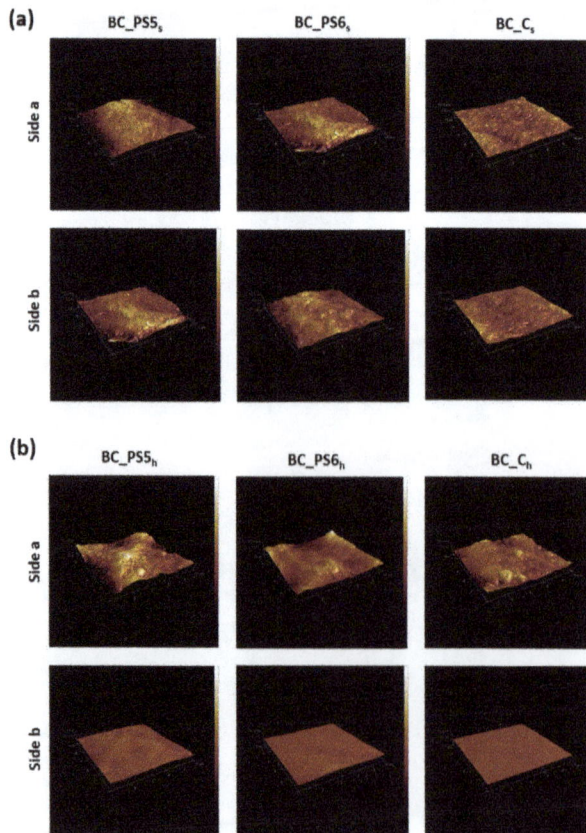

Figure 4. AFM images of samples. (**a**) Samples obtained from non-homogenized BC. (**b**) Samples obtained from homogenized BC. Size of the images: 10 μm × 10 μm × 750 nm.

3.4. Atomic Force Microscopy

AFM was used for studying surface roughness at the nanoscale. The obtained values for Rq are shown in Table 3. It was observed that addition of the BTMAX to the culture medium increases the Rq, having rougher surface when compared to the other samples. When the BTMAXs were added to the homogenized BC, an increment is also observed, but in this case, the increase in side b is less prominent. These results are in agreement with the data obtained in surface free energy determinations, SEM microimages, and gloss values.

Table 3. Roughness values, obtained with AFM, of pure BC and its composites.

	Rq	
	Side a	Side b
BC_C$_s$	55.05	52.25
BC_PS5$_s$	127.00	110.30
BC_PS6$_s$	102.80	87.80
BC_C$_h$	84.80	12.77
BC_PS5$_h$	110.30	38.85
BC_PS6$_h$	88.10	23.95

The qualitative differences between the morphologies of the pure BC samples and those of the nanocomposites can be seen in the AFM images (Figure 4). The images confirm the results obtained by the SEM, the surface free energy measurements, and the gloss values. The polyelectrolytes added to the culture medium (Figure 4a) promote rougher surface formation. On the other hand, the main difference accompanied by polyelectrolytes addition to the homogenized BC (Figure 4b) was the drying method, as it was discussed above.

3.5. Mechanical and Optical Properties

The basic weight and the bulk of the samples are shown in Figure 5. According to several studies, the ratio of the biosynthesis of cellulose by *A. xylinum* is changed depending on the culture conditions, e.g., additives and temperature [44,45]. This observation is consistent with our data, shown in Figure 5a. The specific volume or bulk is the inverse of the density, that is, the volume in cm^3 of 1 g of paper. Bulk provides information on the structure of the sheet, and is related to most of the properties of paper, specially porosity, stiffness, hardness, and strength. Bulk also affects the absorption and the ease of being printed. Bulk can be modified by many factors, as the presence of materials that fill the voids in the sheet, or factors affecting the number of joints between fibers, such as fiber diameter.

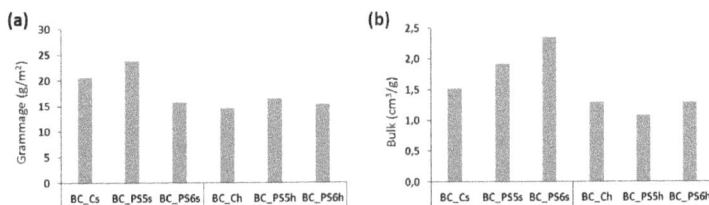

Figure 5. (a) Grammage (g/m^2) and (b) bulk (cm^3/g) of the samples.

When bulk is determined for all samples (Figure 5b), important differences have been found. When composites are made by adding the polyelectrolytes to the homogenized BC, bulk presents similar values in all cases. On the contrary, when the polymers have been added to the culture medium (Figure 5a), resultant samples have higher bulk values, showing a less compact structure, an observation confirmed by SEM images (Figure 3), which showed more compact layers in the case of the samples made from the homogenized BC.

Noticeable results are obtained when mechanical properties (burst and tear) are analyzed, as shown in Figure 6. With both xylan polymers, PS5 and PS6, there is an increment in burst index (Figure 6a), regardless of the strategy followed to obtain the samples (BTMAX addition to culture medium, or addition to the homogenized BC). Similarly, Yano et al. [39] observed an increase in tensile strength by adding silica particles to the BC already formed. Tear index (Figure 6b) remains close to the original value in all cases.

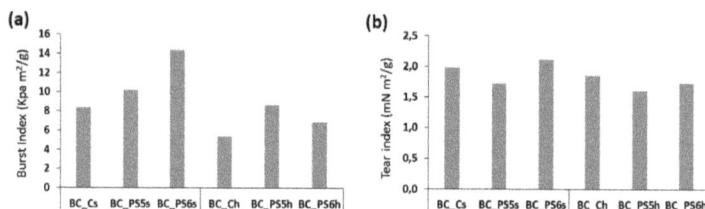

Figure 6. (a) Burst index (KPa m^2/g) and (b) tear index (mN m^2/g) of the samples.

Optical properties of the pure BC and the composites are shown in Table 4. The yellowness is similar in all cases, slightly higher in the case of having added PS5, probably due to the higher amount of polymer. For the same reason, brightness is a little lower when the added polyelectrolyte is PS5. In any case, this variable is a little higher in the case of samples made by adding BTMAXs to homogenized BCs. It should be noted that opacity is twice as high for the samples obtained by adding the polyelectrolytes to the homogenized BC, which may be due to a greater compactness of the layers as observed in SEM micrographs. Santos et al. [46] showed the same effect for aged BC films.

Table 4. Optical properties of the BC and modified samples with PS_5 and PS_6.

	Yellowness (%)	Opacity (%)	Brightness (%)	Gloss (%)	
				Side a	Side b
BC_C$_s$	22.46 ± 1.69	23.61 ± 1.50	50.17 ± 1.24	35.26 ± 10.59	40.69 ± 7.74
BC_PS5$_s$	28.73 ± 0.95	24.25 ± 1.23	41.01 ± 1.05	8.72 ± 2.65	9.93 ± 2.74
BC_PS6$_s$	18.99 ± 0.97	20.72 ± 1.61	53.19 ± 1.14	10.53 ± 2.19	12.36 ± 2.41
BC_C$_h$	19.27 ± 1.12	40.64 ± 2.57	56.89 ± 1.01	13.83 ± 0.39	73.83 ± 4.76
BC_PS5$_h$	25.42 ± 0.78	39.24 ± 4.14	48.79 ± 0.68	14.47 ± 0.33	81.04 ± 4.49
BC_PS6$_h$	19.03 ± 0.89	40.15 ± 2.22	56.70 ± 0.91	13.58 ± 0.18	79.54 ± 2.31

Gloss deserves special attention. If the samples were obtained by adding polyelectrolytes to the culture medium, the resulting gloss of BC composites were lower compared to the control samples, i.e., a drastic (75%) gloss reduction. This result could be of interest in applications requiring a reduced gloss level or no gloss at all, such as paper restoration. Both sides of samples showed similar gloss values. In contrast, when BTMAXs were added to the homogenized BC, there was no difference in the gloss values when compared with the control samples. In all cases, the a-sides of samples show much higher gloss values than the b-sides. This great difference between sides could be due to the drying method; the side that was in contact with the Petri dishes was much smoother than that which was dried in the air. Gloss values do not depend on whether PS5 or PS6 is used.

The influence of BC structure in the properties of the samples is assessed using Gurley permeance. Gurley porosity values were consistently higher than 900 s, so the closed structure of the BC prevents the air flow through it. This agrees with Yousefi et al. findings [47].

Bioengineering **2017**, *4*, 93

4. Conclusions

Incorporation of [4-butyltrimethylammonium]-xylan chloride polyelectrolytes (BTMAXs) on bacterial cellulose (BC) can alter the properties of the cellulose produced, increasing the roughness and the burst index. Gurley porosity values were consistently higher than 900 s, which indicates that the closed structure of the BC prevents the air flow through it. The use of the BTMAXs resulted in materials with less crystallinity index. It also led to a change in the surface free energy, but the behavior depended on the way the biofilms were obtained. The inclusion of BTMAXs in the culture media promotes a remarkable gloss decrease, and the opacity is twice as high in the case of the samples obtained by adding the polyelectrolytes to the homogenized BC. Finally, the described in situ approach proved to be successful for the development of novel nanocomposite materials based on BC and xylan derivatives.

Acknowledgments: The authors wish to thank the Spanish Ministry of Science and Innovation for funding this study via projects CTQ 2010-17702 and CTQ2013-45970-C2-2-R, and the Madrid Regional Government for funding via project RETO-PROSOST S2013/MAE2907. The technical support of Ms. Ana Soubrié (ICTS National Center of Electronic Microscopy in Madrid) in AFM and SEM analysis is gratefully acknowledged. Likewise, we are very grateful to Julian Velázquez, from the DRX research center at Complutense University, for his technical support.

Author Contributions: Sara M. Santos, José M. Carbajo and Juan C. Villar conceived the experiments; Sara M. Santos, José M. Carbajo and Nuria Gómez performed the experiments; Sara M. Santos, José M. Carbajo, Nuria Gómez and Miguel Ladero analyzed the data; all authors contributed writing the paper.

Conflicts of Interest: The authors declare no conflict of interest.

References

1. Iguchi, M.; Yamanaka, S.; Budhiono, A. Bacterial cellulose: A masterpiece of nature's arts. *J. Mater. Sci.* **2000**, *35*, 261–270. [CrossRef]
2. Chawla, P.R.; Bajaj, I.B.; Survase, S.A.; Singhal, R.S. Microbial cellulose: Fermentative production and applications. *Food Technol. Biotechnol.* **2009**, *47*, 107–124.
3. Castro, C.; Zuluaga, R.; Putaux, J.L.; Caro, G.; Mondragon, I.; Gañán, P. Structural characterization of bacterial cellulose produced by *Gluconacetobacter swingsii* sp. from Colombian agroindustrial wastes. *Carbohydr. Polym.* **2011**, *84*, 96–102. [CrossRef]
4. El-Saied, H.; El-Diwany, A.I.; Basta, A.H.; Atwa, N.A.; El-Ghawas, D.E. Production and characterization of economical bacterial cellulose. *Bioresources* **2008**, *3*, 1196–1217.
5. Moon, R.J.; Martini, A.; Nairn, J.; Simonsen, J.; Youngblood, J. Cellulose nanomaterials review: Structure, properties and nanocomposites. *Chem. Soc. Rev.* **2011**, *40*, 3941–3994. [CrossRef] [PubMed]
6. Moniri, M.; Moghaddam, A.B.; Azizi, S.; Rahim, R.A.; Ariff, A.B.; Saad, W.Z.; Navaderi, M.; Mohamad, R. Production and Status of Bacterial Cellulose in Biomedical Engineering. *Nanomaterials* **2017**, *7*, 257. [CrossRef]
7. Klemm, D.; Kramer, F.; Moritz, S.; Lindstrom, T.; Ankerfors, M.; Gray, D.; Dorris, A. Nanocelluloses: A new family of nature-based materials. *Angew. Chem. Int. Ed. Engl.* **2011**, *50*, 5438–5466. [CrossRef] [PubMed]
8. Bae, S.; Sugano, Y.; Shoda, M. Improvement of bacterial cellulose production by addition of agar in a jar fermentor. *J. Biosci. Bioeng.* **2004**, *97*, 33–38. [CrossRef]
9. Ishida, T.; Mitarai, M.; Sugano, Y.; Shoda, M. Role of water-soluble polysaccharides in bacterial cellulose production. *Biotechnol. Bioeng.* **2003**, *83*, 474–478. [CrossRef] [PubMed]
10. Seifert, M.; Hesse, S.; Kabrelian, V.; Klemm, D. Controlling the water content of never dried and reswollen bacterial cellulose by the addition of water-soluble polymers to the culture medium. *J. Polym. Sci. Part A Polym. Chem.* **2003**, *42*, 463–470. [CrossRef]
11. Hirai, A.; Tsuji, M.; Yamamoto, H.; Horii, F. In situ crystallization of bacterial cellulose III. Influence of different polymeric additives on the formation on microfibrils as revealed by transmission electron microscopy. *Cellulose* **1998**, *5*, 201–213. [CrossRef]
12. Yan, Z.; Chen, S.; Wang, H.; Wang, B.; Wang, C.; Jiang, J. Cellulose synthesized by *Acetobacter xylinum* in the presence of multi-walled carbon nanotubes. *Carbohydr. Res.* **2008**, *343*, 73–80. [CrossRef] [PubMed]
13. Joseph, G.; Rowe, G.E.; Margaritis, A.; Wan, W. Effects of polysaccharide-co-acrylic acid on cellulose production by *Acetobacter xylinum*. *J. Chem. Technol. Biotechnol.* **2003**, *78*, 964–970. [CrossRef]

14. Weimer, P.J.; Hackney, J.M.; Jung, H.J.; Hatfield, R.D. Fermentation of bacterial cellulose/xylan composite by mixed ruminal microflora: Implications for the role of polysaccharide matrix interactions in plant cell wall biodegradability. *J. Agric. Food Chem.* **1995**, *48*, 1727–1733. [CrossRef]

15. Whitney, S.E.C.; Brigham, J.E.; Darke, A.H.; Reid, J.S.G.; Gidley, M. In vitro assembly of cellulose/xyloglucan networks: Ultrastructural and molecular aspects. *Plant J.* **1995**, *8*, 491–504. [CrossRef]

16. Tokoh, C.; Takabe, K.; Fujita, M.; Saiki, H. Cellulose synthesized by *Acetobacter xylinum* in the presence of acetyl glucomannan. *Cellulose* **1998**, *5*, 249–261. [CrossRef]

17. Keshk, S. Physical properties of bacterial cellulose sheets produced in presence of lignosulfonate. *Enzyme Microb. Technol.* **2006**, *40*, 9–12. [CrossRef]

18. Cheng, K.C.; Catchmark, M.J.; Demirci, A. Effect of different additives on bacterial cellulose production by *Acetobacter xylinum* and analysis of material property. *Cellulose* **2009**, *16*, 1033–1045. [CrossRef]

19. Linder, Å.; Bergman, R.; Bodin, A.; Gatenholm, P. Mechanism of assembly of xylan onto cellulose surfaces. *Langmuir* **2003**, *19*, 5072–5077. [CrossRef]

20. Köhnke, T.; Brelid, H.; Westman, G. Adsorption of cationized barley husk xylan on Kraft pulp fibres: Influence of degree of cationization on adsorption characteristics. *Cellulose* **2009**, *16*, 1109–1121. [CrossRef]

21. Esker, A.; Becker, U.; Jamin, S.; Beppu, S.; Renneckar, S.; Glasser, W. Self-assembly behavior of some co- and heteropolysaccharides related to hemicelluloses. In *Hemicelluloses: Science and Technology*; Gatenholm, P., Tenkanen, M., Eds.; American Chemical Society: Washington, DC, USA, 2002; pp. 198–219. ISBN 9780841238428.

22. Heinze, T.; Liebert, T.; Koschella, A. *Esterification of Polysaccharides*; Springer: Berlin/Heidelberg, Germany; New York, NY, USA, 2006; p. 86, ISBN 978-3-540-32112-5.

23. Schwikal, K.; Heinze, T.; Saake, B.; Puls, J.; Kaya, A.; Esker, A.R. Properties of spruce sulfite pulp and birch Kraft pulp after sorption of cationic birch xylan. *Cellulose* **2011**, *18*, 727–737. [CrossRef]

24. Vega, B.; Petzold-Welcke, K.; Fardim, P.; Heinze, T. Studies on the fibre surfaces modified with xylan polyelectrolytes. *Carbohydr. Polym.* **2012**, *89*, 768–776. [CrossRef] [PubMed]

25. Hestrin, S.; Schramm, M. Synthesis of cellulose by *Acetobacter xylinum*. 2. Preparation of freeze-dried cells capable of polymerizing glucose to cellulose. *Biochem. J.* **1954**, *58*, 345–352. [CrossRef] [PubMed]

26. Santos, S.M.; Carbajo, J.M.; Villar, J.C. Bacterial Cellulose from *Gluconacetobacter sucrofermentans* CECT 7291 in the Restoration of Degraded Paper: The Effect of Carbon and Nitrogen Sources on Cellulose Production and Properties. *Bioresources* **2013**, *8*, 3630–3645. [CrossRef]

27. Retegi, A.; Gabilondo, N.; Peña, C.; Zuluaga, R.; Castro, C.; Gañan, P.; de La Caba, K.; Mondragon, I. Bacterial cellulose films with controlled microstructure-mechanical property relationship. *Cellulose* **2010**, *17*, 661–669. [CrossRef]

28. Chibowski, E. Surface energy of solid from contact angle hysteresis. *Adv. Colloid Interface Sci.* **2003**, *103*, 149–172. [CrossRef]

29. Tiberg, F.; Daicic, J.; Fröberg, J. Surface chemistry of paper. In *Handbook of Applied Surface and Colloid Chemistry*; Holmberg, K., Ed.; John Wiley & Sons: Chichester, UK, 2001; pp. 123–173, ISBN 0-471-49083-0.

30. Owens, D.K.; Wendt, R.C. Estimation of the surface free energy of polymers. *J. Appl. Polym. Sci.* **1969**, *13*, 1741–1747. [CrossRef]

31. Tåg, C.M.; Pykönen, M.; Rosenholm, J.B.; Backfolk, K. Wettability of model fountain solutions: The influence on topo-chemical and-physical properties of offset paper. *J. Colloid Interface Sci.* **2009**, *330*, 428–436. [CrossRef] [PubMed]

32. Ferreira, P.J.T.; Moutinho, I.M.T.; Figueiredo, M.M.L. How paper topography affects contact angle measurement. In Proceedings of the V Congreso Iberoamericano de Investigación en Celulosa y Papel, Grafisma, Mexico, 20–23 October 2008; pp. 66–69.

33. Wenzel, R.N. Resistance of solid surfaces to wetting by water. *Ind. Eng. Chem.* **1936**, *28*, 988–994. [CrossRef]

34. Barud, H.S.; Assuncao, M.N.; Martines, M.A.U.; Dexpert-Ghys, J.; Marques, R.F.C.; Messaddeq, Y.; Ribeiro, S.J.L. Bacterial cellulose-silica organic-inorganic hybrids. *J. Sol-Gel Sci. Technol.* **2008**, *46*, 363–367. [CrossRef]

35. Huang, H.-C.; Chen, L.-C.; Lin, S.-B.; Hsu, C.-P.; Chen, H.-H. In situ modification of bacterial cellulose network structure by adding interfering substances during fermentation. *Bioresour. Technol.* **2010**, *101*, 6084–6091. [CrossRef] [PubMed]

36. Khan, S.; Ul-Islam, M.; Khattak, W.A.; Ullah, M.W.; Park, J.K. Bacterial cellulose-poly(3,4-ethylenedioxythiophene)-poly(styrenesulfonate) composites for optoelectronic applications. *Carbohydr. Polym.* **2015**, *127*, 86–93. [CrossRef] [PubMed]

37. Kim, S.H.; Lee, C.M.; Kafle, K. Characterization of crystalline cellulose in biomass: Basic principles, applications, and limitations of XRD, NMR, IR, Raman, and SFG. *Korean J. Chem. Eng.* **2013**, *130*, 2127–2141. [CrossRef]

38. Ul-Islam, M.; Shah, N.; Ha, J.H.; Park, J.K. Effect of chitosan penetration on physico-chemical and mechanical properties of bacterial cellulose. *Korean J. Chem. Eng.* **2011**, *28*, 1025–1103. [CrossRef]

39. Yano, S.; Maeda, H.; Nakajima, M.; Hagiwarta, T.; Sawaguchi, T. Preparation and mechanical properties of bacterial cellulose nanocomposites loaded with silica nanoparticles. *Cellulose* **2008**, *15*, 111–120. [CrossRef]

40. Lopes, T.D.; Riegel-Vidotti, I.C.; Grein, A.; Tischer, C.A.; Faria-Tischer, P.C.S. Bacterial cellulose and hyaluronic acid hybrid membranes: Production and characterization. *Int. J. Biol. Macromol.* **2014**, *67*, 401–408. [CrossRef] [PubMed]

41. Harnett, E.M.; Alderman, J.; Wood, T. The surface energy of various biomaterials coated with adhesion molecules used in cell culture. *Colloids Surf. B Biointerfaces* **2007**, *55*, 90–97. [CrossRef] [PubMed]

42. Oliveira, P.; Conceição, S.; Santos, N.F.; Velho, J.; Ferreira, P. The influence on rheological modifiers on coated papers: A comparision between CMC and MHPC. In Proceedings of the III Congreso Iberoamericano de Investigación en Celulosa y Papel, Madrid/Córdoba, Spain, 10–12 November 2004; pp. 354–359.

43. Moutinho, I.M.T.; Ferreira, P.J.T.; Figueiredo, M.L. Impact of surface sizing on inkjet printing quality. *Ind. Eng. Chem. Res.* **2007**, *46*, 6183–6188. [CrossRef]

44. Yamamoto, H.; Horii, F.; Hirai, A. In-situ crystallization of bacterial cellulose II. Influences of polymeric additives with different molecular weights on the formation of Celluloses I_α and I_β at the early stage of incubation. *Cellulose* **1996**, *3*, 229–242. [CrossRef]

45. Yamamoto, H.; Horii, F. In Situ crystallization of bacterial cellulose I. Influences of polymeric additives, stirring and temperature on the formation celluloses I_α and I_β as revealed by cross polarization/magic angle spinning (CP/MAS) ^{13}C NMR spectroscopy. *Cellulose* **1994**, *1*, 57–66. [CrossRef]

46. Santos, S.M.; Carbajo, J.M.; Quintana, E.; Ibarra, D.; Gómez, N.; Ladero, M.; Eugenio, M.E.; Villar, J.C. Characterization of purified bacterial cellulose focused on its use on paper restoration. *Carbohydr. Polym.* **2015**, *116*, 173–181. [CrossRef] [PubMed]

47. Yousefi, H.; Faezipour, S.; Hedjazi, S.; Mousavi, M.M.; Azusa, Y.; Heidaria, A.H. Comparative study of paper and nanopaper properties prepared from bacterial cellulose nanofibers and fibres/ground cellulose nanofibers of canola straw. *Ind. Crops Prod.* **2013**, *43*, 732–737. [CrossRef]

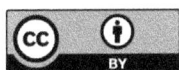

bioengineering

MDPI

Communication

Decoration of Cotton Fibers with a Water-Stable Metal–Organic Framework (UiO-66) for the Decomposition and Enhanced Adsorption of Micropollutants in Water

Marion Schelling [1], Manuela Kim [2,3], Eugenio Otal [2,3] and Juan Hinestroza [1,*

1   Department of Fiber Science, Cornell University, Ithaca, NY 14853, USA; ms2567@cornell.edu
2   Division of Porous Materials, UNIDEF, CITEDEF, CONICET, S. J. B de la Salle 4397, Villa
    Martelli (B1603ALO), Buenos Aires 1603, Argentina; mlkrei@gmail.com (M.K.); Eugenioh@gmail.com (E.O.)
3   Laboratory for Materials Science and Technology, FRSC-UTN, Av. Inmigrantes 555,
    Río Gallegos 9400, Argentina
*   Correspondence: jh433@cornell.edu; Tel.: +1-607-255-7600

Academic Editor: Gary Chinga Carrasco
Received: 15 October 2017; Accepted: 14 January 2018; Published: 12 February 2018

Abstract: We report on the successful functionalization of cotton fabrics with a water-stable metal–organic framework (MOF), UiO-66, under mild solvothermal conditions (80 °C) and its ability to adsorb and degrade water micropollutants. The functionalized cotton samples were characterized by X-ray diffraction (XRD), scanning electron microscopy (SEM), energy-dispersive X-ray spectroscopy (EDX), transmission electron microscopy (TEM), Fourier transform infrared spectroscopy (FTIR), and X-ray photoelectron spectroscopy (XPS). UiO-66 crystals grew in a uniform and conformal manner over the surface of the cotton fibers. The cotton fabrics functionalized with UiO-66 frameworks exhibited an enhanced uptake capacity for methylchlorophenoxypropionic acid (MCPP), a commonly used herbicide. The functionalized fabrics also showed photocatalytic activity, demonstrated by the degradation of acetaminophen, a common pharmaceutical compound, under simulated sunlight irradiation. These results indicate that UiO-66 can be supported on textile substrates for filtration and photocatalytic purposes and that these substrates can find applications in wastewater decontamination and micropollutant degradation.

Keywords: UiO-66; MOF; cotton fabric; functionalized cellulose; methylchlorophenoxypropionic acid; paracetamol

---

1. Introduction

Metal–organic frameworks (MOFs) are highly tunable, porous materials with applications in gas adsorption [1–6], separation [7–9], catalysis [10–13], and filtration [14]. Zirconium-based MOFs in particular are of great interest because of their thermal stability [15] and their robustness over large ranges of pH [16]. UiO-66, a zirconium-based MOF, has excellent stability in water [17], making it an excellent candidate for the removal of micropollutants in aqueous systems [18–20]. However, the fact that these MOFs are synthesized almost exclusively in powder form may hinder their potential in applications requiring the use of large and mechanically stable, yet flexible surfaces. Textiles are mechanically stable and flexible substrates that can be manufactured in large volumes.

While the growth of MOFs on metal oxides has been amply reported, only few of these reports have discussed the coordination of the metal in the MOFs to fibers or textiles [21–27]. In one of these few reports, Zhao et al. [25] describe a method for the formation of MOF–nanofiber kebabs on Nylon-6 nanofibers using atomic layer deposition (ALD). ALD is a highly effective technique for precision coating, but because it requires the use of sophisticated equipment under controlled vacuum conditions, it remains expensive and rather difficult to scale up to large surfaces.

Herein, we report on the growth of UiO-66 on cotton, using methods amenable to existing manufacturing processes used in the textile industry. Figure 1 shows the two-step synthesis pathway followed: The first step is the carboxymethylation of the cotton substrates [21], and the second step is the low-temperature solvothermal synthesis of the MOF on the surface of the carboxymethylated fibers.

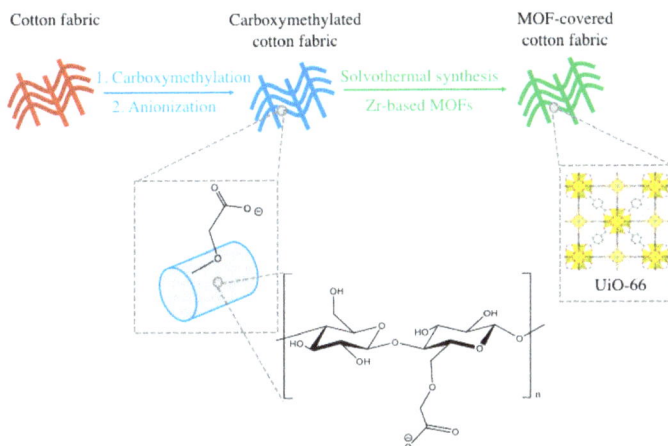

Figure 1. Schematic of the two-step synthesis pathway to grow UiO-66 on the surface of cotton fibers: The first step is the carboxymethylation of cellulose, and the second step is the low-temperature solvothermal synthesis of the metal-organic framework (MOF) on the surface of the carboxymethylated fibers.

Methylchlorophenoxypropionic acid (MCPP) is commonly used as a phenoxyacid herbicide, and it has been frequently detected in groundwater sources [28]. This contaminant can be partially removed by processes such as advanced oxidation and granular activated carbon filtration [29,30]. However, further improvements are needed because of issues related to the effectiveness, cost and environmental sustainability of these processes [31–33]. Seo et al. published promising results showing that the adsorption rate of MCPP onto UiO-66 (powder) was about 70 times faster than the adsorption rate of MCPP onto activated carbon. In the same report, it was shown that the adsorption capacity of UiO-66 was 7 times higher than that of activated carbon, particularly at low concentrations of MCPP [34].

In addition to herbicides, the presence of pharmaceutical products, such as acetaminophen (paracetamol), in natural waters, drinking water, and sewage, as well as in industrial and household waste streams has increased as a result of the growing consumption of antibiotics, anti-inflammatories and other readily available drugs. The long-term effects of exposure to pharmaceutical products in drinking water have not yet been fully determined, and the removal of these micropollutants from water remains a priority. In this manuscript, we evaluate the ability of cotton fabrics decorated with UiO-66 to absorb MCCP and to decompose acetaminophen.

2. Materials and Methods

All reagents were purchased from commercial sources and were used without further purification as follows: zirconium(IV) chloride (ZrCl$_4$, ≥99.5%; Aldrich, St. Louis, MO, USA), terephthalic acid (98%; Alfa Aesar, Haverhill, MA, USA), *N,N*-dimethylformamide (DMF; Mallinckrodt Chemicals, Phillipsburg, NJ, USA), deionized (DI) water, sodium hydroxide (NaOH pellets; Macron), non-ionic surfactant Triton X-100 (0.08%; Electron Microscopy Sciences, Hatfield, PA, USA), isopropyl alcohol (Aldrich), acetic acid (Macron, glacial), sodium chloroacetate (98%; Aldrich), hydrochloric acid (HCl, 36.5–38%; J.T. Baker), methylchlorophenoxypropionic acid (Mecoprop, Santa Cruz Biotechnology, Dallas, TX, USA), and acetaminophen (Spectrum Chemical MFG Corp., New Brunswick, NJ, USA). Standardized cotton fabrics TIC-400 were obtained from Testfabrics, Inc. (West Pittston, PA, USA) and were cut into 2×2 cm^2 squares using a laser cutter.

2.1. Scouring

A scouring solution was prepared by dissolving 5 g of NaOH, 1.5 g of Triton X and 0.75 g of acetic acid in 500 mL of DI water. The cotton swatches were immersed in the scouring solution at 100 °C following a procedure reported by Ozer et al. [35]. After scouring, the swatches were rinsed with DI water and hung to dry at room temperature.

2.2. Carboxymethylation

Carboxymethylation of the cotton swatches was performed by slightly modifying a method reported by Pushpamalar et al. [36]. The scoured cotton swatches were dipped in 100 mL of isopropyl alcohol; 10 mL of 30% (w/v) sodium hydroxide was added drop-wise and stirred for 1 h at room temperature. The solution was heated up to 45 °C, and 6.0 g of sodium monochloroacetate was added the reaction flask. After 3 h of vigorous stirring, the cotton swatches were cured at 85 °C for 30 min. The cotton swatches were washed with DI water and hung to dry at room temperature. Anionization of the substrates was achieved by dipping the modified cotton swatches in a solution of diluted acetic acid (0.2 mL in 100 mL of H$_2$O) for 5 min, followed by washing the swatches with water and hanging at room temperature.

2.3. Growth of UiO-66 on the Surface of Cotton Fabrics

UiO-66 was prepared according to the procedure reported by Katz et al. [37]. The metal precursor solution was prepared by dissolving ZrCl$_4$ (125 mg, 0.54 mmol) in a mixture of 5 mL of DMF and 1 mL of concentrated HCl and sonicating for 10 min. In a separate beaker, terephthalic acid (123 mg, 0.75 mmol) was dissolved in 10 mL of DMF and added to the metal precursor solution. Deprotonated carboxymethylated cotton swatches were dipped into the solution and left overnight at 80 °C in a tightly sealed container. The resulting fabric was washed in DMF (1 h) and H$_2$O (1 h) and was dried at room temperature. UiO-66 in powder form was obtained under the same conditions as are described above but without the addition of the cotton swatches to the reaction vessel.

2.4. Characterization of the Samples

X-ray diffraction (XRD) experiments were performed on a Bruker D8 powder diffractometer with a step size of 0.04°. X-ray photoelectron spectroscopy (XPS) was performed using a Surface Science Instruments SSX-100 with an operating pressure of ~2×10^{-9} Torr. Monochromatic Al Kα X-rays (1486.6 eV) with a 1 mm diameter beam size were used. Photoelectrons were collected at a 55° emission angle. A hemispherical analyzer determined the electron kinetic energy using a pass energy of 150 V for wide/survey scans and of 50 V for high-resolution scans. A flood gun was used for charge neutralization.

Scanning electron microscopy (SEM) and energy-dispersive X-ray spectroscopy (EDX) were performed on a LEO 1550 FESEM (Keck SEM); the specimens were coated with a thin layer of Au-Pd or carbon for SEM and EDX. SEM imaging required an electric potential of 5 keV and an aperture of 30 µm, while EDX was performed using 7 keV and a 240 µm aperture. Transmission electron microscopy (TEM) was performed on a 120 kV field FEI T12 Spirit transmission electron microscope equipped with a LaB$_6$ filament, single and double tilt holders, a SIS Megaview III CCD camera, and a STEM dark field and bright field detector. For the preparation of the TEM samples, the textile samples were immobilized in an epoxy resin mold and cured at 65 °C for 24 h. The immobilized sample was cut into 90 nm thick slides using an ultra-microtome and a diamond knife. Fourier transform infrared spectroscopy (FTIR) spectra were obtained with a Nicolet iS5 FTIR (Thermo Fisher Scientific) in ATR mode.

2.5. MCPP Uptake Experiments

Four cotton swatches functionalized with UiO-66 (0.2341 g) and four cotton swatches that underwent carboxymethylation (0.2349 g) were cut into small pieces using a laser cutter and were dried overnight in an oven at 100 °C. The swatches were immersed into aqueous solutions of MCPP (20 ppm, with a pH of 4.0 adjusted with 0.1 M HCl), which were prepared following the procedure reported by Seo et al. [34]. After 7 h and 24 h of vigorous stirring, the uptake of MCPP was determined using the UV absorbance at 279 nm.

2.6. Degradation of Acetaminophen

Acetaminophen (500 mg) was dissolved in 10 mL ethanol. Unmodified cotton samples (controls) and cotton samples functionalized with UiO-66 were dipped into the acetaminophen solution for 1 min. The wet samples were dried at 80 °C for 20 min and exposed for 10 min to a Xenon lamp to simulate solar conditions.

3. Results

3.1. Characterization of Cotton Fabrics Fucntionalized with UiO-66

3.1.1. X-ray Diffraction

The presence of the highly crystalline structure of the UiO-66 MOF was confirmed using XRD, as shown in Figure 2. The diffraction patterns of functionalized cotton samples (blue) and the pure UiO-66 (red) powder are shown in Figure 2 [15,38]. A clear superposition of the main diffraction peaks can be observed.

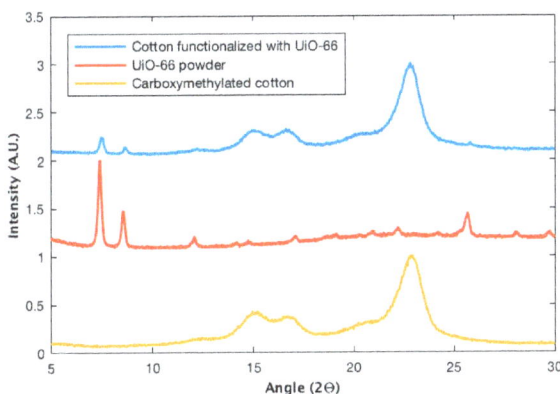

Figure 2. X-ray diffraction patterns for carboxymethylated cotton, UiO-66 powder, and cotton fabric functionalized with UiO-66.

3.1.2. X-ray Photoelectron Spectroscopy

XPS was used to determine the presence of zirconium, which is metal precursor for UiO-66.

In Figure 3, the peaks at 330, 350 and 440 eV are assigned to zirconium's 3p, 3p3/2 and 3s orbital electrons. The peak at 290 eV associated to carbon was used for calibration. This carbon peak can be assigned to both the ligand (terephthalic acid) and the substrate (cellulose). The 1s orbital of oxygen has a binding energy of 530 eV, and oxygen is also present in both the ligand and substrate.

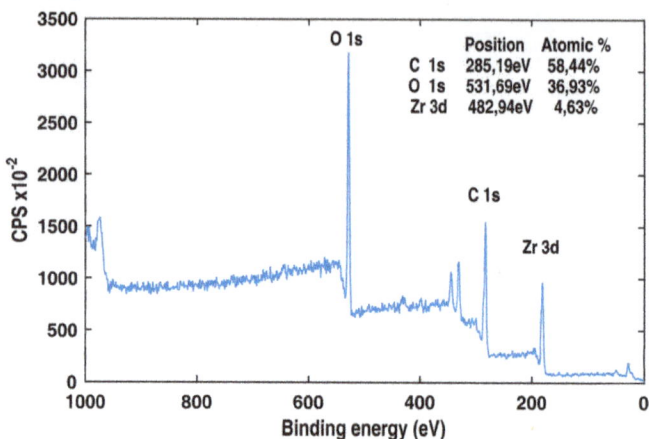

Figure 3. X-ray photoelectron spectroscopy (XPS) of a cotton fabric functionalized with UiO-66.

As cotton samples are non-conductive, a buildup of positive charges on the surface of the sample can be formed immediately after the sample is exposed to X-rays. This charge buildup drags additional electrons from within the sample, hence distorting the spectrum and shifting down the binding energy values. A flood gun was used to neutralize this effect, and the spectrum was recalibrated using the C–C carbon bond at 285 eV. In addition to confirming the presence of Zr, the XPS spectra also indicated the absence of residual chlorine from the $ZrCl_4$ and residual nitrogen that could have originated by the washing of the samples in DMF.

3.1.3. Scanning Electron Microscopy

SEM imaging confirmed the uniformity of the UiO-66 functionalization on the surface of the cotton fabrics, as shown in Figure 4b,c. An SEM image of pristine cotton fibers is shown in Figure 4a for reference [38].

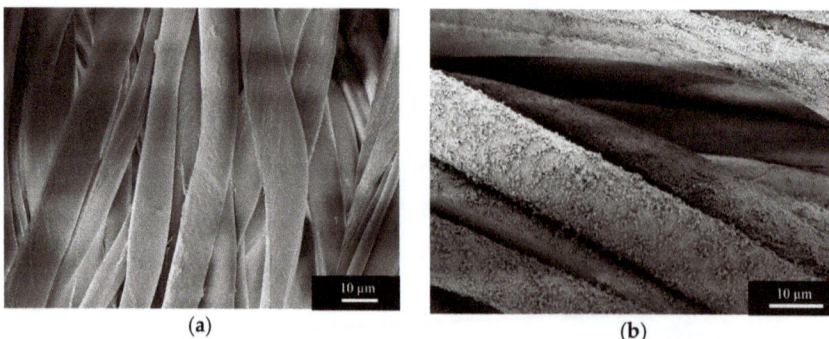

(a)

(b)

Figure 4. *Cont.*

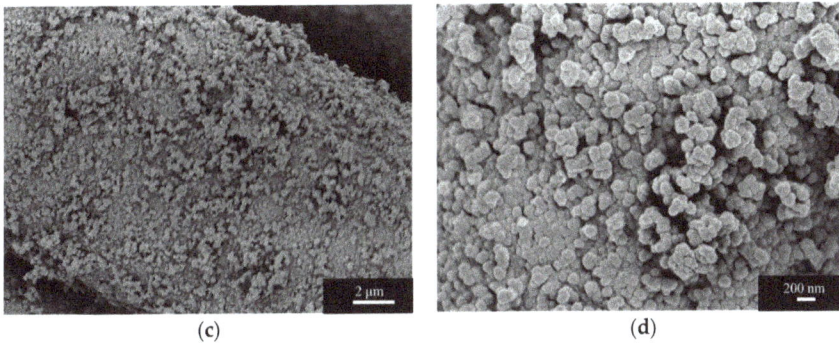

(c)   (d)

Figure 4. Scanning electron microscopy (SEM) images of (**a**) bare cotton fibers, and (**b–d**) cotton fibers functionalized with UiO-66 at different magnifications.

SEM imaging confirmed the presence of crystalline UiO-66. Figure 4d resembles the morphology previously reported for UiO-66 [17] and provides evidence of the homogeneity of the coating.

3.1.4. Energy Dispersive X-ray Spectroscopy

EDX mapping shows the atomic distribution over the surface of a sample. A higher aperture was used to ensure optimal characterization, but this also resulted in cracks in the sample, which are apparent in Figure 5a. Fortunately, once formed, these crevasses did not expand. A uniform distribution of zirconium onto the cotton fibers can be seen in Figure 5b, where the signal attributed to the zirconium channel is highlighted in red. Quantitative analysis of the resulting maps showed an average zirconium atomic percent content of 5% ± 0.7% on the surface of the fibers.

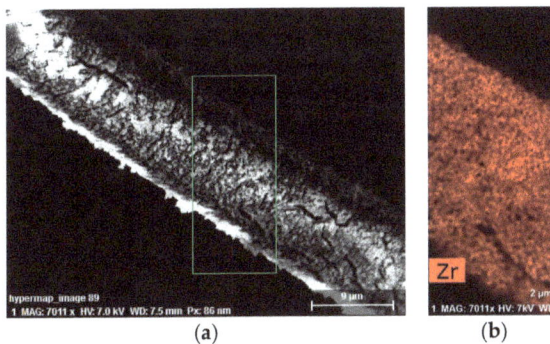

(a)   (b)

Figure 5. (**a**) Scanning electron microscopy (SEM) image of a cotton fiber functionalized with UiO-66 with the energy-dispersive X-ray spectroscopy (EDX) mapped region highlighted in green; (**b**) EDX zirconium map of the highlighted area shown in (**a**).

3.1.5. Transmission Electron Microscopy

TEM imaging allowed to assess the thickness of the UiO-66 coating on the cotton fibers. In Figure 6, the UiO-66 crystals, appearing darker than the cotton substrates because of the presence of Zr ($Z = 40$), formed a conformal coating over the irregular shape of the cotton fiber. These images were used to determine that the thickness of the coating was around 50 nm.

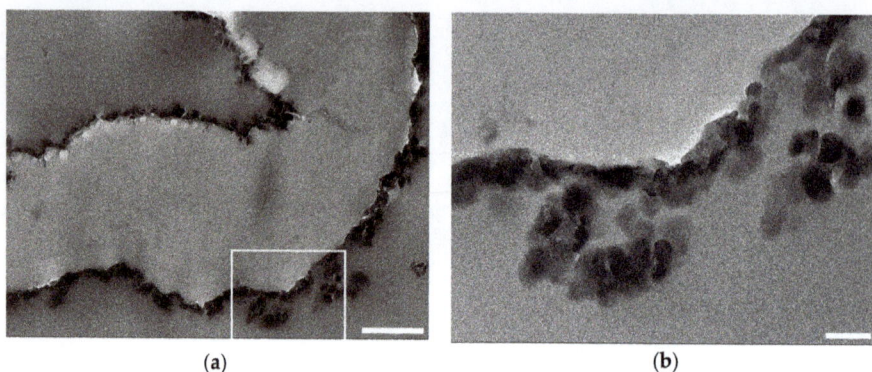

(a)   (b)

Figure 6. Transmission electron microscopy (TEM) image of a cotton fiber functionalized with UiO-66: (a) Cotton fiber cut along its fiber axis. The scale bar corresponds to 500 nm. (b) Magnification of the area delimited by the white square in (a). The scale bar corresponds to 100 nm.

3.1.6. Fourier Transform Infrared Spectroscopy

The degradation of acetaminophen was followed using ATR-FTIR. The ATR-FTIR characterization of the UiO-66-functionalized fabrics is shown in Figure 7.

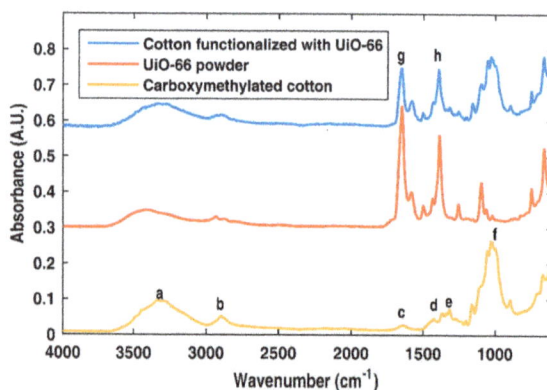

Figure 7. Fourier transform infrared spectroscopy (FTIR) spectra of bare cotton fabric, UiO-66 powder and UiO-66-functionalized cotton fabric.

The labeled FTIR bands in Figure 7 correspond to (a) stretching of hydrogen-bonded O–H, (b) C–H stretching, (c) O–H bending of adsorbed water, (d) CH_2 scissoring, (e) O–H bending (f) OCH–O–CH_2 stretching, (g) asymmetric stretching of the carboxylate band (terephthalic ligand), and (h) carboxylate symmetrical stretching (terephthalic ligand). The powder spectrum and the carboxymethylated cellulose were in quantitative agreement with those previously reported [17,36,39].

3.2. Adsorption of MCPP

The maximum uptake of MCPP by dispersed UiO-66 powders was obtained after about 6 h according to Seo et al. [34]. In our case, the UiO-66 MOF was immobilized onto cotton fabrics. After immersion of the fabrics in the MCPP solution, an aliquot of the MCCP solution was taken after 7 h of vigorous stirring, and another aliquot was taken 24 h later. In both cases, the resulting UV absorption was the same. The calculated removal efficiency for the cotton fibers decorated with UiO-66 was 14.5%. As expected, the removal efficiency for the carboxymethylated cotton samples was 0% for uptake times as large as 24 h.

3.3. Photocatalytic Activity of the UiO-66-Functionalized Fabric

The catalytic activity of the cotton fabrics functionalized with UiO-66 was assessed through degradation of acetaminophen. Figure 8 shows the absorbed and degraded acetaminophen after 10 min of UV exposure.

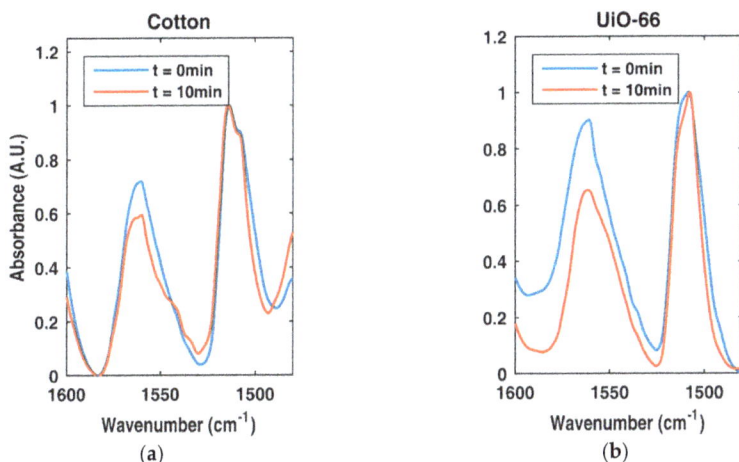

Figure 8. Acetaminophen adsorbed on (**a**) bare cotton fabric and (**b**) cotton fabrics functionalized with UiO-66. The Fourier transform infrared spectroscopy (FTIR) spectra in blue represents time zero and the spectra after 10 min of exposure to UV is shown in red.

The degree of degradation of acetaminophen was evaluated by monitoring the 1560 cm^{-1} peak, which is ascribed to one of the N–H bending modes. The signal was normalized to the 1500 cm^{-1} peak attributed to one of the phenyl C–C stretching modes, a peak that should remain constant during photocatalytic degradation [40,41].

4. Discussion

XRD spectra of cotton samples functionalized with UiO-66 confirmed the crystalline formation of the MOF on the cotton fabric, as shown in Figure 2. Figure 2 also shows that the XRD pattern of the carboxymethylated cotton sample (yellow) exhibited only the characteristic peaks for cellulose (15°, 16° and 23°) [38]. The UiO-66 powder sample (red) matched the peaks reported in the literature [17]. The cotton sample functionalized with UiO-66 (blue) exhibited both the peaks assigned to cellulose and those assigned to UiO-66 in clear superposition, confirming the presence of the crystalline MOF onto the fabric.

XPS (Figure 3) confirmed that the crystalline formation was composed of zirconium, carbon and oxygen. Because of the fact that the substrate, cellulose, was also composed of carbon and oxygen, a quantitative analysis of the MOF content was not possible. The XPS spectra also showed no chlorine, confirming that the zirconium was stoichiometrically coordinated to the oxygen. Moreover, because of the absence of nitrogen in the spectrum, we also concluded that the solvent, DMF, was completely removed from the pores of the UIO-66 framework.

Images obtained via SEM (Figure 4) showed that the coating was uniform across the fabric, and this observation was supported by the EDX map reporting the distribution of zirconium (Figure 5b).

Figure 4c,d show that the UiO-66 MOF completely covered the surface of the fiber, leaving no bare cotton in sight. EDX quantitative analysis indicated a zirconium content on the surface of 5% ± 0.7%.

TEM images (Figure 6) show that the thickness of the coating could be estimated to be around 50 nm and that the coating thickness appeared to be uniform along the fiber's axis.

FTIR (Figure 7) spectra demonstrated the presence of carboxylate and phenyl bonds ascribed to the terephthalic ligands of UiO-66, and the spectra of the powder MOF and cellulose quantitatively agreed with the spectra reported in the literature [17,36]. Moreover, the spectrum of the cotton fabrics functionalized with UiO-66 showed all absorption peaks ascribed to both cellulose and UiO-66, further confirming the presence of this MOF onto the fabric. FTIR characterization was necessary for establishing a baseline for the photocatalytic experiment.

As illustrated by the EDX and XPS results, the amount of MOF immobilized onto the cotton fabric was very small. Therefore, a 14.5% uptake of MCPP is truly remarkable. In their study, Seo et al. reported a maximal adsorption capacity of 370 mg of MCPP/g UiO-66 (powder) [34]. In this study, we used 234.1 mg of a UiO-66-functionalized cotton containing about 5% zirconium on its surface. The mass of MCPP removed from the system was 3 mg, resulting in an adsorption capacity for UiO-66-functionalized cotton of 12.8 mg of MCPP/g functionalized fabric. As expected, the absorption capacity for the functionalized fabric was smaller than the value obtained for the powder sample. Advantages of the fabric sample include its easy recovery and reuse after desorption as well as its mechanical stability and manufacturability.

The catalytic activity of the cotton samples functionalized with UiO-66 MOFs was assessed in the degradation of acetaminophen. The degree of degradation was evaluated via FTIR by monitoring the 1560 cm^{-1} peak, which is ascribed to one of the N–H bending modes in acetaminophen. The signal was normalized to the 1500 cm^{-1} peak, which is ascribed to one of the phenyl C–C stretching modes. This peak should remain constant during the photocatalytic degradation [41]. Experiments were performed with the scoured cotton samples (control) and the cotton samples functionalized with UiO-66. In both experiments, the photocatalytic degradation of acetaminophen was noted (Figure 8). However, when the cotton sample functionalized with UiO-66 was used, the decrease in the N–H band was larger than in the experiments performed with the as-received samples. These results indicate that the presence of the UiO-66 increased the photocatalytic efficiency of the cotton by 63% after only 10 min of UV exposure.

5. Conclusions

Cotton fibers were successfully functionalized with UiO-66, a zirconium-based water-stable MOF. The presence of the crystalline UiO-66 was confirmed via XRD, and the presence of zirconium in the cotton-modified samples was confirmed by XPS and EDX. SEM and TEM imaging confirmed that the UiO-66 crystals uniformly grew on the surface of the cotton fibers and that the MOF layer was 50 nm thick. The reported functionalization did not alter the structure of the textile, hence allowing for the potential use of these materials in protective clothing. The cotton functionalized with UiO-66 exhibited an increased uptake of MCPP as well as enhanced UV degradation capabilities. These results indicate that UiO-66-functionalized textiles can be used as flexible mantles for the photocatalytic decomposition and adsorption of low-concentration pollutants in water streams.

Acknowledgments: This work made use of the Cornell Center for Materials Research Shared Facilities and was supported through the NSF MRSEC program (DMR-1719875). The authors would also like to thank Marcelo Molina and Laura Salvador from the Analytical Chemistry Division, Applied Chemistry Department, CITEDEF for FTIR measurements. This work was supported by the USDA National Institute of Food and Agriculture, **HATCH 329801 project NC-170 NYS.**

Author Contributions: J.H., E.O., M.K. and M.S. conceived the main idea of the study. M.S. synthesized the UiO66-functionalized cotton and characterized it, she also performed the MCPP adsorption experiments. M.K. and E.O. performed experiments regarding acetaminophen degradation and all the authors contributed to the preparation of the manuscript.

Conflicts of Interest: The authors declare no conflicts of interest.

References

1. Rosi, N.L.; Eckert, J.; Eddaoudi, M.; Vodak, D.T.; Kim, J.; O'Keefe, M.; Yaghi, O.M. Hydrogen Storage in Microporous Metal-Organic Frameworks. *Science* **2003**, *300*, 1127–1129. [CrossRef] [PubMed]
2. Férey, G. Hybrid porous solids: Past, present, future. *Chem. Soc. Rev.* **2008**, *37*, 191–214. [CrossRef] [PubMed]
3. Vellingiri, K.; Kumar, P.; Deep, A.; Kim, K.H. Metal-organic frameworks for the adsorption of gaseous toluene under ambient temperature and pressure. *Chem. Eng. J.* **2017**, *307*, 1116–1126. [CrossRef]
4. Cmarik, G.E.; Kim, M.; Cohen, S.M.; Walton, K.S. Tuning the adsorption properties of UiO-66 via ligand functionalization. *Langmuir* **2012**, *28*, 15606–15613. [CrossRef] [PubMed]
5. Sculley, J.; Yuan, D.; Zhou, H.-C. The current status of hydrogen storage in metal-organic frameworks—Updated. *Energy Environ. Sci.* **2011**, *4*, 2721–2735. [CrossRef]
6. Makal, T.A.; Li, J.-R.; Lu, W.; Zhou, H.-C. Methane storage in advanced porous materials. *Chem. Soc. Rev.* **2012**, *41*, 7761–7779. [CrossRef] [PubMed]
7. Fu, Y.-Y.; Yang, C.-X.; Yan, X.-P.; Ma, Q.; Feng, Y.Q.; Chevreau, H.; Serre, C.; Rodrigues, A.E. Incorporation of metal–organic framework UiO-66 into porous polymer monoliths to enhance the liquid chromatographic separation of small molecules. *Chem. Commun.* **2013**, *49*, 7162–7164. [CrossRef] [PubMed]
8. Chang, N.; Yan, X.-P. Exploring reverse shape selectivity and molecular sieving effect of metal-organic framework UiO-66 coated capillary column for gas chromatographic separation. *J. Chromatogr. A* **2012**, *1257*, 116–124. [CrossRef] [PubMed]
9. Vahidi, M.; Rashidi, A.M.; Tavasoli, A. Preparation of piperazine-grafted amine-functionalized UiO-66 metal organic framework and its application for CO$_2$ over CH$_4$ separation. *J. Iran. Chem. Soc.* **2017**, *14*, 2247–2253. [CrossRef]
10. Timofeeva, M.N.; Panchenko, V.N.; Jun, J.W.; Hasan, Z.; Matrosova, M.M.; Jhung, S.H. Effects of linker substitution on catalytic properties of porous zirconium terephthalate UiO-66 in acetalization of benzaldehyde with methanol. *Appl. Catal. A Gen.* **2014**, *471*, 91–97. [CrossRef]
11. Liu, Y.; Howarth, A.J.; Hupp, J.T.; Farha, O.K. Selective Photooxidation of a Mustard-Gas Simulant Catalyzed by a Porphyrinic Metal-Organic Framework. *Angew. Chem. Int. Ed.* **2015**, *54*, 9001–9005. [CrossRef] [PubMed]
12. Cirujano, F.G.; Luz, I.; Soukri, M.; van Goethem, C.; Vankelecom, I.; Lail, M.; de Vos, D.E. Boosting catalytic performance of MOFs for steroid transformations by confinement within mesoporous scaffolds. *Angew. Chem. Int. Ed.* **2017**, *56*, 13302–13306. [CrossRef] [PubMed]
13. Katz, M.J.; Mondloch, J.E.; Totten, R.K.; Park, J.K.; Nguyen, S.T.; Farha, O.K.; Hupp, J.T. Simple and compelling biomimetic metal-organic framework catalyst for the degradation of nerve agent simulants. *Angew. Chem. Int. Ed.* **2014**, *53*, 497–501. [CrossRef] [PubMed]
14. Barea, E.; Montoro, C.; Navarro, J.A.R. Toxic gas removal—Metal-organic frameworks for the capture and degradation of toxic gases and vapours. *Chem. Soc. Rev.* **2014**, *43*, 5419–5430. [CrossRef] [PubMed]
15. Kandiah, M.; Nilsen, M.H.; Usseglio, S.; Jakobsen, S.; Olsbye, U.; Tilset, M.; Larabi, C.; Quadrelli, E.A.; Bonino, F.; Lillerud, K.P. Synthesis and Stability of Tagged UiO-66 Zr-MOFs. *Chem. Mater.* **2010**, *22*, 6632–6640. [CrossRef]
16. Jiang, H.-L.; Feng, D.; Wang, K.; Gu, Z.-Y.; Wei, Z.; Chen, Y.-P.; Zhou, H.-C. An Exceptionally Stable, Porphyrinic Zr Metal–Organic Framework Exhibiting pH-Dependent Fluorescence. *J. Am. Chem. Soc.* **2013**, *135*, 13934–13938. [CrossRef] [PubMed]
17. Cavka, J.H.; Jakobsen, S.; Olsbye, U.; Guillou, N.; Lamberti, C.; Bordiga, S.; Lillerud, K.P. A New Zirconium Inorganic Building Brick Forming Metal Organic Frameworks with Exceptional Stability. *J. Am. Chem. Soc.* **2008**, *130*, 13850–13851. [CrossRef] [PubMed]
18. Chen, C.; Chen, D.; Xie, S.; Quan, H.; Luo, X.; Guo, L. Adsorption Behaviors of Organic Micropollutants on Zirconium Metal-Organic Framework UiO-66: Analysis of Surface Interactions. *ACS Appl. Mater. Interfaces* **2017**, *46*, 41043–41054. [CrossRef] [PubMed]
19. Hasan, Z.; Jhung, H. Removal of hazardous organics from water using metal-organic frameworks (MOFs): Plausible mechanisms for selective adsorptions. *J. Hazard. Mater.* **2015**, *283*, 329–339. [CrossRef] [PubMed]
20. Shang, H.-B.; Yang, C.-X.; Yan, X.-P. Metal–organic framework UiO-66 coated stainless steel fiber for solid-phase microextraction of phenols in water samples. *J. Chromatogr. A* **2014**, *1357*, 165–171. [CrossRef] [PubMed]

21. Da Silva Pinto, M.; Sierra-Avila, C.A.; Hinestroza, J.P. In situ synthesis of a Cu-BTC metal-organic framework (MOF 199) onto cellulosic fibrous substrates: Cotton. *Cellulose* **2012**, *19*, 1771–1779. [CrossRef]

22. Yu, M.; Li, W.; Wang, Z.; Zhang, B.; Ma, H.; Li, L.; Li, J. Covalent immobilization of metal-organic frameworks onto the surface of nylon—A new approach to the functionalization and coloration of textiles. *Sci. Rep.* **2016**, *6*, 22796. [CrossRef] [PubMed]

23. Bunge, M.A.; Ruckart, K.N.; Leavesley, S.; Peterson, G.W.; Nguyen, N.; West, K.N.; Glover, T.G. Modification of Fibers with Nanostructures Using Reactive Dye Chemistry. *Ind. Eng. Chem. Res.* **2015**, *54*, 3821–3827. [CrossRef]

24. Lemaire, P.C.; Zhao, J.; Williams, P.S.; Walls, H.J.; Shepherd, S.D.; Losego, M.D.; Peterson, G.W.; Parsons, G.N. Copper Benzenetricarboxylate Metal–Organic Framework Nucleation Mechanisms on Metal Oxide Powders and Thin Films formed by Atomic Layer Deposition. *ACS Appl. Mater. Interfaces* **2016**, *8*, 9514–9522. [CrossRef] [PubMed]

25. Zhao, J.; Lee, D.T.; Yaga, R.W.; Hall, M.G.; Barton, H.F.; Woodward, I.R.; Oldham, C.J.; Walls, H.J.; Peterson, G.W.; Parsons, G.N. Ultra-Fast Degradation of Chemical Warfare Agents Using MOF-Nanofiber Kebabs. *Angew. Chem. Int. Ed.* **2016**, *55*, 13224–13228. [CrossRef] [PubMed]

26. Lu, A.X.; McEntee, M.; Browe, M.A.; Hall, M.; DeCoste, J.B.; Peterson, G.W. MOFabric: Electrospun Nanofiber Mats from PVDF/UiO-66-NH$_2$ for Chemical Protection and Decontamination. *ACS Appl. Mater. Interfaces* **2017**, *9*, 13632–13636. [CrossRef] [PubMed]

27. Lee, D.T.; Zhao, J.; Peterson, G.W.; Parsons, G.N. A Catalytic 'MOF-Cloth' Formed via Directed Supramolecular Assembly of UiO-66-NH$_2$ Crystals on ALD-coated Textiles for Rapid Degradation of Chemical Warfare Agent Simulants. *Chem. Mater.* **2017**, *29*, 4894–4903. [CrossRef]

28. Ignatowicz, K. Selection of sorbent for removing pesticides during water treatment. *J. Hazard. Mater.* **2009**, *169*, 953–957. [CrossRef] [PubMed]

29. Suty, H.; de Traversay, C.; Cost, M. Applications of advanced oxidation processes: Present and future. *Water Sci. Technol.* **2004**, *49*, 227–233. [CrossRef] [PubMed]

30. SHeijman, G.J.; Siegers, W.; Sterk, R.; Hopman, R. Prediction of breakthrough of pesticides in GAC-filters and breakthrough of colour in ion-exchange-filters. *Water Sci. Technol. Water Supply* **2002**, *2*, 103–108.

31. Godskesen, B.; Zambrano, K.C.; Trautner, A.; Johansen, N.B.; Thiesson, L.; Andersen, L.; Clauson-Kaas, J.; Neidel, T.L.; Rygaard, M.; Kløverpris, N.H.; et al. Life cycle assessment of three water systems in Copenhagen—A management tool of the future. *Water Sci. Technol.* **2011**, *63*, 565–572. [CrossRef] [PubMed]

32. Hedegaard, M.J.; Arvin, E.; Corfitzen, C.B.; Albrechtsen, H.J. Mecoprop (MCPP) removal in full-scale rapid sand filters at a groundwater-based waterworks. *Sci. Total Environ.* **2014**, *499*, 257–264. [CrossRef] [PubMed]

33. Petrović, M.; Gonzalez, S.; Barceló, D. Analysis and removal of emerging contaminants in wastewater and drinking water. *TrAC—Trends Anal. Chem.* **2003**, *22*, 685–696. [CrossRef]

34. Seo, Y.S.; Khan, N.A.; Jhung, S.H. Adsorptive removal of methylchlorophenoxypropionic acid from water with a metal-organic framework. *Chem. Eng. J.* **2015**, *270*, 22–27. [CrossRef]

35. Athauda, T.J.; Hari, P.; Ozer, R.R. Tuning Physical and Optical Properties of ZnO Nanowire Arrays Grown on Cotton Fibers. *ACS Appl. Mater. Interfaces* **2013**, *5*, 6237–6246. [CrossRef] [PubMed]

36. Pushpamalar, V.; Langford, S.J.; Ahmad, M.; Lim, Y.Y. Optimization of reaction conditions for preparing carboxymethyl cellulose from sago waste. *Carbohydr. Polym.* **2006**, *64*, 312–318. [CrossRef]

37. Katz, M.J.; Brown, Z.J.; Colón, Y.J.; Siu, P.W.; Scheidt, K.A.; Snurr, R.Q.; Hupp, J.T.; Farha, O.K. A facile synthesis of UiO-66, UiO-67 and their derivatives. *Chem. Commun.* **2013**, *49*, 9449–9451. [CrossRef] [PubMed]

38. Zhao, H.; Kwak, J.; Conradzhang, Z.; Brown, H.; Arey, B.; Holladay, J. Studying cellulose fiber structure by SEM, XRD, NMR and acid hydrolysis. *Carbohydr. Polym.* **2007**, *68*, 235–241. [CrossRef]

39. Biswal, D.R.; Singh, R.P. Characterisation of carboxymethyl cellulose and polyacrylamide graft copolymer. *Carbohydr. Polym.* **2004**, *57*, 379–387. [CrossRef]

40. Kandiah, M.; Usseglio, S.; Svelle, S.; Olsbye, U.; Lillerud, K.P.; Tilset, M. Post-synthetic modification of the metal–organic framework compound UiO-66. *J. Mater. Chem.* **2010**, *20*, 9848–9851. [CrossRef]

41. Amado, A.M.; Azevedo, C.; Ribeiro-Claro, P.J.A. Conformational and vibrational reassessment of solid paracetamol. *Spectrochim. Acta* **2017**, *183*, 431–438. [CrossRef] [PubMed]

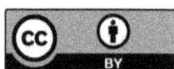

bioengineering

MDPI

Article

Lysine-Grafted MCM-41 Silica as an Antibacterial Biomaterial

María F. Villegas [1], Lorena Garcia-Uriostegui [2], Ofelia Rodríguez [3], Isabel Izquierdo-Barba [4,5], Antonio J. Salinas [4,5], Guillermo Toriz [1], María Vallet-Regí [4,5,*] and Ezequiel Delgado [1,*]

[1]   Departamento de Madera, Celulosa y Papel, Universidad de Guadalajara, Guadalajara 44100, Mexico; ib.fernanda.villegas@gmail.com (M.F.V.); gtoriz@dmcyp.cucei.udg.mx (G.T.)
[2]   CONACYT Research Fellow at Departamento de Madera, Celulosa y Papel, Universidad de Guadalajara, Guadalajara 44100, Mexico; lgarciaur@conacyt.mx
[3]   Laboratorio de Microbiología e Inocuidad de Alimentos, Universidad de Guadalajara, Guadalajara 44100, Mexico; ofelia.rodriguez@cucei.udg.mx
[4]   Departamento de Química Inorgánica y Bioinorgánica, Facultad de Farmacia, Universidad Complutense de Madrid, Instituto de Investigación Sanitaria Hospital 12 de Octubre i+12, Plaza Ramón y Cajal s/n, 28040 Madrid, Spain; ibarba@ucm.es (I.I.-B.); salinas@ucm.es (A.J.S.)
[5]   CIBER de Bioingeniería, Biomateriales y Nanomedicina (CIBER-BBN), 28040 Madrid, Spain
*   Correspondence: vallet@ucm.es (M.V.-R.); ezedelfor@gmail.com (E.D.); Tel.: +52-333-682-0110 (M.V.-R. & E.D.)

Academic Editor: Gary Chinga Carrasco
Received: 23 August 2017; Accepted: 21 September 2017; Published: 26 September 2017

Abstract: This paper proposes a facile strategy for the zwitterionization of bioceramics that is based on the direct incorporation of L-lysine amino acid via the ε-amino group onto mesoporous MCM-41 materials. Fourier transform infrared (FTIR) studies of lysine-grafted MCM-41 (MCM-LYS) simultaneously showed bands at 3080 and 1540 cm^{-1} and bands at 1625 and 1415 cm^{-1} corresponding to $-NH^{3+}/COO^-$ pairs, which demonstrate the incorporation of the amino acid on the material surface keeping its zwitterionic character. Both elemental and thermogravimetric analyses showed that the amount of grafted lysine was 8 wt.% based on the bioceramic total weight. Moreover, MCM-LYS exhibited a reduction of adhesion of *S. aureus* and *E. coli* bacteria in 33% and 50%, respectively at physiological pH, as compared with pristine MCM-41. Biofilm studies onto surfaces showed that lysine functionalization elicited a reduction of the area covered by *S. aureus* biofilm from 42% to only 5% (88%). This research shows a simple and effective approach to chemically modify bioceramics using single amino acids that provides zwitterionic functionality, which is useful to develop new biomaterials that are able to resist bacterial adhesion.

Keywords: lysine grafting; zwitterionization; mesoporous MCM-41 biomaterial; antibacterial adhesion; biofilm formation

---

1. Introduction

Microbial adhesion onto implanted biomaterials and the subsequent formation of biofilms is one of the major causes of failure in biomedical devices. Antimicrobial and non-fouling coatings are two strategies to prevent the attachment and spreading of microorganisms on the surface of implantable materials [1]. The use of hydrophilic or zwitterionic surfaces is among the most useful chemical strategies to avoid bacterial adhesion and biofouling [2–4]. In this sense, zwitterionic polymers such as poly(sulfobetaine methacrylate) (pSBMA) and poly(carboxybetaine methacrylate) (pCBMA), with mixed positively and negatively charged moieties within the same polymer chain and overall charge neutrality, exhibit ultralow fouling ability to resist non-specific protein adsorption, bacterial adhesion and biofilm formation [5,6].

The design of ordered mesoporous materials with resistance to bacterial adhesion is highly desirable, since these materials have unique characteristics such as high surface area and pore volume, tuneable and narrow pore size distributions, as well as ease of functionalization. These materials have been widely used for various applications, i.e., catalysis, carriers for drug storage and delivery, adsorbents [7–10], and as bioceramics for bone tissue regeneration [11,12]. In addition, ordered mesoporous silica materials have excellent properties as drug carriers, such as large loading capacity and low toxicity. Recently, there has been significant research effort on the design of bioceramics functionalized with zwitterions as a promising strategy to develop non-fouling and antibacterial adhesion surfaces [13]. These properties are related to a hydration layer on the surface, since a tightly bound water layer forms a physical and energetic barrier that prevents bacterial adhesion and non-specific protein adsorption [14–17]. It is possible to set up functionalization methods to graft both positively and negatively charged moieties onto the bioceramic surfaces.

Thus, different zwitterionization approaches have been developed so far to prepare non-fouling bioceramics. In general, these strategies include the surface grafting with zwitterionic polymers or with low molecular moieties, involving the surface modification with either carboxylic and/or amine groups in separate steps [15–19]. Recently, it has been reported that the amino acids represent an alternative to provide bioceramics with a zwitterionic character. In this sense, cysteine was grafted to the surface of silica nanoparticles via a two-step procedure, showing high resistance to non-specific protein adsorption [20]. In this sense, the amino acid L-lysine (lysine) is even more attractive to create low-fouling surface owing to its low cost, high biocompatibility, and widespread availability. Lysine is a basic amino acid, which contains two primary amino groups (-NH$_2$) and one carboxylic group (-COOH) with pKa for the α-amino and the carboxylic groups at 9.06 and 2.16, respectively. Consequently, at neutral pH these groups are simultaneously protonated and deprotonated. When the ε-amino group has reacted, the remaining amino group and carboxyl group form an anion-cation pair, i.e., a zwitterion, which exhibits antifouling activity [21–23]. For instance, Shi et al. [24] grafted lysine, glycine, and serine onto the surface of hydrolyzed polyacrylonitrile membrane with a high concentration of carboxylic acid groups. The modified membranes had similar hydrophobicity, as determined from water contact angle measurements, while the lysine-modified membrane showed the least protein fouling. Moreover, Zhi et al. [25] grafted lysine onto polydopamine-coated poly(ethylene terephthalate) that showed improved resistance to non-specific protein adsorption and platelet adhesion.

In the present work, lysine was grafted to silica by means of cyanuric chloride (CC), which acted as a bridging molecule. CC has been shown to be an effective surface coupling agent that can react with a variety of substances, including hydroxyl and amino derivatives, and produce an ether linkage that is chemically and electrochemically stable in organic solvents and in aqueous solution (pH 3–7) [26]. CC has labile chlorine groups that can react both with the hydroxyl groups on the surface of the bioceramics and with ε-amine of lysine. Consequently, the goal of this work was to chemically modify mesoporous silica (MCM-41) using the amino acid lysine, to provide zwitterionic moieties useful for the development of new biomaterials that are able to resist bacterial adhesion and reduce the biofilm formation onto their surface.

2. Materials and Methods

2.1. Materials

L-lysine monohydrochloride (98%), tetraethyl orthosilicate (TEOS, 98%), 2,4,6-Trichloro-1,3,5-triazine (Cyanuric chloride, CC) (99%), hexadecyl trimethylammonium bromide (CTAB), and glutaraldehyde (50 wt.%) were purchased from Sigma-Aldrich (St. Louis, MI, USA). Sodium hydroxide (NaOH, 98.9%), ethylenediamine tetra acetic acid (EDTA, 98%), and copper (II) sulfate (CuSO$_4$·5H$_2$O, 98%) were purchased from Analytyka (Guadalajara, Mexico). Tryptic soy agar (TSA, BIOXON, Mexico City, Mexico), Tryptic soy broth (TSB, BIOXON, Mexico City, Mexico) and Todd Hewitt Broth (THB, Fluka analytical, Toluca, Mexico) were used as received. The microorganisms *Escherichia coli* (ATCC 25922), and

Staphylococcus aureus (ATCC 29213) were obtained from the American Type Culture Collection (Manassas, VA, USA). All the other reagents were analytical grade and used without further purification.

2.2. Preparation of MCM-41 with Zwitterionic Moieties

MCM-41 silica was synthesized by the sol-gel method according to Cai et al. [27]. In brief, CTAB (1 g) was dissolved in 480 mL of distilled water, and then 3.5 mL of NaOH (2 M) were added, the temperature raised to 85 °C and stirred for 30 min. TEOS (5.0 mL) was then introduced drop-wise to the surfactant solution. Once the addition of TEOS was completed, the mixture was stirred for 2 h at 85 °C. The white precipitates were filtered, washed with ethanol, dried under vacuum at room temperature for 48 h, and calcined in air at 550 °C for 4 h with a heating rate of 1 °C/min.

The resulting bioceramic was functionalized with the amino acid lysine (MCM-LYS) to confer its zwitterionic character. The modification of MCM-41 with the amino acid lysine was carried out following the procedure reported by Delgado et al. [28]. In brief, L-lysine hydrochloride was first converted into the copper complex as it follows: lysine (2.32 g in 12.72 mL NaOH 1 M) and copper sulfate (1.59 g $CuSO_4 \cdot 5H_2O$ in 30 mL H_2O) were brought together and stirred into a homogeneous solution. The pH of the solution was adjusted to 7.0 with NaOH (1 M) and cooled to 0 °C. MCM-41 was grafted with CC as follows: 1 g MCM-41 was placed in a water–acetone mixture (80 mL, 75/25) under constant stirring and cooled at 0 °C. Afterwards, the CC (2.34 g) solution in p-dioxane (40 mL) was added under magnetic stirring. Subsequently, NaCl (1.5 g) was added in two equivalent portions, and the pH of the mixture was adjusted to 12 with NaOH (6 M) and kept at 0 °C for 30 min under constant stirring. The coupling of lysine to the grafted MCM-41 was achieved by immediately adding the lysine-copper complex under vigorous stirring and leaving it to react for 15 min. Then, the reaction mixture was removed from the ice bath and placed in a water bath at room temperature, followed by a slow increase of temperature until it reached 65 °C, and then kept stable for 40 min. The functionalized bioceramic was filtered off and washed with water and p-dioxane several times to remove CC residues. The copper was completely eliminated from the lysine copper complex by suspending the functionalized bioceramic in 40 mL distilled water with 1.18 g EDTA (twice, the second time adding 0.1% triton X-100 detergent), boiled at 100 °C for 10 min, filtered, treated with 0.05 M acetic acid (30 mL) and extensively washed with water and dried overnight under vacuum at 60 °C.

2.3. Characterization

The structural characteristics of the resulting materials were determined by powder X-ray diffraction (XRD) in a Siemens D500 diffractometer (Siemens, Eindhoven, The Netherlands) equipped with Cu Kα (40 kV, 20 mA) over the range from 2° to 10° with a step of 0.005 and a contact time of 4 s. The nitrogen adsorption isotherms were measured at −196 °C with a Micromeritics ASAP 2020 analyzer (Micromeritics, Norcross, GA, USA). In all cases, the samples were degassed at 60 °C for 24 h before analysis. Electron microscopy was carried out in a JEOL JEM-220FS transmission electron microscope (JEOL, Tokyo, Japan) operating at 300 kV. The chemical composition and the presence of functional groups on the synthesized materials was determined using Fourier transform infrared (FTIR) spectroscopy in a Thermo Nicolet Nexus spectrometer equipped with a Goldengate attenuated total reflectance (ATR) device (Thermo scientific, Waltham, MA, USA) from 4000 to 400 cm^{-1}. Quantitative determination of chemical composition of the samples was carried out by elemental chemical analysis in a LECO CHNS-932 microanalyzer (Saint Joseph, MI, USA). Thermogravimetric analyses (TGA) were carried out in nitrogen between 30 and 600 °C (flow rate of 50 mL/min, heating rate of 10 °C/min) using a Perkin Elmer TGA Diamond analyzer (PerkinElmer, Akron, OH, USA). Zeta-potential (ζ) measurements were performed on a Malvern Zetasizer Nano Series instrument (Malvern Instruments Ltd., Malvern, UK) with 55 mg of each sample in 30 mL of 10 mM KCl (used as the supporting electrolyte), the mixture was vigorously stirred to reach a homogenous suspension and the pH adjusted by adding appropriate volumes of 0.1 M HCl or 0.1 M KOH solutions.

2.4. Bacterial Adhesion Assays

Bacterial adhesion assays on MCM-41 and MCM-LYS were tested using gram negative *E. coli* (assay A) and gram positive *S. aureus* (assay B) by using an established methodology [29–33]. In brief, disk-shaped pieces of 6 mm diameter and 1 mm height were prepared by compacting fractions of 30 mg of dried powders using 2.75 and 3 MPa uniaxial and isostatic pressure, respectively. Before the adhesion assay, samples were sterilized by UV irradiation for 10 min on each side of the piece and then stabilized in sterile phosphate-buffered saline (PBS) for 2 h.

Assay A: *S. aureus* strain was grown to a mid-logarithmic phase in THB medium at 37 °C under orbital stirring at 100 rpm until the optical density measured at 600 nm reached 0.5 in an UV/VIS spectrometer (UV-530, Bonsai technologies, Madrid, Spain). Bacteria from the culture were collected by centrifugation (Labofuge 400 centrifuge, Thermo Scientific, Waltham, MA, USA) at 1500 rpm for 10 min at room temperature, washed three times with sterile PBS (pH 7.4), and re-suspended in 12 mL of PBS. In this study (Assay A), PBS solutions with pH 3.6 and 7.8 were also used.

Assay B: *E. coli* was grown in TSB at 37 °C under orbital stirring at 100 rpm until the optimal density, as measured at 600 nm, reached 0.5. At this point, bacteria from the culture were collected by centrifugation at 1500 rpm for 10 min at room temperature, washed three times with sterile PBS (pH 7.4), and subsequently re-suspended in 12 mL of sterile PBS.

Then, different disk-shaped samples were soaked in 1 mL of each bacterial suspension (A or B) and incubated at 37 °C under orbital stirring at 100 rpm for 90 min.

The quantification of bacteria attached to the biomaterial surfaces after the bacterial adhesion assays (A and B) was performed by a method described elsewhere [29,30]. The bioceramic samples were aseptically removed and rinsed three times with sterile PBS to eliminate any free bacteria [32]. Each disk was placed in 1 mL sterile PBS in Eppendorf vials (Nirco, Madrid, Spain), followed by 10 min sonication in a low-power bath sonicator (Selecta, Madrid, Spain). This sonication process was carried out three times, assuming then that 99.9% of adhered bacteria were removed. Thereafter, 100 μL of each sonication product were cultivated on TSA plates, followed by incubation at 37 °C overnight. Determination of the number of colony forming units (CFU) resulting from the overall sum of the three sonication stages allowed the determination of the number of bacteria initially adhered onto the disks. The experiments were performed in duplicate. Surface characterization of the samples after 90 min in *E. coli* bacterial incubation was performed by SEM in a JEOL model JSM-6335F microscope (JEOL, Tokyo, Japan). Before the SEM studies, the attached bacteria were fixed with 2.5 vol. % glutaraldehyde in PBS, pH 7.4 and dehydrated by slow water replacement using a series of graded ethanol solutions (10%, 30%, 50%, 70% and 100%) in deionized water, with a final dehydration step in absolute ethanol before critical point drying (Baltec AG, Balzers, Liechtenstein) [33]. The materials were mounted on stubs and gold plated in a vacuum using a sputter coater (Baltec AG, Balzers, Liechtenstein) and visualized by SEM.

2.5. S. aureus Bacterial Biofilm Formation

Biofilm growth onto MCM-41 and MCM-LYS surfaces was determined. Briefly, *S. aureus* biofilms were developed by suspending the disks of each material in a bacteria solution of 10^8 bacteria per mL during 48 h at 37 °C and orbital stirring at 100 rpm. In this case, the medium used was 66% tryptic soy broth TSB (BioMerieux, Marcy L'Etoile, France) +0.2% glucose to promote robust biofilm formation. After 90 min of incubation, the disks were washed three times with sterile PBS, stained with a 3 μL/mL of Live/Dead® Bacterial Viability Kit BaclightTM (Thermo Fisher Scientific, Waltham, MA, USA) and 5 μL/mL of Calcofluor solution to specifically determine the biofilm formation, staining the mucopolysaccharides of the biofilm (extracellular matrix in blue). Both reactants were incubated for 15 min at room temperature. Biofilm formation was examined in an Olympus FV1200 confocal microscope (Olympus, Tokyo, Japan), by taking eight photographs of each sample (60× magnification) [34]. The surface area covered with adhered bacteria was calculated using ImageJ software (National Institutes of Health, Bethesda, MD, USA). The experiments were performed in triplicate, and the results were expressed as the mean ± standard deviation.

3. Results

MCM-41 was successfully synthesized by the sol-gel methodology, as shown in the following analyses. In Figure 1, the XRD pattern exhibits a strong (100) reflection peak with three small peaks (110), (200), and (210) typical of MCM-41 material [35]; the formation of MCM-41 particles with diameters of around 0.2 µm with the ordered 2D hexagonal array and straight structural features of MCM-41 are clearly revealed by TEM, as observed in Figure 2a,b. It is worth noticing that the synthesized MCM-41 did not present intergrowth or intertwinned aggregations.

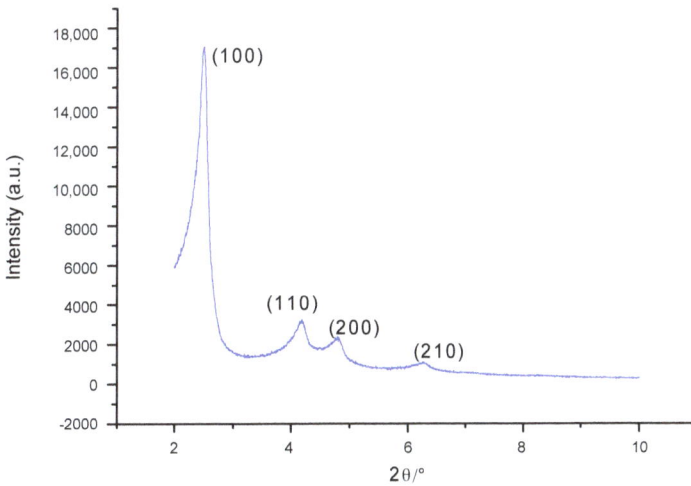

Figure 1. XRD patterns of pristine mesoporous silica (MCM-41). Characteristic diffraction patterns of ordered mesoporous silica corresponding to 2D hexagonal structure, p6mm plain group is observed.

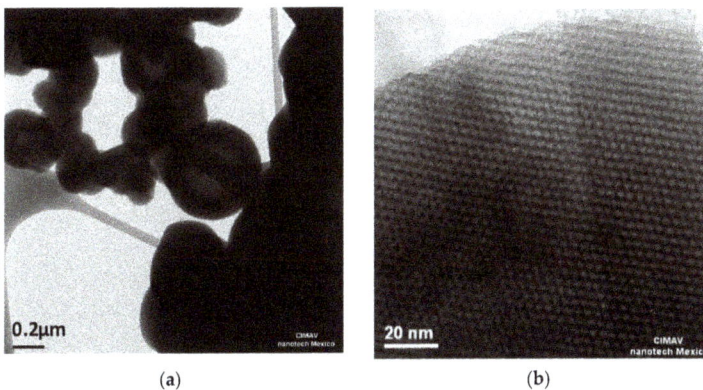

(a)   (b)

Figure 2. Transmission electron microscope (TEM) images of MCM-41: (**a**) The image shows aggregates of circular particles between 200–500 nm; (**b**) The image shows the surface of a particle demonstrating a honeycomb array with a regular pore size of about 2 nm.

Lysine was grafted onto MCM-41 silica using CC as linking agent, as shown in Scheme 1. The surface hydroxyl groups of MCM-41 react with chlorine atoms of CC in a first stage. The remaining chlorine atoms in CC can react with the ε-amino group of lysine (Compound **1**) in a second stage. The protection of α-amino and carboxyl groups is achieved by complexing them with Cu^{2+} (Compound **2**); the free ε-amino groups of the copper complex reacted with Compound **1** to obtain the MCM-LYS material.

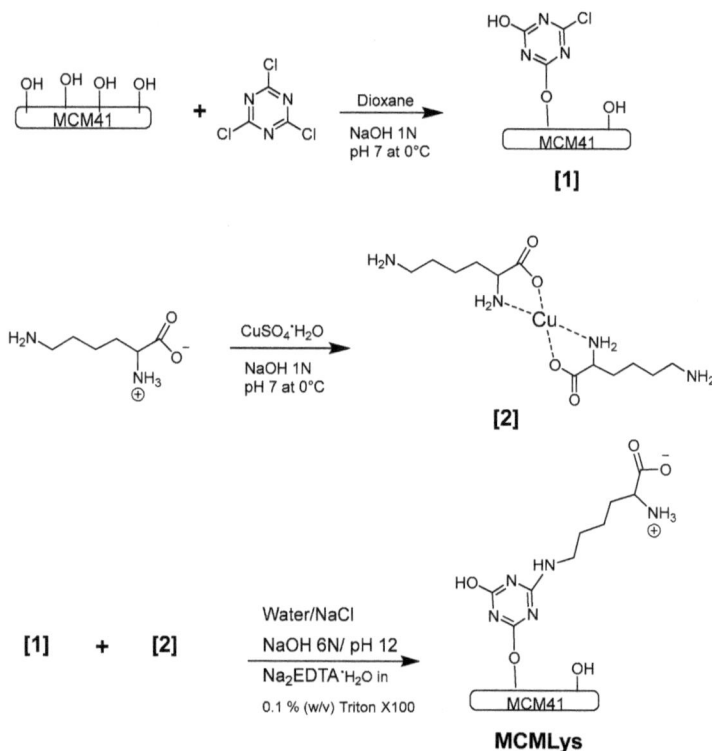

Scheme 1. Lysine grafting via coupling with cyanuric chloride (CC) onto MCM-41. Silanol groups on MCM-41 first react with CC, which in turn react with the ε-amino group of a Cu^{2+} lysine complex. After treatment of the product of [1] and [2] with EDTA to remove copper, the proper zwitterionic function on the bioceramic is achieved.

Figure 3 shows the FTIR spectra of pristine MCM-41 and MCM-LYS. MCM-41 shows the characteristic band of the siloxane group (-Si-O-Si-) at 1060 cm^{-1}, whereas the bands at 955 and 795 cm^{-1} correspond to -Si-OH and -Si-O, respectively [14]. The new bands, shown in the inset, at 3204 and 1399 cm^{-1}, originate from N-H stretching and deformation frequencies, respectively. Furthermore, the presence of zwitterionic pairs can be demonstrated by observing the peaks at 3080 and 1540 cm^{-1}, which correspond to $-NH_3^+$ stretching and deformation frequencies, respectively, and the bands at 1625 and 1415 cm^{-1}, which are typical of the antisymmetric and symmetric frequencies of ionic carboxyl (COO^-). The carbonyl group of lysine is observed in 1715 cm^{-1}, while the bands observed in 2971 and 2874 cm^{-1} correspond to $-CH_2-$ of the amino acid chain. It was therefore established that MCM-41 was successfully modified with lysine, and that the samples exhibit a zwitterion moieties due to the presence of NH_3^+ and COO^- groups (see insets in Figure 3).

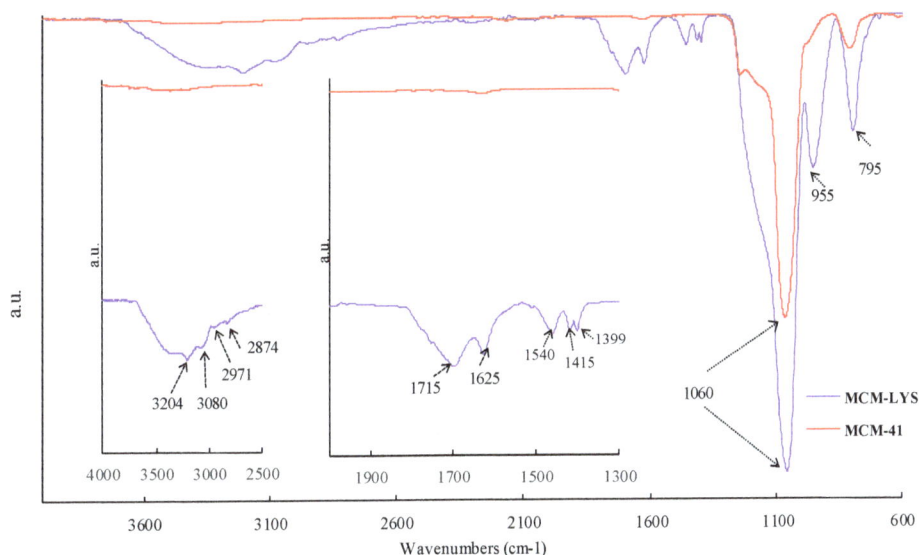

Figure 3. Fourier transform infrared (FTIR) spectra of MCM-41 and lysine-grafted MCM-41 (MCM-LYS). The insets show regions from 4000–2500 cm^{-1} (**left**) and 2000–1300 cm^{-1} (**right**) to better appreciate the changes arising from the grafting of pristine MCM-41.

The textural properties and the organic elemental analysis of MCM-41 and MCM-LYS are summarized in Table 1. It can be seen that the surface area and pore volume of MCM-LYS considerably decreased to 62% and 55%, respectively, in comparison with pristine MCM-41. This reduction of surface area and pore volume is due to the blocking of pores as mesoporous silica is being functionalized. Furthermore, the organic elemental analysis showed that MCM-LYS had 2.47, 2.53, and 5.95 wt.% N, H, and C content, respectively, whereas pristine MCM-41 showed no organic elements (except for hydrogen) in its composition. These facts indicate that lysine was successfully attached onto the bioceramic. The amount of lysine attached to the bioceramic was calculated by taking into account the amount of CC that was previously attached for coupling. In parallel, TGA of MCM-LYS and MCM-41 was carried out up to 600 °C. It was found that the TGA curve of MCM-LYS, which is shown in Figure 4, had two step changes: one at 100–140 °C, which corresponding to the loss of water molecules entrapped in the bioceramic, and the other at 200–300 °C from lysine decomposition. Then, the curve drifted, showing the decomposition of the remaining organic matter that must correspond to CC, which is attached to the bioceramic. From these transitions, it was found that lysine was attached in about 8 wt.%, and that CC was attached in about 7 wt.%, with a decrease in organic material for about 15 wt.%. These numbers are in agreement with the result of the elemental analysis presented in Table 1, which showed an organic content of about 11%.

Table 1. Textural data and elemental analysis of MCM-41 and MCM-LYS.

Sample	S_{BET} (m^2/g)	Vp (cm^3/g)	Dp (nm)	Elemental Analysis			% CC/Lys
				C (%)	H (%)	N (%)	
MCM-41	954	0.95	4.96	—	0.79	—	—
MCM-Lys	359	0.43	4.80	5.95	2.53	2.47	11

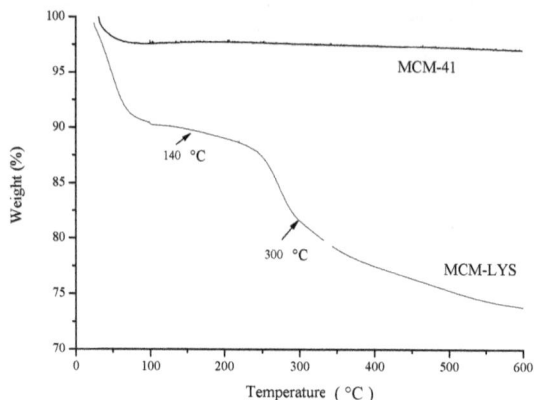

Figure 4. Thermogravimetric analyses (TGA) curves of MCM-41 and MCM-LYS. The thermogram of MCM-LYS shows weight loss in three different regions: 25–140 °C, 140–300 °C, and 300–600 °C.

It is noteworthy that MCM-LYS retained up to 10% of the weight of water, as opposed to bare MCM-41, which indicates that the grafted zwitterions were capable to form a layer of water on the surface of the material that in turn might inhibit the adhesion of bacteria [4].

ζ-potential was measured to determine the isoelectric point (IEP) and the electrostatic behavior of MCM-41 and modified MCM-41 at physiological pH in PBS (pH = 7.4). Figure 5 shows that MCM-41 has a near zero charge at pH 3, whereas MCM-LYS has an IEP at pH 3.6. At physiological pH 7.4, MCM-41 and MCM-LYS show a ζ-potential of −35 and −28 mV, respectively. In the case of MCM-41, this is due to ionized silanol groups (–Si–O–), whereas in the case of MCM-LYS, it is owed to the presence of –Si–O– groups unreacted in the grafting process, since lysine is in its zwitterionic form. Similar behavior was observed by Shi et al. [24], when lysine was grafted onto polyacrylonitrile membrane.

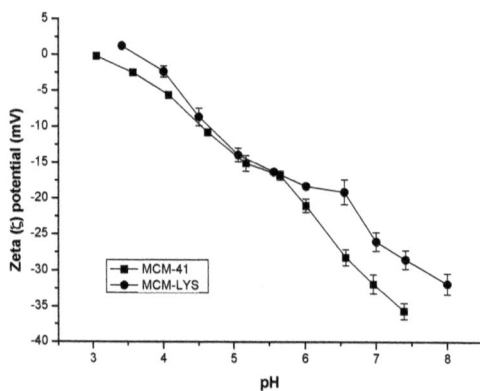

Figure 5. ζ-Potential vs. pH of MCM 41 and MCM-LYS.

To evaluate the *S. aureus* adhesion on the bioceramics, *in vitro* assays were carried out at 37 °C for 90 min at different pH levels (assay A). Figure 6 shows the CFU adhered to the different bioceramics as a function of pH. It can be seen that MCM-LYS had the lowest bacterial adhesion regardless of pH, showing a decrease of about of 77%, 33%, and 15% as compared with pristine MCM-41, at pH of 3.6, 7.4, and 7.8 respectively. It is noteworthy that at pH 3.6, MCM-LYS showed the lowest bacterial adhesion, which corresponds to its isoelectric point, i.e., the pH at which the electric charges are neutralized.

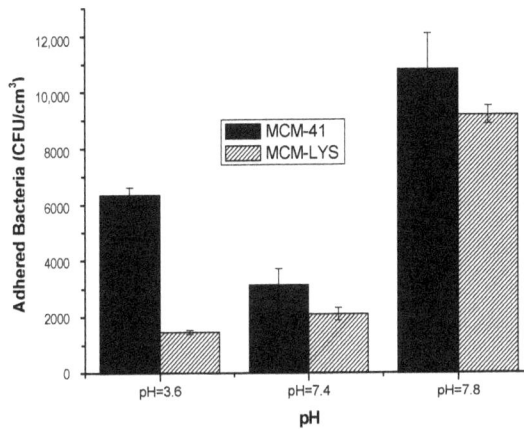

Figure 6. *S. aureus* CFU/cm^3 after 90 min cultivation in the presence of MCM-41 and MCM-LYS at the studied pHs.

Studies of *E. coli* adhesion onto the samples were carried out only at the physiological pH of 7.4. Figure 7a shows that MCM-LYS has the lowest bacterial adhesion, which decreased 50% as compared with pristine MCM-41. Moreover, Figure 7b depicts SEM images of the adhesion of *E. coli* on the surface of both materials, which confirm the results obtained by counting the CFU. SEM micrographs of a MCM-LYS sample show a lower amount of *E. coli* bacteria as compared with MCM-41. In addition, the SEM images show that bacteria are interconnected in MCM-41. In contrast, in MCM-LYS bioceramic, the amount of bacteria observed is smaller, and they appear isolated without apparent communication between them. These results show that zwitterionic moieties on the surface of MCM-LYS, provided by lysine, decreased the initial attachment of both bacteria [31]. In absolute terms, the adhesion of *E. coli* was higher on MCM materials, as compared with *S. aureus*; however, the relative effectiveness of the zwitterionic pair was more pronounced on *E. coli*, which was shown as a reduction of 50% adhesion on MCM-LYS.

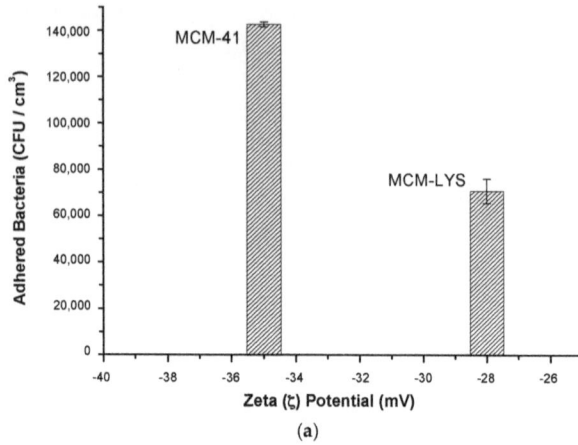

(a)

Figure 7. *Cont.*

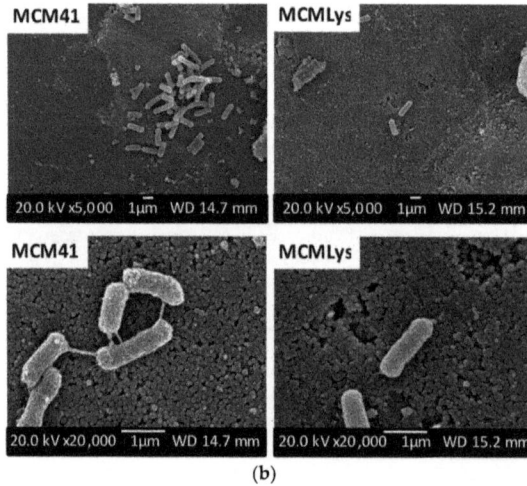

(b)

Figure 7. (a) *E. coli* colony forming units (CFU)/cm^3 after 90 min cultivation in the presence of MCM-41 and MCM-LYS at physiological pH (7.4); (b) SEM micrographs at 5000× and 20,000× of MCM-41 and MCM-LYS after 90 min cultivation of *E. coli*.

Confocal microscopy was carried out to characterize the biofilm formation onto MCM-LYS and bare MCM-41 after 48 h of incubation using Syto-9/propidium iodide dyes (to stain alive and dead bacteria in green and red, respectively), and Calcofluor fluorescent stains (to stain the extracellular matrix of biofilms in blue). The thickness of the biological material attached to both surfaces was determined by analyzing eight different areas of each piece by confocal microscopy. The measured thickness was 30.3 ± 3.3 µm for the bare MCM-41 substrate ($n = 8$ and $p < 0.001$, Kruskal-Wallis test), while the measured thickness was 15.3 ± 7.8 µm for MCM-LYS. Moreover, Figure 8 depicts a compact biofilm layer formed by large colonies with a size >500 µm for MCM-41. However, for the MCM-LYS sample, the scenario is completely different, showing smaller colonies (<50 µm). These results reveal the limited ability of *S. aureus* to form biofilm onto a lysine-functionalized surface as compared with bare MCM-41.

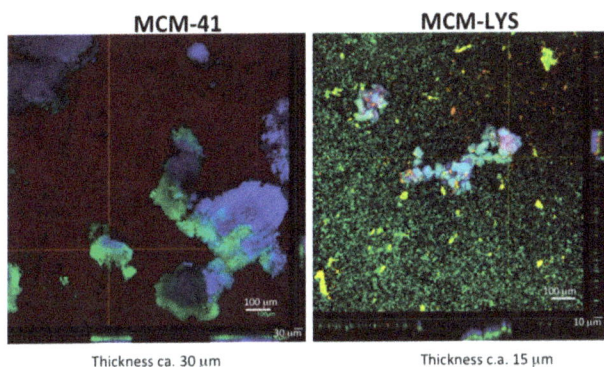

Figure 8. *S. aureus* biofilm grown on MCM-41 and MCM-LYS samples, respectively; the images were collected by confocal microscopy after 48 h of incubation (the larger scale bars correspond to the area of the figure, whereas the smaller scale bar refers to the thickness).

4. Discussion

Different zwitterionization approaches have been developed to prepare non-fouling bioceramics, which include surface grafting with zwitterionic polymers, separately grafting low molecular moieties containing carboxylic and/or amine groups, or with cysteine [15–20]. In this contribution, a facile strategy for creating a non-fouling, antibacterial bioceramic surface is reported. MCM-41 bioceramic was synthesized, and thereafter functionalized with lysine in order to create surface zwitterionic pairs. The use of cyanuric chloride as a coupling agent between MCM-41 and the amino acid warrants mild reaction conditions, and also acts as a bridge to effectively connect the copper complexed L-lysine through its ε-amino group. A battery of analytical techniques was used to confirm that L-lysine was covalently attached to the surface of the bioceramic while maintaining its zwitterionic character. For example, ATR–FTIR analysis established that the zwitterionic pair was present, as demonstrated by the simultaneous appearance of bands at 3080, 1540 cm^{-1} (NH^{3+}), and at 1625 and 1415 cm^{-1} (COO^{-}). The pristine bioceramic had a large surface area and pore volume, which after functionalization were significantly reduced due to pore blockage. Organic elemental analysis corroborated the presence of organic elements such as C, H, N, whereas neat MCM-41 contained only hydrogen; the approximate amount of grafted lysine was 8 wt.%, which was confirmed both with TGA and elemental analysis. TGA revealed a very important fact: the amount of water retained by the modified bioceramic was 10 wt.%, whereas bare MCM-41 only retained about 2 wt.%. This fact indicates that the grafted zwitterions allow the surface to retain five-fold more water as compared with bare MCM-41. This layer of water elicits a resistance to bacterial adhesion [36,37], which is critical for biofilm formation. It has been shown that a single compact layer of mixed charged groups, such as zwitterions, play a dominant role in surface resistance to non-specific protein adsorption due to strong binding of water molecules, which form a physical and energetic barrier that prevents bacterial adhesion [14–17,38]. ζ-potential revealed that both surfaces were negatively charged at physiological pH, due to ionized silanol groups, and that the IEP was slightly increased for the modified bioceramic. MCM-LYS showed the lowest adhesion of *S. aureus*, especially at the IEP. At physiological pH, MCM-LYS showed even lower adhesion for *E. coli* (50%) as compared with unmodified MCM-41. These results showed that the zwitterionic moieties on the modified bioceramic, provided by lysine, decreased the initial attachment of both bacteria [31]. Confocal microscopy images confirmed the limited ability of *S. aureus* to form a biofilm (88% less) in the lysine-modified bioceramic. The facile method here described for incorporation of zwitterionic functions onto bioceramics opens up a great opportunity to develop new biomaterials resistant to bacterial adhesion.

Acknowledgments: María F. Villegas acknowledges the Mexican Council of Science and Techonology (CONCACYT) for financial support of her Master Studies (Scholarship #270469). Guillermo Toriz and Ezequiel Delgado thank the support of Ayudas Santander 2010 for academic exchange to Universidad Complutense de Madrid. María Vallet-Regí acknowledges funding from the European Research Council (Advanced Grant VERDI; ERC-2015-AdG Proposal No.694160) and MINECO MAT2015-64831-R; Antonio J. Salinas thanks the support of Instituto de Salud Carlos III PI15/00978 project co-financied with the European Union FEDER funds; Isabel Izquierdo-Barba thanks also funding from MINECO (MAT2013-43299-R and MAT2016-75611-R AEI/FEDER, UE). The authors wish to thank the ICTS Centro Nacional de Microscopia Electrónica (Spain) and CAI Flow Cytometry and Fluorescence Microscopy of the Universidad Complutense de Madrid (Spain) for the assistance.

Author Contributions: Ezequiel Delgado, Guillermo Toriz, Ofelia Rodríguez and María Vallet-Regí conceived the experiments; María F. Villegas, Isabel Izquierdo-Barba and Lorena Garcia-Uriostegui performed the experiments; Ezequiel Delgado, Guillermo Toriz, Antonio J. Salinas, María Vallet-Regí and Ofelia Rodríguez analyzed the data; all authors contributed writing the paper.

Conflicts of Interest: The authors declare no conflict of interest.

References

1. Nejadnik, M.R.; Olsson, A.L.; Sharma, P.K.; van der Mei, H.C.; Norde, W.; Busscher, H.J. Adsorption of pluronic F-127 on surfaces with different hydrophobicities probed by quartz crystal microbalance with dissipation. *Langmuir* **2009**, *25*, 6245–6249. [CrossRef] [PubMed]

2. Ding, X.; Yang, C.; Lim, T.P.; Hsu, L.Y.; Engler, A.C.; Hedrick, J.L.; Yang, Y.Y. Antibacterial and antifouling catheter coatings using surface grafted PEG-b-cationic polycarbonate diblock copolymers. *Biomaterials* **2012**, *33*, 6593–6603. [CrossRef] [PubMed]

3. Eshet, I.; Freger, V.; Kasher, R.; Herzberg, M.; Lei, J.; Ulbricht, M. Chemical and physical factors in design of antibiofouling polymer coatings. *Biomacromolecules* **2011**, *12*, 2681–2685. [CrossRef] [PubMed]

4. Cheng, G.; Li, G.; Xue, H.; Chen, S.; Bryers, J.D.; Jiang, S. Zwitterionic carboxybetaine polymer surfaces and their resistance to long-term biofilm formation. *Biomaterials* **2009**, *30*, 5234–5240. [CrossRef] [PubMed]

5. Cheng, G.; Xue, H.; Zhang, Z.; Chen, S.; Jiang, S. A switchable biocompatible polymer surface with self-sterilizing and nonfouling capabilities. *Angew. Chem. Int. Ed.* **2008**, *47*, 8831–8834. [CrossRef] [PubMed]

6. Jiang, S.; Cao, Z. Ultralow-fouling, functionalizable, and hydrolyzable zwitterionic materials and their derivatives for biological applications. *Adv. Mater.* **2010**, *22*, 920–932. [CrossRef] [PubMed]

7. Kalbasi, R.J.; Kolahdoozan, M.; Rezaei, M. Synthesis and characterization of PVAm/SBA-15 as a novel organic-inorganic hybrid basic catalyst. *Mater. Chem. Phys.* **2011**, *125*, 784–790. [CrossRef]

8. Rosenholm, J.M.; Sahlgren, C.; Lindén, M. Towards multifunctional, targeted drug delivery systems using mesoporous silica nanoparticles—Opportunities & challenges. *Nanoscale* **2010**, *2*, 1870–1883. [PubMed]

9. Wu, Z.; Zhao, D. Ordered mesoporous materials as adsorbents. *Chem. Commun.* **2011**, *47*, 3332–3338. [CrossRef] [PubMed]

10. Kumar, P.; Guliants, V.V. Periodic mesoporous organic-inorganic hybrid materials: applications in membrane separations and adsorption. *Microporous Mesoporous Mater.* **2010**, *132*, 1–14. [CrossRef]

11. Vallet-Regí, M. Nanostructured mesoporous silica matrices in nanomedicine. *J. Int. Med.* **2010**, *267*, 22–43. [CrossRef] [PubMed]

12. Vallet-Regí, M.; Balas, F.; Arcos, D. Mesoporous materials for drug delivery. *Angew. Chem. Int. Ed.* **2007**, *46*, 7548–7558. [CrossRef] [PubMed]

13. Izquierdo-Barba, I.; Colilla, M.; Vallet-Regí, M. Zwitterionic ceramics for biomedical applications. *Acta Biomater.* **2016**, *40*, 201–211. [CrossRef] [PubMed]

14. Colilla, M.; Izquierdo-Barba, I.; Sánchez-Salcedo, S.; Fierro, J.L.; Hueso, J.L.; Vallet-Regí, M. Synthesis and characterization of zwitterionic SBA-15 nanostructured materials. *Chem. Mater.* **2010**, *22*, 6459–6466. [CrossRef]

15. Izquierdo-Barba, I.; Sánchez-Salcedo, S.; Colilla, M.; Feito, M.J.; Ramírez-Santillán, C.; Portolés, M.T.; Vallet-Regí, M. Inhibition of bacterial adhesion on biocompatible zwitterionic SBA-15 mesoporous materials. *Acta Biomater.* **2011**, *7*, 2977–2985. [CrossRef] [PubMed]

16. Sánchez-Salcedo, S.; Colilla, M.; Izquierdo-Barba, I.; Vallet-Regí, M. Design and preparation of biocompatible zwitterionic hydroxyapatite. *J. Mater. Chem. B* **2013**, *1*, 1595–1606. [CrossRef]
17. Vallet-Regí, M.; Izquierdo-Barba, I.; Colilla, M. Structure and functionalization of mesoporous bioceramics for bone tissue regeneration and local drug delivery. *Philos. Trans. R. Soc. A* **2012**, *370*, 1400–1421. [CrossRef] [PubMed]
18. Alswieleh, A.M.; Cheng, N.; Canton, I.; Ustbas, B.; Xue, X.; Ladmiral, V.; Xia, S.; Ducker, R.E.; Zubir, O.E.; Cartron, M.L.; et al. Zwitterionic Poly (amino acid methacrylate) Brushes. *J. Am. Chem. Soc.* **2014**, *136*, 9404–9413. [CrossRef] [PubMed]
19. Colilla, M.; Martínez-Carmona, M.; Sánchez-Salcedo, S.; Ruiz-González, M.L.; González-Calbet, J.M.; Vallet-Regí, M. A novel zwitterionic bioceramic with dual antibacterial capability. *J. Mater. Chem. B* **2014**, *2*, 5639–5651. [CrossRef]
20. Rosen, J.E.; Gu, F.X. Surface functionalization of silica nanoparticles with cysteine: A low-fouling zwitterionic surface. *Langmuir* **2011**, *27*, 10507–10513. [CrossRef] [PubMed]
21. Khatayevich, D.; Gungormus, M.; Yazici, H.; So, C.; Cetinel, S.; Ma, H.; Jen, A.; Tamerler, C.; Sarikaya, M. Biofunctionalization of materials for implants using engineered peptides. *Acta Biomater.* **2010**, *6*, 4634–4641. [CrossRef] [PubMed]
22. Meyers, S.R.; Khoo, X.; Huang, X.; Walsh, E.B.; Grinstaff, M.W.; Kenan, D.J. The development of peptide-based interfacial biomaterials for generating biological functionality on the surface of bioinert materials. *Biomaterials* **2009**, *30*, 277–286. [CrossRef] [PubMed]
23. Chen, S.; Cao, Z.; Jiang, S. Ultra-low fouling peptide surfaces derived from natural amino acids. *Biomaterials* **2009**, *30*, 5892–5896. [CrossRef] [PubMed]
24. Shi, Q.; Su, Y.; Chen, W.; Peng, J.; Nie, L.; Zhang, L.; Jiang, Z. Grafting short-chain amino acids onto membrane surfaces to resist protein fouling. *J. Membr. Sci.* **2011**, *366*, 398–404. [CrossRef]
25. Zhi, X.; Li, P.; Gan, X.; Zhang, W.; Shen, T.; Yuan, J.; Shen, J. Hemocompatibility and anti-biofouling property improvement of poly (ethylene terephthalate) via self-polymerization of dopamine and covalent graft of lysine. *J. Biomater. Sci. Polym. Ed.* **2014**, *25*, 1619–1628. [CrossRef] [PubMed]
26. Yacynych, A.M.; Kuwana, T. Cyanuric chloride as a general linking agent for modified electrodes: Attachment of redox groups to pyrolytic graphite. *Anal. Chem.* **1978**, *50*, 640–645. [CrossRef]
27. Cai, Q.; Luo, Z.S.; Pang, W.Q.; Fan, Y.W.; Chen, X.H.; Cui, F.Z. Dilute solution routes to various controllable morphologies of MCM-41 silica with a basic medium. *Chem. Mater.* **2001**, *13*, 258–263. [CrossRef]
28. Delgado, E.; Lopez-Dellamary, F.A.; Allan, G.G.; Andrade, A.; Contreras, H.; Regla, H. Zwitterion modification of fibres: Effect of fibre flexibility on wet strength of paper. *J. Pulp Pap. Sci.* **2004**, *30*, 141–144.
29. An, Y.H.; Friedman, R.J. (Eds.) *Handbook of Bacterial Adhesion: Principles, Methods, and Applications*; Springer Science & Business Media: Berlin, Germany, 2000; Volume 204.
30. Bauer, S.M.; Santschi, E.M.; Fialkowski, J.; Clayton, M.K.; Proctor, R.A. Quantification of Staphylococcus aureus adhesion to equine bone surfaces passivated with Plasmalyte™ and hyperimmune plasma. *Vet. Surg.* **2004**, *33*, 376–381. [CrossRef] [PubMed]
31. Cheng, G.; Zhang, Z.; Chen, S.; Bryers, J.D.; Jiang, S. Inhibition of bacterial adhesion and biofilm formation on zwitterionic surfaces. *Biomaterials* **2007**, *28*, 4192–4199. [CrossRef] [PubMed]
32. Kinnari, T.J.; Esteban, J.; Martin-de-Hijas, N.Z.; Sanchez-Munoz, O.; Sanchez-Salcedo, S.; Colilla, M.; Vallet-Regí, M.; Gomez-Barrena, E. Influence of surface porosity and pH on bacterial adherence to hydroxyapatite and biphasic calcium phosphate bioceramics. *J. Med. Microbiol.* **2009**, *58*, 132–137. [CrossRef] [PubMed]
33. Izquierdo-Barba, I.; Vallet-Regí, M.; Kupferschmidt, N.; Terasaki, O.; Schmidtchen, A.; Malmsten, M. Incorporation of antimicrobial compounds in mesoporous silica film monolith. *Biomaterials* **2009**, *30*, 5729–5736. [CrossRef] [PubMed]
34. Izquierdo-Barba, I.; García-Martín, J.M.; Álvarez, R.; Palmero, A.; Esteban, J.; Pérez-Jorge, C.; Arcos, D.; Vallet-Regí, M. Nanocolumnar coatings with selective behavior towards osteoblast and Staphylococcus aureus proliferation. *Acta Biomater.* **2015**, *15*, 20–28. [CrossRef] [PubMed]
35. Wagner, V.E.; Koberstein, J.T.; Bryers, J.D. Protein and bacterial fouling characteristics of peptide and antibody decorated surfaces of PEG-poly (acrylic acid) co-polymers. *Biomaterials* **2004**, *25*, 2247–2263. [CrossRef] [PubMed]

36. Gottenbos, B.; Grijpma, D.W.; van der Mei, H.C.; Feijen, J.; Busscher, H.J. Antimicrobial effects of positively charged surfaces on adhering Gram-positive and Gram-negative bacteria. *J. Antimicrob. Chemother.* **2001**, *48*, 7–13. [CrossRef] [PubMed]

37. He, Y.; Chang, Y.; Hower, J.C.; Zheng, J.; Chen, S.; Jiang, S. Origin of repulsive force and structure/dynamics of interfacial water in OEG–protein interactions: a molecular simulation study. *Phys. Chem. Chem. Phys.* **2008**, *10*, 5539–5544. [CrossRef] [PubMed]

38. Zheng, J.; Li, L.; Tsao, H.K.; Sheng, Y.J.; Chen, S.; Jiang, S. Strong repulsive forces between protein and oligo (ethylene glycol) self-assembled monolayers: A molecular simulation study. *Biophys. J.* **2005**, *89*, 158–166. [CrossRef] [PubMed]

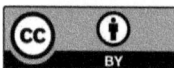

bioengineering

MDPI

Article

Chitosan–Cellulose Multifunctional Hydrogel Beads: Design, Characterization and Evaluation of Cytocompatibility with Breast Adenocarcinoma and Osteoblast Cells

Poonam Trivedi [1], Tiina Saloranta-Simell [2], Uroš Maver [3], Lidija Gradišnik [3], Neeraj Prabhakar [4], Jan-Henrik Smått [5], Tamilselvan Mohan [6], Martin Gericke [7], Thomas Heinze [8] and Pedro Fardim [1,8,*]

[1] Laboratory of Fibre and Cellulose, Åbo Akademi University, 20500 Turku, Finland; ptrivedi@abo.fi
[2] Johan Gadolin Process Chemistry Centre, Laboratory of Organic Chemistry, Åbo Akademi University, 20500 Turku, Finland; tiina.saloranta-simell@abo.fi
[3] Faculty of Medicine, University of Maribor, 2000 Maribor, Slovenia; uros.maver@um.si (U.M.); lidija.gradisnik@um.si (L.G.)
[4] Pharmaceutical Sciences Laboratory, Åbo Akademi University, 20500 Turku, Finland; Neeraj.Prabhakar@abo.fi
[5] Laboratory of Physical Chemistry and Center for Functional Materials, Åbo Akademi University, 20500 Turku, Finland; Jan-Henrik.Smatt@abo.fi
[6] Institute of Chemistry, Karl-Franzens-University Graz, Heinrichstraße 28, 8010 Graz, Austria; tamilselvan.mohan@gmail.com
[7] Institute of Organic Chemistry and Macromolecular Chemistry, Centre of Excellence for Polysaccharide Research, Friedrich Schiller University of Jena, Humboldtstraße 10, D-07743 Jena, Germany; martin.gericke@uni-jena.de
[8] Department of Chemical Engineering, KU Leuven, Celestijnenlaan 200F, B-3001 Leuven, Belgium; thomas.heinze@uni-jena.de
* Correspondence: pfardim@abo.fi; Tel.: +358-(0)5-0409-6424

Academic Editor: Gary Chinga Carrasco
Received: 15 November 2017; Accepted: 5 January 2018; Published: 9 January 2018

Abstract: Cytocompatible polysaccharide-based functional scaffolds are potential extracellular matrix candidates for soft and hard tissue engineering. This paper describes a facile approach to design cytocompatible, non-toxic, and multifunctional chitosan-cellulose based hydrogel beads utilising polysaccharide dissolution in sodium hydroxide-urea-water solvent system and coagulation under three different acidic conditions, namely 2 M acetic acid, 2 M hydrochloric acid, and 2 M sulfuric acid. The effect of coagulating medium on the final chemical composition of the hydrogel beads is investigated by spectroscopic techniques (ATR–FTIR, Raman, NMR), and elemental analysis. The beads coagulated in 2 M acetic acid displayed an unchanged chitosan composition with free amino groups, while the beads coagulated in 2 M hydrochloric and sulfuric acid showed protonation of amino groups and ionic interaction with the counterions. The ultrastructural morphological study of lyophilized beads showed that increased chitosan content enhanced the porosity of the hydrogel beads. Furthermore, cytocompatibility evaluation of the hydrogel beads with human breast adenocarcinoma cells (soft tissue) showed that the beads coagulated in 2 M acetic acid are the most suitable for this type of cells in comparison to other coagulating systems. The acetic acid fabricated hydrogel beads also support osteoblast growth and adhesion over 192 h. Thus, in future, these hydrogel beads can be tested in the in vitro studies related to breast cancer and for bone regeneration.

Keywords: chitosan; cellulose; coagulation; hydrogel; scaffolds; cytocompatibility; tissue engineering

1. Introduction

Polymers, derived from plant and animal sources, such as cellulose and chitosan, have functional groups that provide the unique characteristics, physicochemical properties, and are responsible for their cytocompatibility [1]. Chitosan is the glucosamine polymer obtained after deacetylation of chitin, which results in free amino groups along with abundant hydroxyl groups [2]. Cellulose, on the other hand, possesses already in its main structure abundant hydroxyl groups, leading to extensive hydrogen bonding and stereoregularity in the polymeric chain [3]. Both mentioned naturally derived polymers are non-toxic and cytocompatible [4]. Chitosan and cellulose had been previously successfully processed in the form of beads, fibres, films, nanoparticles, hydrogels, cryogels, and are used in various pharmaceutical and tissue engineering applications [5,6].

Scaffolds prepared from various biomaterials have been used in hard (bone) and soft tissue (skin) engineering [7]. The key requirements for such biomaterial-based scaffolds are cytocompatibility, potential biodegradability, nontoxicity of degradation products, and porosity that suits the chosen cell type [8]. All of these factors altogether contribute to mimicry of the role of the extracellular matrix, by which the scaffolds act as an adhesive substrate, support for cell survival, aids cell migration, and promotes the preservation of the desired cell type [9,10].

Chitosan-based composite hydrogels, such as chitosan/alginate and chitosan/silica, have been tested to promote bone regeneration [11,12]. Similarly, Chitosan-based sponges prepared by lyophilization of chitosan hydrogels, have also been proven to be effective as a bone tissue engineering material [13]. In recent studies, the preparation of highly porous scaffolds from nano-fibrillated cellulose was also investigated [14,15]. The method of designing a biomaterial scaffold has a direct impact on its application in tissue engineering. Thus, when considering the method of preparation of chitosan-cellulose composite hydrogels, these can be classified as physical or chemical hydrogels. In physical hydrogels, the interactions between polymeric chains are van der Waals forces, chain entanglements, hydrogen bonding, and hydrophobic or electronic associations. In the case of chemical hydrogels, the interpolymer interactions are due to crosslinking agents, such as glutaraldehyde, genipin, and tripolyphosphate [16–21]. A related well-known fact about chitosan is that its glucosamine residues protonate in diluted acidic solutions and form ionic complexes with anionic species [22,23].

In case of chitosan-cellulose-based hydrogel beads design, the solvent system plays a key role in the resulting properties such as chemical constitution, porosity, size, water retention capacity, which ultimately governs the application. Until now acetic acid, N-methylmorpholine-N-oxide (NNMO), ionic liquids, and NaOH/urea/water solvent system are used to design chitosan-cellulose hydrogel beads of varying properties [24]. Nevertheless, the hydrogel beads previously developed had been tested for different applications, like the adsorption and removal of metal ions, such as copper, iron, and nickel [25–27].

We aimed to design chitosan-cellulose hydrogel beads in an environment-friendly medium with variable ionic interactions of the protonated amino groups with the counter ions generated from the coagulating solvent systems. The cytocompatibility of novel materials to be used in biomedical applications is considered as the most crucial initial requirement for their potential application. Therefore, an effort was put to evaluate the same in our study. For this purpose, the novel hydrogel beads were tested towards human breast adenocarcinoma (MDA-MB-231) cells as an example of a soft tissue and towards human osteoblast cells as an example of hard tissue. Initially, we tested the basic cytocompatibility of the novel hydrogel beads, while based on the positive results, additional attachment testing was performed in the case of the osteoblast cells. Finally, a multi-day exposure of the cells to the developed materials was performed to evaluate their potential for tissue engineering applications.

In a previous study, the NaOH/urea/water solvent system was used to prepare the chitosan-cellulose composite solution by freeze-thaw cycles at low temperatures [28]. Thus, we choose the 7% NaOH/12% urea/ 81% water solvent system to prepare the polymer blends. The polymer solution was coagulated in the form of hydrogel beads in 2 M acetic acid, hydrochloric acid, and sulfuric acid, respectively. The effect of polymer concentration and the nature of coagulating acid on the hydrogel beads were investigated by Nuclear Magnetic Resonance (NMR), Infrared (IR) and Raman spectroscopy as well as by X-ray Diffraction (XRD) and Scanning Electron Microscopy (SEM) techniques. These hydrogel beads could be easily transformed into cryogels via lyophilization technique. The designed hydrogel beads coagulated in 2 M acetic acid showed the optimal cytocompatibility and could be used in the future for bone tissue engineering studies that are related to the treatment of bone injuries.

2. Materials and Methods

2.1. Materials

Enoalfa cellulose pulp with alpha cellulose content >93.5% was provided by Enocell pulp mill, Finland. Low molecular weight chitosan (190–310 kDa with 75–85% degree of deacetylation) was purchased from Aldrich, sodium hydroxide (NaOH, 97% purity) was purchased from Fluka. Urea ($CO(NH_2)_2$, 99.5% purity), sulfuric acid (H_2SO_4, 98%), acetic acid (CH_3COOH, 98%), and hydrochloric acid (HCl, 37%) were obtained from Merck. Ethanol (92%) was purchased from VWR. Deionized water was obtained from the Milli-Q system (0.2 µm filters). MDA-MB-231 cells (Human breast adenocarcinoma), Dulbecco's modified Eagle's medium (DMEM) supplemented with 10% fetal bovine serum, 2 mM L-glutamine, and 1% penicillin, streptomycin (v/v) were purchased from Life Technologies, ThermoFisher Scientific Inc., Darmstadt Germany. WST-1 cell proliferation reagent was from Roche Diagnostics, Germany. 10% DMSO, Human bone osteoblasts (ATCC CRL-11372), DMEM with 5 wt.% FBS were purchased from Life Technologies, ThermoFisher Scientific Inc., Darmstadt, Germany and 3-(4,5-dimethylthiazol-2-yl)-2,5-diphenyltetrazolium bromide (MTT) assay was purchased from Sigma-Aldrich, Hamburg, Germany.

2.2. Methods

2.2.1. Preparation of Chitosan-Cellulose Hydrogel Beads

To prepare chitosan–cellulose hydrogel beads, varying proportions of chitosan (10–90%) were mixed with HyCelSol [29] treated cellulose pulp keeping 5% final polymer concentration in the solution. The polymer mixture was added to the NaOH/urea/water (7/11/81) solvent system and stirred for 1 h at room temperature, followed by cooling at −13 °C for 1 h. The obtained composite solution was extruded through a 0.8 mm needle in the form of beads into 250 mL 2 M acetic acid, hydrochloric acid, and sulfuric acid solutions, respectively. The beads formed were kept in the coagulation medium for 2 h, followed by subsequent washing with deionized water until neutral conditions were achieved. The beads extruded in 2 M acetic acid, hydrochloric acid, and sulfuric acids were named as **A**, **B**, and **C** type with the initial chitosan percentage in the blend, respectively. (For example **0A**, **0B** and **0C** had 0% initial chitosan concentration). The pH value of coagulating medium was recorded after hydrogel beads gelation of the **70A**, **70B**, and **70C** (hydrogel beads coagulated in 2 M acetic, hydrochloric, and sulphuric acid, respectively with initial chitosan concentration of 70%) samples. Finally, the hydrogel beads were stored in deionized water.

2.2.2. Ftir and Raman Spectroscopy

Nicolet iS 50 FT-IR spectrometer with Raman module from Thermo Scientific (Darmstadt, Germany) was used for spectrometric measurements. FT-IR spectra were collected using tungsten-halogen source and DLaTGS-KBr detector splitter setup with 4.00 cm^{-1} resolution and 64 scans. Raman spectra were collected using a diode laser (power–0.5 W). The detector was InGaAs with CaF$_2$ splitter, resolution 8.0 cm^{-1}, aperture size 200, and number of scans 64,000. Lyophilized hydrogel beads were cross-sectioned and were analysed.

2.2.3. Solid State ^{13}C and ^{15}N NMR Spectroscopy

The solid-state ^{13}C and ^{15}N NMR spectra were recorded with 400 MHz Bruker AVANCE-III NMR spectrometer, equipped with a 4 mm Cross-Polarisation Magic Angle Spinning CP-MAS probe operating frequencies 100.52 MHz (^{13}C) and 40.51 MHz (^{15}N). The spectra were recorded at the spinning rate of 5 kHz and a contact time of 2 ms (^{13}C) and 3.5 ms (^{15}N).

2.2.4. Elemental Analysis

A VARIO EL III CHNS analyser (Elementar Analysensysteme GmbH, Langenselbold, Germany) was used for elemental analysis according to standardised procedures. The chlorine content was determined subsequently by combustion of the organic samples and potentiometric titration with $AgNO_3$ using a chloride-sensitive electrode.

2.2.5. XRD Analysis

XRD measurements were performed on a Bruker D8 Discover instrument (Bruker, Karlsruhe, Germany) with a Cu K_α X-ray source and an HI-STAR area detector. The incident angle was kept at $6°$, while the detector angle (2θ) was $25°$.

2.2.6. Scanning Electron Microscopy-Energy Dispersive Spectroscopy

The qualitative composition analysis of beads was performed with JEOL JSM-6335F (JEOL Ltd., Tokyo, Japan) with accelerating voltage 15 kV, Working Distance (WD) = 15 mm. Air dried cross-sectioned beads were moulded into the epoxy resin in a gelatinous capsule. The resin was allowed to cure at RT for 24 h. Trimming was performed with a microtome. After trimming, the sample was sputtered with platinum and a fresh surface exposed by slicing a thin layer off of the surface with the microtome. A spot analysis was taken with a COMPO image detector from two places representing different phases of the sample denoted as shades of lighter and darker grey.

The cross-section analysis of beads was performed with LEO Gemini 1530. A Thermo Scientific Ultra Silicon Drift Detector (SDD) equipped with secondary electron backscattered electron and In lens, detector was used. The chitosan-cellulose hydrogel beads were frozen in liquid nitrogen and were lyophilized. The beads were further cross-sectioned, coated with carbon and analyzed. The magnification of the images corresponds to a Polaroid 545 print with the image size of 8.9×11.4 cm^2.

2.2.7. Cytocompatibility Evaluation of Chitosan-Cellulose Hydrogel Beads Coagulated in Different Acids with MDA-MB-231 (Human Breast Adenocarcinoma) Cells

The cell studies were performed under standard conditions in a humidified, 37 °C, 5 wt.% CO_2 environment using MDA-MB-231 cells. MDA-MB-231 cells (Human breast adenocarcinoma) were cultured in Dulbecco's modified Eagle's medium (DMEM) supplemented with 10 wt.% fetal bovine serum (FBS), 2 mM L-glutamine, and 1% penicillin–streptomycin (v/v). **0A**, **70A**, **0B**, **70B**, and **0C**, **70C**, hydrogel beads that were previously soaked in cell culture medium were placed in a 96 well cell culture plate. MDA-MB-231 cells were added to each type of hydrogel beads for evaluation of attachment and proliferation for 48 h. After incubating the cells with hydrogel beads for 48 h at 37 °C, 5 wt.% CO_2, 10 μL of WST-1 cell proliferation reagent (Roche Diagnostics, Mannheim, Germany) was added to the respective wells containing 100 μL of cell growth media, and the plate was again allowed to incubate for 3 h at 37 °C, 5 wt.% CO_2. After the incubation period, the absorbance was read at 430 nm by Tecan Ultra microplate reader (MTX Lab Systems, Inc.) from Bradenton, FL, USA. The number of viable cells was correlated with the observed absorbance from each sample. 10 wt.% DMSO (toxin) was added as a negative control, whereas wells without beads (tissue culture plastic (TCP)) were used as positive control cells and were allowed to grow without any cellulose beads.

2.2.8. Cytocompatibility Evaluation of Chitosan-Cellulose Hydrogel Beads Coagulated in 2 M Acetic Acid with Osteoblast Cells

The **0A**, **50A**, and **70A** hydrogel bead samples suspended in ultrapure water obtained from Milli-Q were used for the osteoblast cells adhesion and proliferation studies. The number of hydrogel beads used was three **0A** and two **50A** and **70A** respectively. The beads were sterilised using UV light (for 30 min) followed by soaking in 1 mL of the cell culture medium (advanced DMEM) with 5 wt.% FBS for 30 min. Human bone osteoblasts (ATCC CRL-11372), were seeded on a P96 well microtiter plate at a concentration of 20.000 cells/cm^2. Allowing the cells to attach for 24 h, the hydrogel beads samples were added in four repetitions. For this purpose, we used the as-prepared samples, and their dilutions of 1:2, 1:4, and 1:8 in Advanced DMEM with 5 wt.% FBS. After one, four, six, and 192 h of incubation at 37 °C and 5 wt.% CO$_2$, the sample cytocompatibility/cytotoxicity was assessed using the MTT assay (Sigma-Aldrich, Germany). The media was changed every other day. Cell viability was determined via the reduction reaction of the tetrazolium salt MTT (3(4,5-dimethylthiazolyl-2)-2,5-diphenyltetrazolium bromide), as determined by measuring the absorbance (using Varioskan, Thermo Fisher Scientific Inc., Germany) at 570 nm [30].

2.2.9. Cell Attachment Testing of Chitosan-Cellulose Hydrogel Beads Coagulated in 2 M Acetic Acid with Osteoblast Cells

The **0A**, **50A**, and **70A** hydrogel bead samples were stored in ultrapure water obtained from Milli-Q. Four beads of sample **70A**, and five beads of samples **0A** and **50A** were poured with 1 mL of Advanced DMEM medium with 5 wt.% FBS and left to culture with it for 30 min. Since the beads were of different sizes and had therefore different weights, as well as different surface to volume rations, our experiments were based on using same weights of the beads instead of the same number. Consequently, the number of beads for respective samples used for the experiments is different. The samples were transferred to a chamber with eight wells (8 well glass slide, slide Chamber, Nunc, Thermo Fisher Scientific, USA) and combined in the cell suspension with a cell density of 17,500 cells/well. The same cell density was used for the control well (as the control we used Advanced DMEM medium with 5 wt.% FBS without beads in tissue culture plastic plates (TCP)). Samples were prepared in duplicates. The obtained cells with beads were cultured at 37 °C, using an atmosphere of 5 wt.% CO$_2$. The growth medium was replaced after 72 h cells seeding. After 192 h the samples were stained using the crystal violet dye (0.1 wt.% crystal violet in 20 wt.% ethanol). For this purpose, the medium was pipetted from respective wells, followed by washing of the samples twice with PBS (phosphate buffered saline, Sigma, Darmstadt, Germany), poured with 300 μL of the as-prepared dye solution and left for 5 min at room temperature. The dye was consequently pipetted away, and the samples were washed three times with ultrapure water obtained from Milli-Q system. This was followed by observing the surface of the beads with a Leica DM2500 microscope (Leica, Germany).

2.2.10. Statistical Analysis

The data obtained for both the cell-based tests is presented as mean values ± standard deviation of the mean. Statistical analysis of the significance for the cytocompatibility testing on both cell types was performed using a one-way analysis of variance (ANOVA test) against respective control samples. A $p < 0.05$ (and lower) was considered as significant. All of the statistical tests were performed using Excel 2016.

3. Results and Discussions

3.1. Effect of Coagulating Medium on the Mechanism of the Chitosan-Cellulose Hydrogel Beads Formation

Chitosan and cellulose were blended in the ratio of 0/100, 10/90, 30/70, 50/50, 70/30, 90/10 in NaOH/urea/water (7/12/81) solvent system. The beads were extruded in 2 M acetic acid, hydrochloric acid, and sulfuric acid, and named as **A**, **B**, and **C**, respectively (Figure 1). The hydrogel beads with a chitosan-cellulose ratio up to 70/30 were stable, and further increasing chitosan content to 90/10 did not result in stable entities. Thus 90/10 beads were not characterized. The chosen coagulating acidic medium affected the final composition of the resulting hydrogel beads. The measured pH value of the coagulating medium after hydrogel formation was 5.0, 1.0, and <1.0 in case of **A**, **B** and **C** systems, respectively.

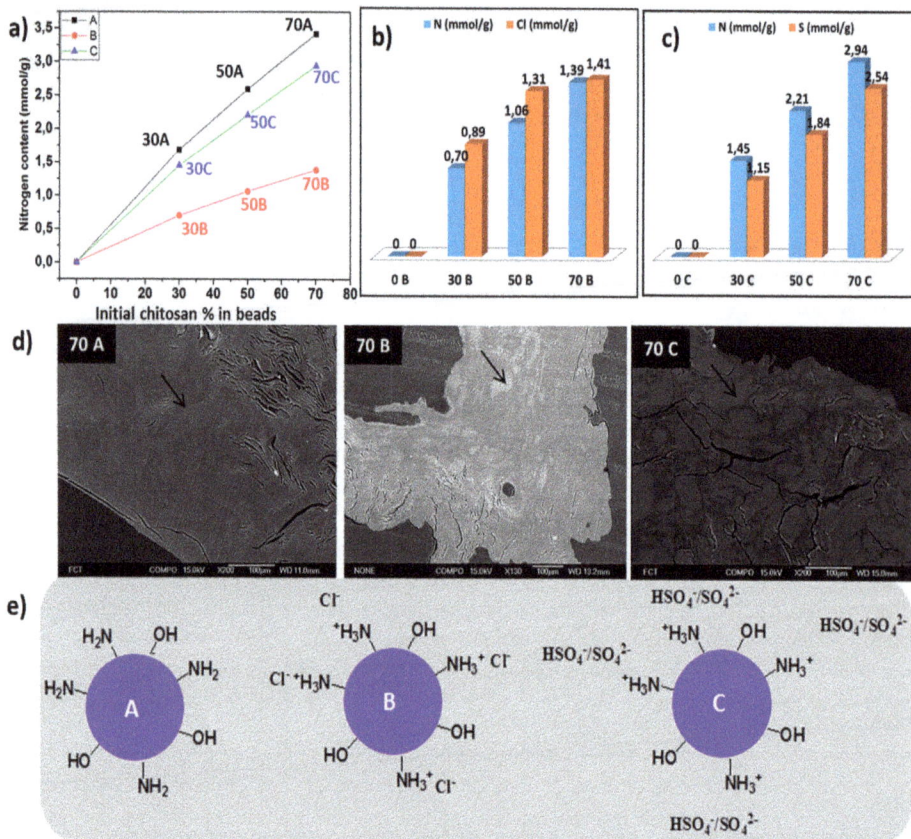

Figure 1. (**a**) Total nitrogen content present in beads with varying chitosan composition coagulated in 2 M acetic acid (**A**), 2 M hydrochloric acid (**B**) and 2 M sulfuric acid (**C**). (**b,c**) A comparison of chlorine and sulphur with the nitrogen content in **B** and **C** type. (**d**) Nitrogen element distribution measured via spot analysis in **70A**, **70B**, and **70C** and (**e**) Presentation of possible ionic interactions in **A**, **B** and **C** type.

Further elemental analysis of the samples was performed to understand the mechanism of hydrogel formation in each type of acidic medium. A detailed elemental composition analysis of the dried beads coagulated in 2 M acetic acid (**A**) type, hydrochloric (**B**) type, and sulfuric acid (**C**) type, respectively shows an increasing trend in the nitrogen content, which corresponds to the chitosan content in hydrogel beads from initial 0 to 70% composition. The **70A** has the highest nitrogen content equivalent to 3.4 mmol/g, while **70B** has 1.2 mmol/g and **70C** 2.9 mmol/g, respectively. The beads coagulated in 2 M hydrochloric acid had the lowest nitrogen content in comparison to the two other systems (Figure 1a). The beads coagulated in hydrochloric and sulfuric acid also showed the presence of chlorine and sulphur atoms, respectively (Figure 1b,c). In the case of beads coagulated in 2 M hydrochloric acid and 2 M sulfuric acid, the amino group of chitosan were protonated (NH_3^+) and had ionic interactions with the chloride (Cl^-) and hydrogen sulphate (HSO_4^-) or sulphate (SO_4^{2-}) ions. The qualitative analysis of the beads via SEM-EDS displayed shades of lighter and darker grey corresponding to different positions in the bead samples, which has been indicated by arrow in (Figure 1d). Spot analysis of **70A** revealed a homogeneous distribution of chitosan, while in the case of **70B** and **70C**, a non-homogenous chitosan composition was observed. The EDS spectra are included in (Supplementary Figure S1). The elucidated chemistry of the designed beads has been proposed, as shown in Figure 1e. The presence of higher chitosan content in **A**-type of hydrogel beads can be explained by the fact that at pH value of 5, chitosan exhibits reduced solubility, resulting in an irreversible interaction with the cellulose and the enhanced chitosan deposition [31].

In the case of **B**-type, the final coagulating medium had a pH value of 1. Even at low concentrations, HCl is a strong acidic solvent for the dissolution of chitosan. Therefore the maximum dissolution of chitosan in the beads is presumed. In **C**-type, the pH value was <1.0, and sulfuric acid does not lead to the dissolution of chitosan even after the protonation of amino groups (NH_3^+). It could be explained by the study by Cui et al., which showed that in the presence of sulfuric acid, the amino groups of chitosan are protonated (NH_3^+), but are in strong electrostatic interaction with the sulfonate (SO_4^{2-}) anions [32]. Therefore, the coagulating medium dictates the final chemistry and composition of the chitosan-cellulose hydrogel beads.

3.2. Attenuated Total Reflectance–Fourier Transform Infra-Red (ATR–FTIR) and Raman Spectroscopic Analysis

In the IR spectra of pristine chitosan and cellulose, broad bands are visible in the region 3700–3000 cm^{-1}, corresponding to O–H stretching and N–H vibrations. The presence of amide I band at 1651 cm^{-1} due to the carbonyl stretching vibrations, and a bifurcated band with peaks at 1590 cm^{-1} due to amide II, corresponding to N–H bending vibrations and at 1560 cm^{-1}, due to free NH_2 bending vibrations are present in chitosan. A slight variation in the CHx deformations region at 1425 and 1374 cm^{-1}, C–O–C and C–O stretching vibration region at 1200–950 cm^{-1} are also apparent (Figure 2a). The chitosan-cellulose hydrogel beads coagulated in 2 M acetic, hydrochloric and sulfuric acid displayed significant variations in the region 4000–1450 cm^{-1} and in the fingerprint region 1450–500 cm^{-1} when compared to the pristine chitosan and cellulose biopolymers. In chitosan-cellulose beads, the 3600–3000 cm^{-1} region in **70C** is broader than the **70A** and **70B**. In the 1700–1500 cm^{-1} region corresponding to amide and amino group vibrations, significant variations are observed. In **70A**, **70B**, and **70C**, the peak due to amide I (at 1641 cm^{-1}) overlaps with the water absorbance peak. Also, in the band corresponding to free amino groups clear variations are observed. In **70A**, the band appears in the chitosan in the same region at 1555 cm^{-1}, while in **70B**, a band with lower intensity exhibiting a slight shift towards right at 1525 cm^{-1} is visible. In the case of **70C** beads, a peak at 1532 cm^{-1} of equal intensity exhibiting a small shift towards the right, is present. The shift in peaks towards the right in the case of **70B** and **70C** is presumably related to the protonated amino (NH_3^+) groups bending vibrations having interaction with the counterions [33]. A slight variation in the CHx deformations that correspond to peaks at 1425 and 1374 cm^{-1} can also be observed (Figure 2a).

Similarly, in the region 3600–3100 cm^{-1} of the Raman spectra, the sharp O-H and N-H stretching vibrations in chitosan and broad O–H stretching vibrations in cellulose are visible. In chitosan, the peak due to alkyl groups shows slight bifurcation, which is not apparent in cellulose (Figure 2b). In **70A**, the 3600–3100 cm^{-1} region matches with that of chitosan, and as such, displaying sharp peaks, whereas **70B** and **70C** show broader bands in the same region. The amide and the amino region in **70A** matches with the natural chitosan, indicating the presence of unchanged chitosan. A comparatively less intensity band in **70B** and broadband in **70C** is evident. The band broadening in **70C** could be due to strong ionic interactions between the protonated amino groups and hydrogen sulphate or sulfonate anion. The appearance of a new distinct peak at 974 cm^{-1} in **70C** is due to the presence of SO_4^{2-} ions [33]. The effect of sulfuric acid has also been explained by the fact that first, the sulfuric acid protonates the amino group, and then acts as a crosslinking agent between the protonated amino groups by sulfate (SO_4^{2-}) ions [33]. Hence, the spectroscopic data confirms the protonation of amino groups and interaction between the amino groups and negatively charged species in case of **70B** and **70C** hydrogel beads, while in **70A** beads, no such evidence was observed.

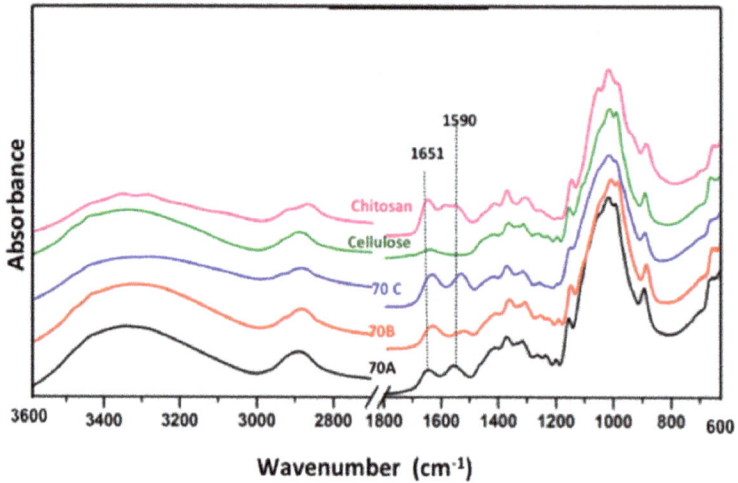

(a)

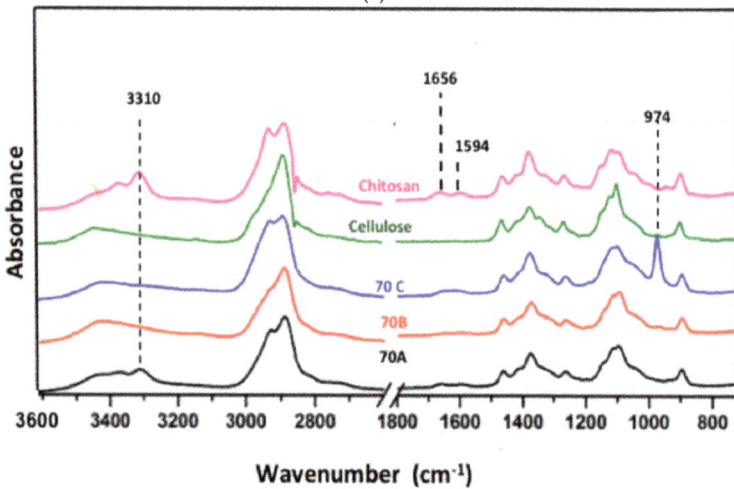

(b)

Figure 2. (a) Attenuated Total Reflectance–Fourier Transform Infra-Red (ATR-FTIR) and (b) Raman spectra of chitosan cellulose and **70A, 70B** and **70C** lyophilized hydrogel beads.

3.3. Solid-State ^{13}C and ^{15}N Nuclear Magnetic Resonance

In order to study the hydrogel beads further, chitosan, cellulose, H_2SO_4 treated chitosan reference samples, as well as the lyophilized hydrogel beads **70A, 70B,** and **70C,** were analysed by solid-state

CP-MAS ^{13}C- and ^{15}N NMR spectroscopy. The characteristic signals observed in the CP-MAS ^{13}C NMR spectra of cellulose and chitosan (Figure 3a) have been reported in the literature [34,35]. The main difference between the CP-MAS ^{13}C NMR spectra of cellulose and chitosan is the C-2 signal that is shifted to the higher field in chitosan (56 ppm) when compared to cellulose (73 ppm). Moreover, the signals corresponding to residual acetyl groups are observed in the CP-MAS ^{13}C NMR spectrum of chitosan, i.e., the signals at 22 ppm (CH_3) and 173 ppm (C=O), respectively. When chitosan was treated with sulfuric acid, the NH_2-groups are converted to NH_3^+-groups and are ionically interacting with sulfonate ions. This resulted in broadening of all the signals observed in CP-MAS ^{13}C NMR spectra and shift of C1- and C4-signals (supporting information).

The **70A**, seems to be a physical mixture of cellulose and chitosan with no changes in the chemical structure. While **70B** consisted of the low amount of chitosan, therefore based on this analysis, it is impossible to comment on possible changes in the chitosan part. The **70C** is a mixture of cellulose and ionically crosslinked chitosan. These observations are further supported by CP-MAS ^{15}N NMR spectra (Figure 3b). The NH_2-signal in unmodified chitosan resonates at 22.6 ppm, whereas the nitrogen atoms in the NHOAc-groups resonates at 121.7 ppm. When chitosan is treated with sulfuric acid, the nitrogen atoms in the corresponding NH_3^+- groups resonates at 32.0 ppm, which is regarded as a clear indication of the modification of chitosan (Supplementary Figure S2).

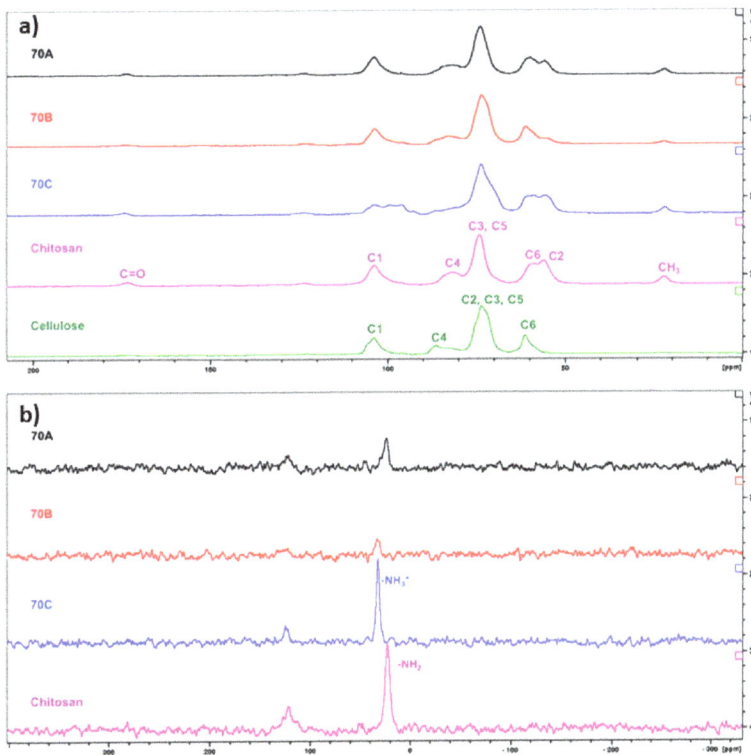

Figure 3. (a) CP-MAS ^{13}C NMR spectra (b) CP-MAS ^{15}N NMR spectra of chitosan, cellulose, **70A**, **70B**, and **70C** chitosan-cellulose lyophilized hydrogel beads.

In the **70C** and **70B**, the main signal in the CP-MAS ^{15}N NMR spectra corresponds to the resonance frequency of NH_3^+- groups further strengthening the conclusion on ionic crosslinking of chitosan in these hydrogel beads. The corresponding signal in the CP-MAS ^{15}N NMR spectra of **70A** is at 22.6 ppm, indicating that chitosan in this sample is not in ionic interaction with any counterion. Hence, the CP-MAS ^{13}C and ^{15}N NMR spectra support the results from IR and Raman spectroscopy.

3.4. XRD Analysis

The XRD analysis of pristine chitosan, regenerated cellulose, as well as **70A**, **70B**, and **70C** lyophilized hydrogel beads shows that chitosan has a different diffraction pattern when compared to the regenerated cellulose. In the case of pure chitosan, a sharp reflection at $2\theta = 19°$ and a broad reflection at $10°–11°$ are present, while in cellulose broad reflections at $2\theta = 22°$ and $12°–13°$ are observed. Since the beads are composites of chitosan and cellulose, an overlap of the chitosan ($19°$) and cellulose ($22°$) reflections in the beads is apparent. However, the relative peak intensities in the $10°–13°$ 2θ region can be used to distinguish the pattern of composite beads equivalent to chitosan or cellulose. The **70A** sample shows a pattern closer to the pure chitosan pattern, while **70B** and **70C** have patterns closer to cellulose. These observations could be explained by the fact that in **70A**, the chitosan has not undergone any changes during coagulation in 2 M acetic acid, while in **70B**, lower content of chitosan is present due to dissolution and leaching out from the hydrogel beads during gelation. In **70C**, the peak shapes resemble more the regenerated cellulose. This behaviour could be due to ionic interactions between chitosan and sulphuric acid. Therefore, the coagulating medium affects the crystallinity and the final composition of the beads, as shown in (Figure 4).

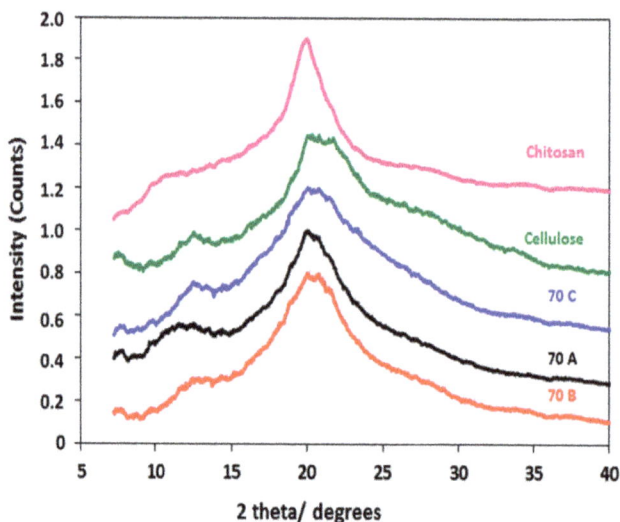

Figure 4. XRD diffraction patterns of chitosan, regenerated cellulose, 70A, 70B and 70C chitosan-cellulose hydrogel beads.

3.5. Scanning Electron Microscopic Analysis (SEM)

The qualitative morphological analysis of hydrogel beads was done by scanning electron microscopy (Figure 5). The pore size of the hydrogels is dependent on the polymer concentration, processing conditions, and the drying procedure. In the present study, liquid nitrogen was used to freeze the water in the hydrogel beads before the lyophilization. A considerable variation in the morphology and ultrastructure of all the samples was observed. A comparison of surface morphology of **0A**, **70A**, and **0B**, **70B** shows that the hydrogel beads have a porous surface with slightly larger pores in the case of **70A** and **70B**. In the case of **0C**, a highly compact ultrastructure is observed while the morphology is loose and porous for the **70C** sample. The cross-section ultrastructure evaluation of hydrogel beads has shown that **70A**, **70B**, and **70C** have increased porosity in comparison to the **0A**, **0B**, and **0C**, respectively. An unusual behaviour was observed in the hydrogel beads, namely fine fibrillary deposits were found on the surface of hydrogel beads in some regions. Thus, the variation in morphology of the hydrogel beads shows that the presence of chitosan and the coagulating medium governs the ultrastructure of the entities prepared.

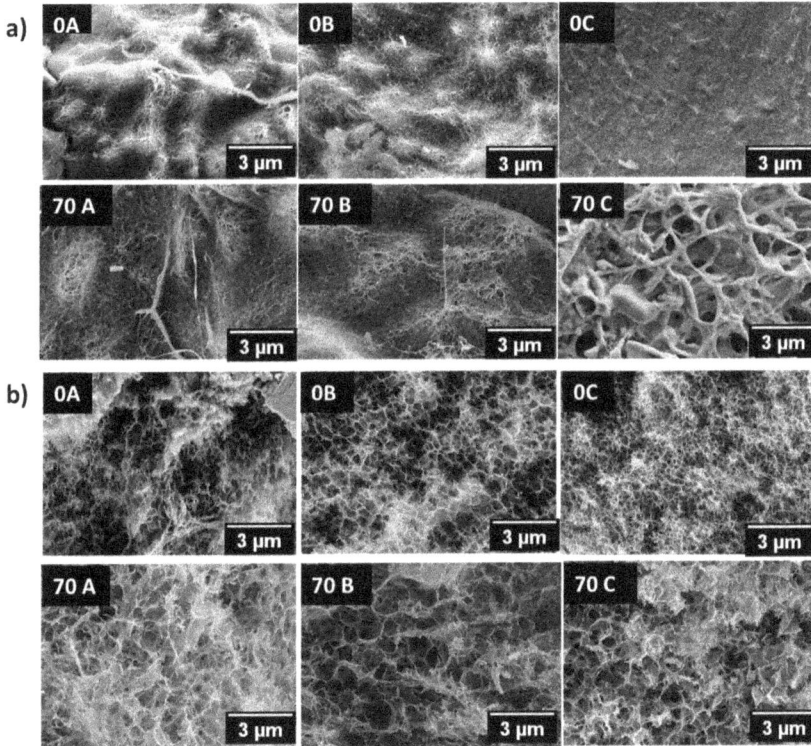

Figure 5. (**a**) Surface and (**b**) core morphology of **0A**, **0B**, **0C**, **70A**, **70B**, and **70C** chitosan–cellulose hydrogel beads with the scale bar 3 μm.

3.6. Cytocompatibility Evaluation of Chitosan-Cellulose Hydrogel Beads with MDA-MB-231 Cells (Human Breast Adenocarcinoma—A Soft Tissue Organ)

The human breast adenocarcinoma cells originate from the human female breast (a soft tissue organ), making them appropriate model cells for evaluating the potential of the developed materials for soft tissue engineering applications. For this purpose, we performed a cell viability testing. The cytocompatibility of the **70A**, **70B**, and **70C** hydrogel beads with MDA-MB-231 cells (human breast adenocarcinoma) over 48 h was evaluated using the WST-1 cell proliferation assay. A comparison between positive control and **0A**, **70A**, **0B**, **70B**, **0C**, **70C** was performed, as shown in (Figure 6). DMSO was used as positive control for cellular toxicity because at higher concentration it is toxic to the cells. As expected, all the groups showed higher cell proliferation as compared to DMSO. However, a comparison of all groups with negative control showed variable cytocompatibility amongst all of the hydrogel beads. The hydrogel beads **0A**, **0B**, **70B**, **0C**, and **70C** displayed less than 70% viability of the cells, which could be due to potential degradation products of the beads that could have eroded from the beads during their soaking. These could in turn partially hinder the growth of cells in the early stages of the experiment, resulting in lower viabilities when compared to the negative control. Thus further testing of these beads for any application is insignificant. Interestingly, a comparison between **0A–70A** showed that **70A** type has improved cytocompatiblity than the **0A** type, while we did not observe such difference between **0B–70B** and **0C–70C**. Further, between **70A–70B**, no significant difference was observed, but in case of **70A–70C**, the **70A** type was more cytocompatible than the **70C** type, possibly due to the presence of higher content of chitosan in the **70A** hydrogel beads where no counterions were present to interact with the amino groups, thus making them available to interact with the cells [2]. While in case of **70B** and **70C**, the amino groups are ionically crosslinked with the chloride and sulfonate or hydrogen sulphate groups, respectively, thus making amino groups unavailable to interact with the cells. Overall, **70A** type was comparatively more cytocompatible than the other hydrogel bead types with the model cells qualifying their use for soft tissue engineering.

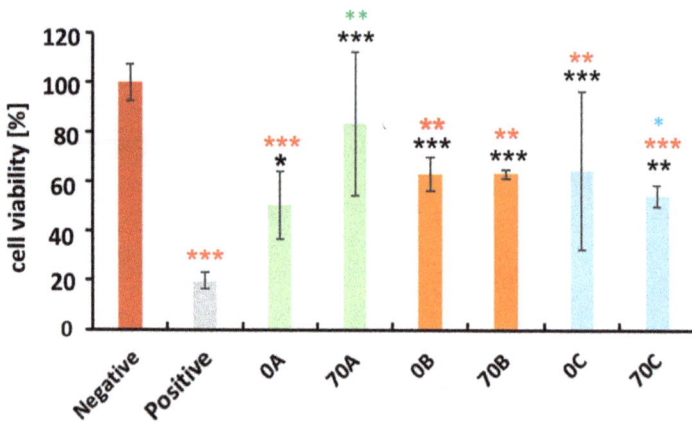

Figure 6. Human breast adenocarcinoma (MDA-MB-231) cytocompatibility with **0A**, **70A**, **0B**, **70B**, and **0C**, **70C** chitosan–cellulose hydrogel beads over the timeframe of 48 h. Values are expressed as percentage of the means ± SD ($n = 4$). Statistical significance was defined as * $p < 0.05$, ** $p < 0.01$, *** $p < 0.005$ compared to control samples (ANOVA test). Black * and red * indicates sample comparison to positive and negative control respectively. While green * shows comparison between **0A** and **70A**, **0B** and **70B**, **0C** and **70C**; blue * shows between **70A** and **70B**, **70A** and **70C**, **70B** and **70C**.

3.7. Cytocompatibility Evaluation of Chitosan-Cellulose Beads Coagulated in Acetic Acid with Osteoblast Cells (Hard Tissue)

Proven cytocompatibility is the prerequisite for any scaffold to be used in bone tissue engineering. The main objective of this study was to evaluate the cytocompatibility of the chitosan cellulose hydrogel beads coagulated in acetic acid with human bone-derived osteoblast cells, as shown in (Figure 7).

The results show a comparative cytocompatibility study between the control sample, i.e., Advanced DMEM, **0A**, **50A**, and **70A** at various times of exposure (up to 192 h). It is clear that the prepared beads affect the growth of the used cells, especially in comparison to the cell growth after each of the time intervals. After 24 h, we see a lower viability of the cells grown together with the bead groups, whereas already after 48 h, all of the prepared samples (**0A**, **50A**, and **70A**) show an increased viability, when compared to the control. Both samples that included chitosan (**50A** and **70A**) also showed a higher viability than the beads prepared from pure cellulose. Between them, the difference was in the range of rerpoted error for respective samples. After 96 h the viability was comparable to the control sample, whereas the samples **50A** and **70A** again outperformed the control sample after 144 h. Since at this time period, the sample **50A** showed the highest viability of all the samples, this might indicate that a modest number of free amino groups (from chitosan) has the most positive influence of the growth of osteoblast cells, whereas an even hugher number of free amino groups could potentially lead to a higher surface charge, which seems still suits the cells, but to a smaller extent. Regardless of the respective viabilities, these results definitely show that all of the tested (**0A**, **50A** and **70A**) beads are suitable for growth of osteoblast cells at least up to 144 h.

After 192 h, we observed a decrease in the viability of the cells exposed to the bead samples, when compared to the control. Examination of the optical micrographs of the cells after the mentioned time period (not shown) showed no negative effect of the beads that could be observed in comparison with the control (no changes in cell morphology or shape etc.). It seems that the lower viabilities might be related to the fact that the cells have overgrown the experimental environment of the well in the P96 plate. In comparison with the control, where we do not see this decrease in viability, this effect is mainly due to the faster growth of cells in the case of sample exposure, potentially leading to contact inhibition. Further studies are of course necessary to confirm the latter via other methods, yet this is out of the scope of the present study.

A crystal violet dye viability/cytocompatibility assay was also performed to check the cytocompatibility of the hydrogel beads. The result is summarized in (Supplementary Figure S3). Finally, from Figure 7, we can also see that in the timeframe, where we observed an increased viability after exposure to the beads, in comparison with the control samples. The chitosan modified hydrogel bead outperform the pure cellulose beads, making these promising for future testing and development of such materials for bone tissue engineering applications.

Since our intention was not only to assess if the proposed hydrogel beads degrade in the cells native environment, which could hinder cell growth (Figure 7—cytocompatibility assessment), but also to evaluate the viability of the osteoblast cell culture directly on the as-prepared samples (attachment or direct contact test). However, we could not find any literature source that would describe an efficient method for direct visualization of grown cells on such hydrogel beads.

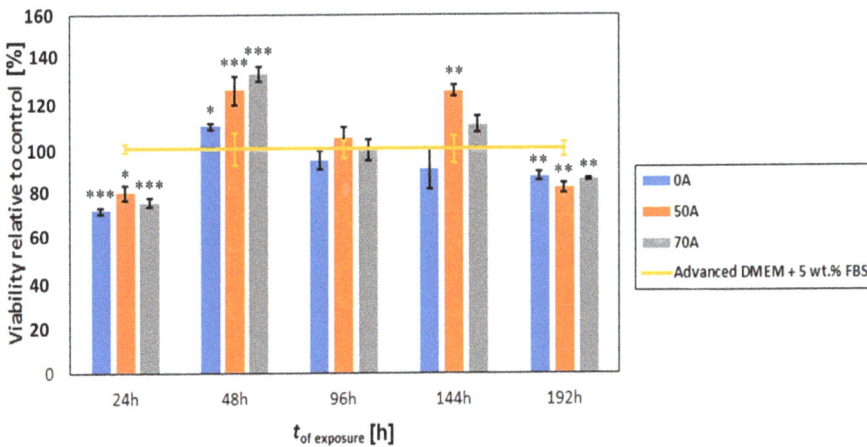

Figure 7. Osteoblast cytocompatibility (proliferation behaviour) with **0A**, **50A** and **70A** chitosan–cellulose hydrogel beads based on the MTT assay over the timeframe of 192 h. Values are expressed as percentage of the means $\pm$ SD ($n = 4$). Statistical significance was defined as * $p < 0.05$, ** $p < 0.005$, *** $p < 0.001$ as compared to control sample (ANOVA test).

4. Conclusions

Cytocompatible chitosan-cellulose hydrogel beads were prepared with varying chitosan content and chemistry along the amino group. The hydrogel beads coagulated in 2 M acetic acid (**70A**)

Bioengineering **2018**, *5*, 3

showed higher chitosan retention with free amino groups. Whereas, in case of a 2 M hydrochloric acid (**70B**), low amount of chitosan was present and the amino groups are ionically interacting with Cl^- ions. While in 2 M sulfuric acid (**70C**), although high chitosan was present, amino groups were involved in ionic interactions with HSO_4^-/SO_4^{2-} ions. The cytocompatibility evaluation of the hydrogel bead groups with breast adenocarcinoma cell lines displayed **70A** type has the maximum cytocompatibility in comparison to other groups. Similarly, in the case of beads coagulated in 2 M acetic acid, the osteoblast cells showed effective adhesion to the bead surface, as well as an increased viability, when compared to the positive control. These results are presumably related to the form of amino groups present in the hydrogel beads. Concretely, the chitosan-cellulose hydrogel beads exhibiting free amino groups, led to a higher cell viability, when compared to the prepared samples, where the amino groups were involved in ionic interactions with the anions as in the case of Cl^- and HSO_4^-/SO_4^{2-}. Herein, we propose the chemistry and the mechanism behind the hydrogel beads coagulation in different acidic media, cytocompatibility with model soft and hard tissue cell lines and their future potential use in the bone tissue engineering applications.

Supplementary Materials: The following are available online at www.mdpi.com/2306-5354/5/1/3/s1, Figure S1: SEM-EDS spectra of **70A**, **70B** and **70C** hydrogel beads, Figure S2: CP-MAS ^{13}C and ^{15}N NMR spectra of chitosan and chitosan treated with sulfuric acid, Figure S3: Crystal violet (CV) staining of beads with attached osteoblasts. Black spots and clusters show healthy cells (typical cells on all bead samples are marked with red circles). The darker the spots, the more viable the cells are (according to CV dyeing protocol). Control sample was dyed with CV for comparison as well.

Acknowledgments: We thank the PShapes project of WoodWisdom.net and the Academy of Finland for the financial support. The authors acknowledge also the financial support from the Slovenian Research Agency (grant numbers: P-0036 and I0-0029).

Author Contributions: Poonam Trivedi, Pedro Fardim: Conceived, designed and wrote the paper. Tiina Saloranta-Simell helped with NMR characterisation and analysis, Uroš Maver and Lidija Gradišnik performed the osteoblast studies. Neeraj Prabhakar did breast adenocarcinoma cell studies, Jan-Henrik Smått performed XRD experiments. Martin Gericke and Thomas Heinze were involved in elemental analysis.

Conflicts of Interest: The authors declare no conflict of interest.

References

1. Mano, J.; Silva, G.; Azevedo, H.; Malafaya, P.; Sousa, R.; Silva, S.; Boesel, L.F.; Oliveira, J.M.; Santos, T.C.; Marques, A.P.; et al. Natural origin biodegradable systems in tissue engineering and regenerative medicine: Present status and some moving trends. *J. R. Soc. Interface* **2007**, *4*, 999–1030. [CrossRef] [PubMed]
2. Cheung, R.; Ng, T.; Wong, J.; Chan, W. Chitosan: An update on potential biomedical and pharmaceutical applications. *Mar. Drugs* **2015**, *13*, 5156–5186. [CrossRef] [PubMed]
3. Malmström, E.; Carlmark, A. Controlled grafting of cellulose fibres—An outlook beyond paper and cardboard. *Polym. Chem.* **2012**, *3*, 1702–1713. [CrossRef]
4. Vieira, M.; da Silva, M.; dos Santos, L.; Beppu, M. Natural-based plasticizers and biopolymer films: A review. *Eur. Polym. J.* **2011**, *47*, 254–263. [CrossRef]
5. Gericke, M.; Trygg, J.; Fardim, P. Functional Cellulose Beads: Preparation, Characterization, and Applications. *Chem. Rev.* **2013**, *113*, 4812–4836. [CrossRef] [PubMed]
6. Ravi Kumar, M. A review of chitin and chitosan applications. *React. Funct. Polym.* **2000**, *46*, 1–27. [CrossRef]
7. Chaudhari, A.; Vig, K.; Baganizi, D.; Sahu, R.; Dixit, S.; Dennis, V.; Singh, S.R.; Pillai, S.R. Future prospects for scaffolding methods and biomaterials in skin tissue engineering: A Review. *Int. J. Mol. Sci.* **2016**, *17*, 1974. [CrossRef] [PubMed]
8. Guo, Z.; Yang, C.; Zhou, Z.; Chen, S.; Li, F. Characterization of biodegradable poly(lactic acid) porous scaffolds prepared using selective enzymatic degradation for tissue engineering. *RSC Adv.* **2017**, *7*, 34063–34070. [CrossRef]
9. Pääkkö, M.; Vapaavuori, J.; Silvennoinen, R.; Kosonen, H.; Ankerfors, M.; Lindström, T.; Berglundc, L.A.; Ikkala, O. Long and entangled native cellulose I nanofibers allow flexible aerogels and hierarchically porous templates for functionalities. *Soft Matter* **2008**, *4*, 2492–2499. [CrossRef]

10. Kim, I.; Seo, S.; Moon, H.; Yoo, M.; Park, I.; Kim, B.; Cho, C. Chitosan and its derivatives for tissue engineering applications. *Biotechnol. Adv.* **2008**, *26*, 1–21. [CrossRef] [PubMed]
11. Rodríguez-Vázquez, M.; Vega-Ruiz, B.; Ramos-Zúñiga, R.; Saldaña-Koppel, D.; Quiñones-Olvera, L. Chitosan and its potential use as a scaffold for tissue engineering in regenerative medicine. *BioMed Res. Int.* **2015**, *2015*, 821279. [CrossRef] [PubMed]
12. Finšgar, M.; Uzunalić, A.; Stergar, J.; Gradišnik, L.; Maver, U. Novel chitosan/diclofenac coatings on medical grade stainless steel for hip replacement applications. *Sci. Rep.* **2016**, *6*. [CrossRef] [PubMed]
13. Al-Munajjed, A.; Plunkett, N.; Gleeson, J.; Weber, T.; Jungreuthmayer, C.; Levingstone, T.; Hammer, J.; O'Brien, F.J. Development of a biomimetic collagen-hydroxyapatite scaffold for bone tissue engineering using a SBF immersion technique. *J. Biomed. Mater. Res. Part B Appl. Biomater.* **2009**, *90B*, 584–591. [CrossRef] [PubMed]
14. VandeVord, P.; Matthew, H.; DeSilva, S.; Mayton, L.; Wu, B.; Wooley, P. Evaluation of the Cytocompatibility of a chitosan scaffold in mice. *J. Biomed. Mater. Res.* **2001**, *59*, 585–590. [CrossRef] [PubMed]
15. Costa-Pinto, A.; Reis, R.; Neves, N. Scaffolds based bone tissue engineering: The role of chitosan. *Tissue Eng. Part B Rev.* **2011**, *17*, 331–347. [CrossRef] [PubMed]
16. Ma, L. Collagen/chitosan porous scaffolds with improved biostability for skin tissue engineering. *Biomaterials* **2003**, *24*, 4833–4841. [CrossRef]
17. Mwale, F.; Iordanova, M.; Demers, C.; Steffen, T.; Roughley, P.; Antoniou, J. Biological evaluation of chitosan salts cross-linked to genipin as a cell scaffold for disk tissue engineering. *Tissue Eng.* **2005**, *11*, 130–140. [CrossRef] [PubMed]
18. Hsieh, C.; Tsai, S.; Ho, M.; Wang, D.; Liu, C.; Hsieh, C.; Tseng, H.; Hsieh, H. Analysis of freeze-gelation and cross-linking processes for preparing porous chitosan scaffolds. *Carbohydr. Polym.* **2007**, *67*, 124–132. [CrossRef]
19. Zhang, Q.; Wu, Q.; Lin, D.; Yao, S. Effect and mechanism of sodium chloride on the formation of chitosan–cellulose sulfate–tripolyphosphate crosslinked beads. *Soft Matter* **2013**, *9*, 10354–10363. [CrossRef]
20. Chan, B.; Leong, K. Scaffolding in tissue engineering: General approaches and tissue-specific considerations. *Eur. Spine J.* **2008**, *17*, 467–479. [CrossRef] [PubMed]
21. Cai, H.; Sharma, S.; Liu, W.; Mu, W.; Liu, W.; Zhang, X.; Deng, Y. Aerogel Microspheres from Natural Cellulose Nanofibrils and Their Application as Cell Culture Scaffold. *Biomacromolecules* **2014**, *15*, 2540–2547. [CrossRef] [PubMed]
22. Jayakumar, R.; Prabaharan, M.; Sudheesh Kumar, P.; Nair, S.; Tamura, H. Biomaterials based on chitin and chitosan in wound dressing applications. *Biotechnol. Adv.* **2011**, *29*, 322–337. [CrossRef] [PubMed]
23. Madihally, S.; Matthew, H. Porous chitosan scaffolds for tissue engineering. *Biomaterials* **1999**, *20*, 1133–1142. [CrossRef]
24. Shen, X.; Shamshina, J.L.; Berton, P.; Gurau, G.; Rogers, R.D. Hydrogels based on cellulose and chitin: Fabrication, properties, and applications. *Green Chem.* **2016**, *18*, 53–75. [CrossRef]
25. Li, N.; Bai, N. Copper adsorption on chitosan-cellulose hydrogel beads: Behaviors and mechanisms. *Sep. Purif. Technol.* **2005**, *42*, 237–247. [CrossRef]
26. Twu, Y.K.; Huang, H.I.; Chang, S.Y.; Wang, S.L. Preparation and sorption activity of chitosan/cellulose blend beads. *Carbohydr. Polym.* **2003**, *54*, 425–430. [CrossRef]
27. Liu, Z.; Wang, H.; Liu, C.; Jiang, Y.; Yu, G.; Mu, X.; Wang, X. Magnetic cellulose–chitosan hydrogels prepared from ionic liquids as reusable adsorbent for removal of heavy metal ions. *Chem. Commun.* **2012**, *48*, 7350–7352. [CrossRef] [PubMed]
28. Zhou, D.; Zhang, L.; Zhou, J.; Guo, S. Cellulose/chitin beads for adsorption of heavy metals in aqueous solution. *Water Res.* **2004**, *38*, 2643–2650. [CrossRef] [PubMed]
29. Trygg, J.; Fardim, P. Enhancement of cellulose dissolution in water-based solvent via ethanol–hydrochloric acid pretreatment. *Cellulose* **2011**, *18*, 987–994. [CrossRef]
30. Van de Loosdrecht, A.A.; Beelen, R.H.J.; Ossenkoppele, G.J.; Broekhoven, M.G.; Langenhuijsen, M.M.A.C. A tetrazolium-based colorimetric MTT assay to quantitate human monocyte mediated cytotoxicity against leukemic cells from cell lines and patients with acute myeloid leukemia. *J. Immunol. Methods* **1994**, *174*, 311–320. [CrossRef]
31. Myllytie, P.; Salmi, J.; Laine, J. The influence of pH on the adsorption and interaction of chitosan with cellulose. *Bioresources* **2009**, *4*, 1647–1662.

32. Cui, Z.; Xiang, Y.; Si, J.; Yang, M.; Zhang, Q.; Zhang, T. Ionic interactions between sulfuric acid and chitosan membranes. *Carbohydr. Polym.* **2008**, *73*, 111–116. [CrossRef]

33. Larkin, P. *Infrared and Raman Spectroscopy: Principles and Spectral Interpretation;* Elsevier: Amsterdam, The Netherlands, 2011; pp. 110–130.

34. Kono, H.; Yunoki, S.; Shikano, T.; Fujiwara, M.; Erata, T.; Takai, M. CP/MAS13C NMR Study of cellulose and cellulose derivatives. 1. Complete assignment of the CP/MAS13C NMR spectrum of the native cellulose. *J. Am. Chem. Soc.* **2002**, *124*, 7506–7511. [CrossRef] [PubMed]

35. Heux, L.; Brugnerotto, J.; Desbrières, J.; Versali, M.; Rinaudo, M. Solid state NMR for determination of degree of acetylation of chitin and chitosan. *Biomacromolecules* **2000**, *1*, 746–751. [CrossRef] [PubMed]

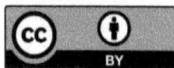

bioengineering

MDPI

Article

An Approach to In Vitro Manufacturing of Hypertrophic Cartilage Matrix for Bone Repair

Bach Quang Le [1,*], Clemens van Blitterswijk [1,2] and Jan de Boer [1,3,*]

[1] Department of Tissue Regeneration, MIRA Institute for Biomedical Technology and Technical Medicine, University of Twente, Postbus 217, 7500 AE Enschede, The Netherlands; c.vanblitterswijk@maastrichtuniversity.nl

[2] Department of Complex Tissue Regeneration, MERLN Institute, University of Maastricht, P.O. Box 616, 6200 MD Maastricht, The Netherlands

[3] Laboratory for Cell Biology-inspired Tissue Engineering, MERLN Institute, University of Maastricht, P.O. Box 616, 6200 MD Maastricht, The Netherlands

* Correspondence: Lequangbach@gmail.com (B.Q.L.); jan.deboer@maastrichtuniversity.nl (J.d.B.)

Academic Editor: Gary Chinga Carrasco
Received: 20 February 2017; Accepted: 18 April 2017; Published: 20 April 2017

Abstract: Devitalized hypertrophic cartilage matrix (DCM) is an attractive concept for an off-the-shelf bone graft substitute. Upon implantation, DCM can trigger the natural endochondral ossification process, but only when the hypertrophic cartilage matrix has been reconstituted correctly. In vivo hypertrophic differentiation has been reported for multiple cell types but up-scaling and in vivo devitalization remain a big challenge. To this end, we developed a micro tissue-engineered cartilage (MiTEC) model using the chondrogenic cell line ATDC5. Micro-aggregates of ATDC5 cells (approximately 1000 cells per aggregate) were cultured on a 3% agarose mold consisting of 1585 microwells, each measuring 400 μm in diameter. Chondrogenic differentiation was strongly enhanced using media supplemented with combinations of growth factors e.g., insulin, transforming growth factor beta and dexamethasone. Next, mineralization was induced by supplying the culture medium with beta-glycerophosphate, and finally we boosted the secretion of proangiogenic growth factors using the hypoxia mimetic phenanthroline in the final stage of in vivo culture. Then, ATDC5 aggregates were devitalized by freeze/thawing or sodium dodecyl sulfate treatment before co-culturing with human mesenchymal stromal cells (hMSCs). We observed a strong effect on chondrogenic differentiation of hMSCs. Using this MiTEC model, we were able to not only upscale the production of cartilage to a clinically relevant amount but were also able to vary the cartilage matrix composition in different ways, making MiTEC an ideal model to develop DCM as a bone graft substitute.

Keywords: Hypertrophic cartilage; ATDC5; decellularized matrix; devitalized matrix; tissue engineering; bone regeneration

---

1. Introduction

Endochondral ossification is a fascinating phenomenon in which a cartilage template is remodeled into bone tissue by a highly regulated mechanism. During embryonic development, endochondral ossification occurs in parallel to intramembranous ossification to build the skeletal system. In fracture healing, the process very much recapitulates embryonic development and thus usually results in complete restoration of the skeletal organ [1–3]. However, when bone defects reach critical sizes or when systemic factors such as osteoporosis presents, clinical intervention is necessary to augment bone healing [4]. Current options to treat bone defects range from autologous bone to synthetic osteoinductive materials with/without growth factors e.g., bone morphogenetic proteins [5]. Until now, there is no clinical treatment that utilizes endochondral ossification, specifically from a hypertrophic cartilage graft.

Previously, we have demonstrated the feasibility of tissue-engineering hypertrophic cartilage from mouse embryonic stem cells (mESCs) in vivo which then remodeled into new bone in vivo [6]. To this end, mESCs were chondrogenically differentiated for 2 to 3 weeks, followed by subcutaneous implantation in immunodeficient mice for 4 weeks. A high correlation was observed between the amount of hypertrophic cartilage created in vivo and the amount of bone detected in vivo. Similarly, Scotti et al. subcutaneously implanted bone marrow-derived human mesenchymal stromal cells (hMSCs) at various stages of chondrogenic differentiation [7]. They observed bone trabeculae only when the hMSCs differentiated in vivo into hypertrophic cartilage-like tissue. Weiss et al. differentiated ATDC5 pellets into hypertrophic cartilage in vivo before implantation in nude mice for 8 weeks [8]. They found mineralized tissue with active osteoclast resorption and neo-angiogenesis throughout the implants. These experiments and others [9–12] show proof of concept that in vivo cultured hypertrophic cartilage can continue endochondral ossification in vivo.

Live hypertrophic cartilage will form bone in vivo, but it has long been realized that even non-living tissues still contain bioactive components that can induce ossification. The most relevant example is demineralized bone matrix (DBM) developed by Urist in 1960. DBM is allogenic or xenogeneic bone processed to remove immunogenicity and preserve the osteoinductive bone morphogenetic proteins [13]. The chemistry of the remaining extracellular matrix (ECM), not the living cells, is sufficient to induce bone formation upon implantation and DBM is widely used as a bone graft substitute. Interestingly, hypertrophic cartilage tissue which is devitalized under certain conditions can also form bone in vivo. Bridge and Pritchard showed that epiphyseal plate or fracture callus devitalized with alcohol, acetone, HCl or heated to 55 °C consistently formed bone when implanted subcutaneously in the ear of rabbits [14]. Urist also observed bone formation when devitalized fracture callus was implanted into the anterior chamber of the eye of rats [15–17]. More recently, Bourgine et al. proved that hMSC-derived hypertrophic cartilage which was devitalized by inducible apoptosis could efficiently remodel to form de novo bone tissue of host origin, including mature vasculature and a hematopoietic compartment [18]. Cunniffe et al. created a porous scaffold by freeze-drying SDS-decellularized hMSC-engineered hypertrophic cartilage tissue. The scaffold induced vascularization and de novo mineral accumulation in a mouse ectopic model and formed full bridging (4 out of 8 animals) in a rat critically-sized femoral defect model [19]. Taken all together, these experiments demonstrated the feasibility of an osteoinductive material made of devitalized hypertrophic cartilage matrix (DCM), either harvested from biological sources or cultured in the lab.

A problem that will eventually hinder the utilization of DCM in the clinic is the ability to manufacture a great amount of this material in a reproducible and cost-effective manner. Making DCM from allografts or xenografts will not yield sufficient amounts since hypertrophic cartilage only presents in small amounts at the ends of long bones before adulthood. Thus, producing DCM from hypertrophic cartilage cultured in vivo seems to be a plausible answer. For this matter, choosing a cell type is the most critical step. One could start with undifferentiated stem cells, for examples embryonic (ES) cells or hMSCs, then induce chondrogenic differentiation until the cells reach the hypertrophic stage. The disadvantages of stem cells are, apart from the cost of maintaining stemness during storage and expansion, chondrogenic differentiation of ES cells is often heterogeneous [20] and donor variation in hMSCs is inevitable [21]. Starting with mature cells such as chondrocytes poses another problem; the cells have limited proliferation capacity before becoming senescent. While the choice of cell types remains to be elucidated, it is worth mentioning that the ideal cell type should have the following properties: (1) already committed to the chondrogenic lineage and (2) have unlimited capacity to divide. In the current study, although we do not claim to have the ideal cell type, we chose a cancer cell line—ATDC5—which has both mentioned properties to demonstrate our hypertrophic cartilage in vivo culturing model. The cell line ATDC5, derived from a mouse teratocarcinoma, is an excellent model to study skeletal development and has been utilized in over 200 studies to date [22]. ATDC5 has an intrinsic property to sequentially undergo hypertrophic chondrogenic differentiation [22–24]. Previously, we developed a spheroid culture system which allows us to assemble 3D, free-standing tissues with an intermediate complexity between 2D cell cultures and model organisms [25]. The advantages of this system and its application to date has been reviewed by Fennema et al. [26]. Here, we cultured ATDC5 in aggregates of approximately 1000–10,000 cells, which we named Micro Tissue-Engineered Cartilage (MiTEC). Compared to 2D culture models, MiTEC offers better cell-cell contacts and chondrogenic differentiation. Compared to traditional micro-mass or pellet models (of about 100,000 to 1,000,000 cells), MiTEC allows better diffusion of nutrients and growth factors. This model does not require additional scaffolding material but can be easily upscaled to produce a large amount of tissue mass applicable for all clinical purposes. Our long-term goal is to create an osteoinductive material made of devitalized ATDC5-derived hypertrophic cartilage that offers the ideal micro-environment for en route endochondral ossification. To reach this goal, in this study we optimized the in vivo production of MiTEC qualitatively and quantitatively. Medium composition and culture time was optimized to maximize hypertrophy; endogenous growth factor (VEGF) secretion was enhanced by treatment with hypoxia mimic molecules; and mineralization was induced with beta-glycerophosphate. MiTEC were devitalized either by freeze/thawing or by sodium dodecyl sulfate (SDS) treatment. Upon co-culturing with hMSCs, the SDS treated MiTEC had a strong effect on hMSC chondrogenic differentiation. Thus, we demonstrated the usability of the MiTEC model in optimizing and upscaling the in vivo culture of hypertrophic cartilage.

2. Materials and Methods

2.1. Cell Culture

ATDC5 cells (RIKEN cell bank, Ibaraki, Japan) were maintained in basic medium (BM) consisting of DMEM/F-12 GlutaMAX, 5% v/v fetal bovine serum (FBS, Lonza, Breda, Netherlands), 0.2 mM L-ascorbic acid-2 phosphate (ASAP), 100 U/mL penicillin and 100 µg/mL streptomycin (PS). Cells were grown at 37 °C in a humid atmosphere with 5% CO_2. The medium was refreshed 2–3 times per week and the cells were used for further subculturing or cryopreservation upon reaching near confluence.

3% agarose (Life Technologies, Bleiswijk, Netherlands) chips were produced by replica molding from elastomeric stamps of poly(dimethylsiloxane) (PDMS; Sylgard 184, Dow Corning, Seneffe, Belgium); the stamps were replicated from either etched silicon wafers or SU-8/silicon wafers [25]. An agarose chip contains 1585 micro-wells, each measuring 400 µm in diameter and fitting in a well of a 12-well plate. To make aggregates, 1.5 million cells were seeded per agarose chip and centrifuged for 1 min at 300 G to collect the cells at the bottom of the micro-wells. This seeding density created an aggregate size of about 1,000 cells per aggregate, which was optimized for our 400 µm diameter micro-wells. The medium was changed every 1–2 days by pipetting from the side of the agarose chips without disturbing the aggregates. To optimize medium composition, 4 different formulations were used: (1) basic medium (BM); (2) BM supplemented with 1× insulin-transferrin-selenium (ITS) solution (IM); (3) BM supplemented with 0.1 µM dexamethasone (Dex) and 10 ng/mL transforming growth factor beta 3 (TGFβ3, R&D systems, 243-B3-010) (BC); and BM supplemented with 1× ITS, 0.1 µM Dex and 10 ng/mL TGFβ3 (IC).

Primary human mesenchymal stem cells (hMSCs) were obtained and isolated as described previously [27]. The use of bone marrow aspirates was approved for this whole study by the Medical Ethics Committee of Medisch Spectrum Twente and written informed consent was obtained from all patients. hMSCs were expanded at an initial seeding density of 1000 cells/cm^2 in proliferation medium consisting of α-MEM, 10% v/v FBS (Lonza), 2 mM L-glutamine, 0.2 mM ASAP, PS, and 1 ng/mL recombinant human basic fibroblast growth factor (AbD Serotec, Kidlington, UK). For pellet mix-culture of hMSCs with devitalized or decellularized ATDC5 aggregates, a cell suspension of 2.5×10^5 hMSCs (passage 2–5) was mixed with aggregates taken from 1 agarose chip in a 10-mL tube (Greiner, Kremsmünster, Austria) and was centrifuged for 3 min at 300 G to form a pellet. As a control, 2.5×10^5 hMSCs alone were used to form a pellet in the same way. The chondrogenic medium for pellet co-culture consisted of DMEM high glucose, 100 µg/mL sodium pyruvate, 0.2 mM ASAP, PS, 1× ITS,

0.1 μM Dex, and 10 ng/mL TGFβ3 [28]. The basic medium for pellet co-culture was chondrogenic medium without Dex and TGFβ3. The pellets were cultured for 4 weeks and the medium was changed 2–3 times per week. All media and medium supplements were purchased from Life Technologies; all chemicals were purchased from Sigma-Aldrich (Zwijndrecht, Netherland), unless otherwise stated.

2.2. Devitalization and Decellularization

ATDC5 aggregates were cultured for 2 weeks in IC medium before devitalization by liquid nitrogen freeze/thawing or decellularization by sodium dodecyl sulfate (SDS). For devitalization, aggregates were collected and washed once with PBS followed by submersion in liquid nitrogen for 30 s and then in a 45°C water bath for 30 s, which was repeated 10 times. Decellularization was based on a protocol described by Kheir et al. [29]. Briefly, aggregates were subjected to 2 cycles of dry freeze/thaw followed by another 2 cycles of freeze/thaw in hypotonic buffer consisting of 10 mM Tris-HCl (pH 8.0) supplemented with 1× halt proteinase inhibitor cocktail (Thermo Scientific). Samples were frozen at $-20\,°C$ until crystal formation and were then thawed on the bench for 4 h. Then, aggregates were incubated in hypotonic buffer, 45 °C for 24 h, followed by 0.1% w/v SDS in hypotonic buffer at 45 °C for 24 h, with agitation. After washing with PBS twice for 30 min twice and incubation for 24 h at 45 °C, the aggregates were treated with a nuclease solution consisting of 50 mM Tris (pH 7.5), 10 mM magnesium chloride, 50 μg/mL bovine serum albumin, DNase (Sigma-Aldrich, 50 U/mL) and RNase (Sigma-Aldrich, 1U/mL), for 3 h at 37 °C. Finally, the aggregates were washed in PBS twice for 30 min and incubated for 24 h at 45 °C. All chemicals were purchased from Sigma-Aldrich unless otherwise stated.

2.3. Histological Staining and Immunostaining

Samples were fixed in 4% paraformaldehyde (Merck) in PBS. To avoid loss during histology processing, aggregates were incorporated in 0.5% agarose. Molten agarose (0.5% in ddH$_2$O) was poured into 10 mL tubes containing aggregates followed by a quick centrifugation to collect all the aggregates at the bottom of the tubes. After solidification, the agarose portions holding all the aggregates were cut off for processing. Samples were dehydrated using sequential ethanol series, embedded in paraffin and 7 μm sections were cut using a microtome. Cartilage formation was visualized by 1% Alcian Blue staining in 3% acetic acid and 0.1% Nuclear Fast Red in 5% aluminum sulfate, which stained sulfated glycosaminoglycans blue and cell nuclei red. Mineralization was visualized by 2% Alizarin Red S, which stained calcium deposits orange-red. All chemicals were purchased from Sigma-Aldrich unless otherwise stated.

For immunostaining, the VECTASTAIN®Elite ABC-Peroxidase kit (Vector laboratories, Burlingame, CA, USA) was employed following the manufacturer's protocol with some modifications. Briefly, antigen retrieval was performed by incubating sections with 0.1% w/v hyaluronidase (Sigma, H3506) and 0.1% w/v protease (Sigma, P5147) in PBS for 30 min at 37 °C. Sections were washed with 0.1% Tween-PBS and blocked with 0.3% H$_2$O$_2$-PBS for 10 min followed by 5% BSA-PBS for 30 min both at room temperature. Sections were incubated with primary antibody anti-collagen type 2 (1:100; Abcam; ab34712) or anti-collagen type 10 antibody (1:100; Abcam; ab58632), overnight at 4 °C in a humidified chamber. After washing, sections were incubated with biotinylated secondary antibody (1:100) followed by VECTASTAIN®ABC Reagent for 30 min each at RT. Brown staining was developed by incubating sections with peroxidase substrate solution for 5 min. Sections were rinsed with tap water and counterstained with haematoxylin (Sigma). Histological sections were analyzed by light microscopy (E600 Nikon).

2.4. Mineralization, Calcium Assay and Hydroxyproline Assay

Aggregates were cultured in IC medium for 2 or 3 weeks before switching to mineralization medium consisting of α-MEM, 5% v/v FBS, PS, 1× ITS, and 10 mM β-glycerophosphate. After 1 week culture in mineralization medium, the aggregates were collected for histological analysis, hydroxyproline assay and calcium assay. Samples were transferred to pressure-tight, teflon capped vials and hydrolyzed with 100 μL of 12 M HCl for 3 h at 120 °C. Five μL of the lysate was used for calcium analysis using the QuantiChrom Calcium Assay Kit (DICA-500) according to the manufacturer's protocol. Briefly, free calcium specifically forms a stable blue colored complex with the phenolsulphonephthalein dye in the kit. The color intensity, measured at 612 nm, is directly proportional to the calcium concentration in the sample. A standard curve was generated using the Ca^{2+} standard. For hydroxyproline analysis, the Hydroxyproline Assay Kit (Biovision-K555) was used. Briefly, 10 μL of the hydrolyzed sample lysate was transferred to a 96-well plate and evaporated to dryness under vacuum. Next, chloramine T and 4-(dimethylamino)benzaldehyde (DMAB) reagent was added to each sample and incubated for 90 min at 60 °C. The reaction resulted in a colorimetric (560 nm) product, proportional to the hydroxyproline present. A standard curve was generated using 4-hydroxyproline as indicated in the manufacturer's protocol.

2.5. Gene Expression Analysis

Cell aggregates or pellets were collected and washed once with PBS and then homogenized in Trizol reagent (Life Technologies) by crushing with a pestle and mortar under liquid nitrogen. After adding 20% v/v chloroform and centrifugation for 15 min at 11,000 g at 4 °C, the aqueous phase containing RNA was transferred to a new Eppendorf tube, combined with an equal volume of 70% ethanol, and then was loaded onto the RNA binding column of the RNA II nucleospin RNA isolation kit (Machery Nagel). The rest of the RNA isolation followed the kit protocol. RNA concentrations were measured using a ND100 spectrophotometer (Nanodrop1000). cDNA was synthesized from 1 μg of RNA, using iScript (BioRad) according to the manufacturer's protocol. qPCR was performed using 50 ng of cDNA, 0.4 μM of each forward and reverse primer (Sigma Genosys), and 1× SensiMix SYBR&Fluorescein master mix (Bioline). Primer sequences are shown in Table 1. Real-time qPCR was performed in a Biorad My IQ5 machine (Biorad). Data was analyzed using the fit point method of the My IQ5 software. The baseline was calculated automatically by the software at the lower log-linear part above baseline noise and the crossing temperature (Ct value) was determined. Ct values were normalized to the Beta-2 microglobulin (B2M) housekeeping gene and ΔCt (Ct, control—Ct, sample) was used to calculate the up-regulation in gene expression.

Table 1. Primer sequence.

Name	Primer Sequence
Mouse beta-2 microglobulin	5′-CATGGCTCGCTCGGTGACC-3′ 5′-AATGTGAGGCGGGTGGAACTG-3′
Mouse collagen 2 alpha	5′-CAAGGCCCCCGAGGTGACAAA-3′ 5′-GGGGCCAGGGATTCCATTAGAGC-3′
Mouse collagen 10 alpha	5′-CATAAAGGGCCCACTTGCTA-3′ 5′-TGGCTGATATTCCTGGTGGT-3′
Mouse aggrecan	5′-AGAACCTTCGCTCCAATGACTC-3′ 5′-AGGGTGTAGCGTGTGGAAATAG-3′
Mouse Sry-related HMG box 9 (SOX9)	5′-CCACGGAACAGACTCACATCTCTC-3′ 5′-CTGCTCAGTTCACCGATGTCCACG-3′
Mouse hypoxia-inducible factors 1 alpha (HIF1α)	5′-TGCTCATCAGTTGCCACTTC-3′ 5′-TGGGCCATTTCTGTGTGTAA-3′
Mouse hypoxia-inducible factors 2 alpha (HIF2α)	5′-TGAGTTGGCTCATGAGTTGC-3′ 5′-CTCACGGATCTCCTCATGGT-3′
Mouse alkaline phosphatase (ALP)	5′-AACCCAGACACAAGCATTCC-3′ 5′-GAGACATTTTCCCGTTCACC-3′
Mouse matrix metalloproteinases 13 (MMP13)	5′-AGGCCTTCAGAAAAGCCTTC-3′ 5′-TCCTTGGAGTGATCCAGACC-3′
Human B2M	5′-GACTTGTCTTTCAGCAAGGA-3′ 5′-ACAAAGTCACATGGTTCACA-3′
Human collagen 2 alpha	5′-CGTCCAGATGACCTTCCTACG-3′ 5′-TGAGCAGGGCCTTCTTGAG-3′
Human aggrecan	5′-AGAATCCACCACCACCAG-3′ 5′-ATGCTGGTGCTGATGACA-3′
Human SOX9	5′-TGGGCAAGCTCTGGAGACTTC-3′ 5′-ATCCGGGTGGTCCTTCTTGTG-3′

2.6. ELISA

ATDC5 aggregates were cultured for 2 or 3 weeks in different media (BM, IM, BC or IC). Medium was changed every 2 days, with only half of the volume (1 mL) changed to avoid loss of the aggregates. VEGF was allowed to accumulate in medium for 2 days before the collection point. To boost VEGF secretion, ATDC5 aggregates were cultured in IC medium for 2 or 3 weeks, then the medium was supplemented with 50 µM phenanthroline (1,10-Phenanthroline monohydrate, Sigma-Aldrich) [30] and VEGF was allowed to accumulate for 2 days, 3 days or 6 days (with 1 medium change after 3 days) before the collection point. 1 mL of medium was collected from each chip and 50µL was assayed in duplicate using a mouse VEGF quantikine ELISA kit (R&D, MMV00) following the kit protocol.

2.7. Statistics

One-way or two-way ANOVA with Bonferroni post-test were performed using GraphPad Prism version 6.02 for Windows, GraphPad Software, La Jolla California USA, www.graphpad.com.

3. Results

3.1. Bulk Production of Micro-Tissue Engineered Cartilage (MiTEC)

ATDC5 micro-aggregates were cultured in basic medium (BM) or basic medium supplemented with 1× ITS (IM medium) for 4 weeks on agarose chips. Cell aggregates formed within 24 h after seeding (Figure 1A). Over longer times, the aggregates in IM medium grew bigger and firmer than those in BM medium. After 4 weeks, the aggregates in IM medium developed a very firm appearance whereas those in BM appeared to break down. Scanning electron microscopy of aggregates cultured in IM medium showed a uniform size distribution (Figure 1B). After an even longer culture time, clusters of up to 10 aggregates were observed. The exterior of these aggregates were covered by thick layers of extracellular matrix, while inside them lay many lacunae where the cells resided. Gene expression analysis of the aggregates cultured in BM and IM medium for 4 weeks was performed; expression levels were compared to that of BM medium at week 1 (Figure 1C and Figure S1A). Genes related to early chondrogenesis such as collagen type 2, aggrecan, hypoxia-inducible factors 1 alpha (HIF1α) and Sry-related HMG box (SOX9) as well as late chondrogenesis and hypertrophy such as collagen type 10, matrix metalloproteinases 13 (MMP13), hypoxia-inducible factors 2 alpha (HIF2α) and alkaline phosphatase (ALP) were studied. Expression of all the early markers peaked at week 2 in both BM and IM conditions, although with higher expression in IM medium, then declined in the following weeks. Hypertrophic markers collagen type 10 and ALP expression peaked at week 2, with expression in IM condition double that of the BM condition. MMP13 and HIF2α expression peaked at week 3 and 4 respectively, with expression in the IM always higher than BM condition. This characterization has demonstrated the feasibility of using our spheroid culture system to grow and differentiate ATDC5 in vivo.

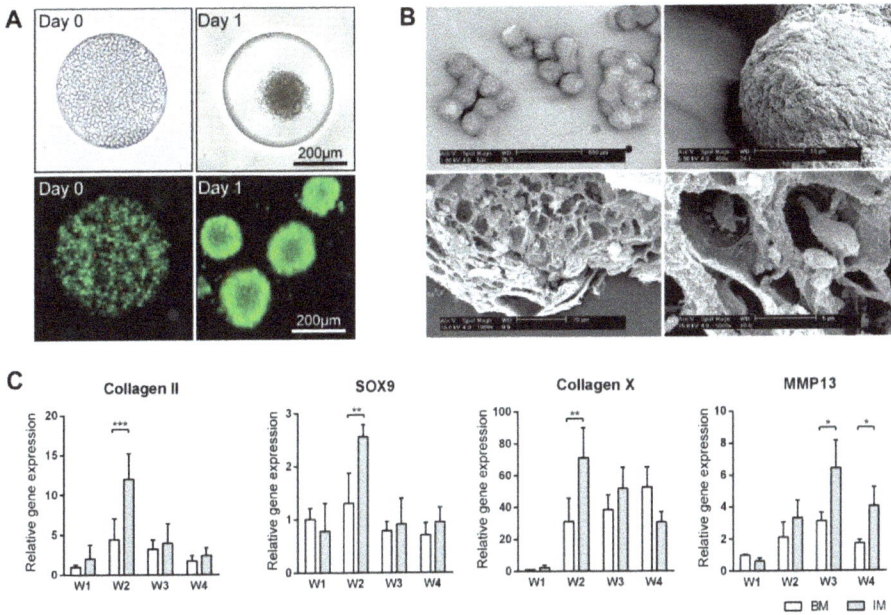

Figure 1. Production of micro-tissue engineered cartilage (MiTEC). Cells were seeded on day 0 and the aggregate formed on day 1; the panel shows brightfield images (top row) and fluorescent images (bottom row) of cells staining with calcein (green) and ethidium homodimer-1 (red) (**A**). Scanning electron microscope images of MiTEC showed uniform size aggregates and cartilage-like lacunae (**B**). Gene expression profile of MiTEC cultured in basic medium (BM—white bar) and basic medium + ITS (IM—gray bar) at week 1–4 (**C**). Error bars represent standard deviation (n = 3). (*) denotes $p < 0.05$, (**) denotes $p < 0.01$, (***) denotes $p < 0.001$.

3.2. Optimization of Chondrogenic Differentiation of MiTEC

Improved chondrogenic differentiation of aggregates in IM medium showed that it is possible to manipulate the expression of chondrogenic genes. Since the amount of hypertrophic cartilage matrix is known to correlate to in vivo bone formation [6,7], we next maximized the extracellular matrix (ECM) deposition in MiTEC by optimizing medium composition [28]. Four different medium compositions were tested: basic medium (BM); BM supplemented with ITS (IM); BM supplemented with TGFβ3 and Dex (BC); and BM supplemented with ITS, TGFβ3 and Dex (IC). After only 1 week in culture, the difference in size of MiTECs was apparent by light microscopy (Figure 2, top row). In ascending order, BC, IM and IC medium had a positive effect on the size of MiTEC over BM. Histological analysis with Alcian Blue staining for glycosaminoglycan in cartilage (Figure 2) clearly shows that BM was not a good medium to culture MiTEC, with disintegration of the aggregates and very poor Alcian Blue staining. In the IM medium condition, spots with blue stain were visible in week 2 which became bigger and more intense in week 3. Hypertrophic chondrocytes, recognized by their large lacunae, appeared to reside within the intensely blue stained extracellular matrix. Interestingly, the use of both TGFβ3 and Dex (BC condition) resulted only in a faint Alcian Blue stain at both week 2 and 3. The aggregates in the BC condition were also smaller in size compared to the IM condition (just ITS added to the basic medium). Finally, when cultured in the presence of TGFβ3, Dex and ITS (IC condition), a uniform and intense blue stain was observed in all aggregates.

Gene expression analysis for early and late chondrogenic markers at week 2 and 3 was performed; expression levels were compared to that of BM at week 2 (Figure 3 and Figure S1B). For early markers (collagen type 2, aggrecan, SOX9, and HIF1α), gene expression in BC and IC conditions (both contained TGFβ3 and Dex) was always higher than those of BM and IM conditions (except for HIF1α where the expression in the BC condition was similar to those of BM and IM). For late markers, collagen type 10 expression in the BC and IC conditions was particularly high (300 times at week 2 and 500–1500 times at week 3) compared to BM and IM. MMP13 expression was only high in the IM and IC conditions (both contained ITS), 5-12 times at week 2 and 5–70 times at week 3 compared to the BM condition respectively. Interestingly, HIF2α, ALP and VEGF expression was highest in the IM condition at both week 2 and 3. Overall, in term of aggregate size, extracellular matrix stain for Alcian Blue and certain gene markers, IC is the most potent medium to induce extracellular matrix deposition and hypertrophic differentiation of MiTEC. Thus we chose the IC medium to continue with for the next experiments.

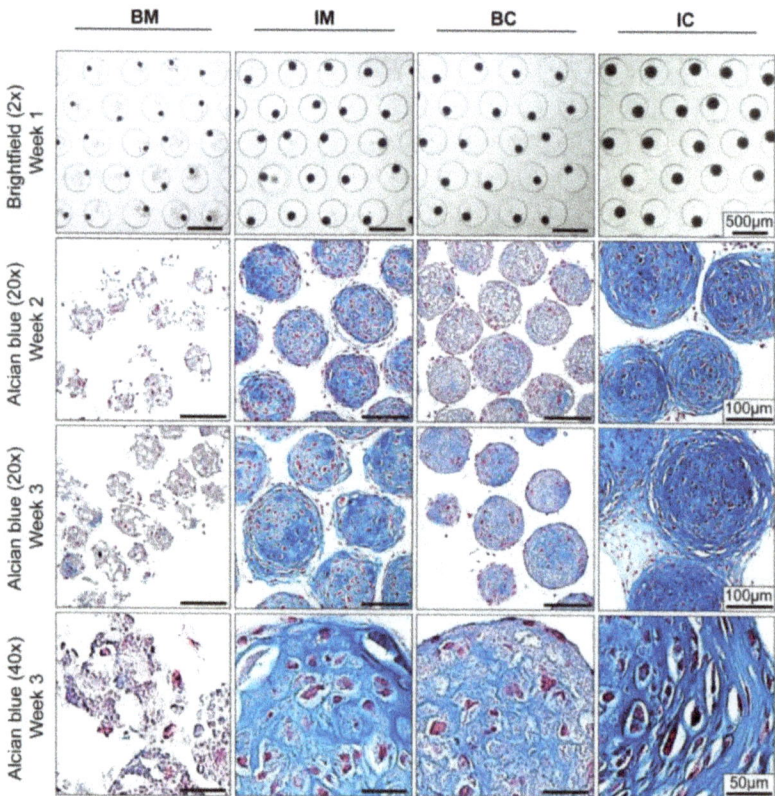

Figure 2. Effect of different media on MiTEC morphology. Aggregates were cultured for 3 weeks in different media: basic medium (**BM**), BM supplemented with 1×ITS (**IM**), BM supplemented with 0.1 μM dexamethasone (Dex) and 10 ng/mL transforming growth factor beta 3 (TGFβ3) (**BC**) and BM supplemented with 1× ITS, 0.1 μM Dex, and 10 ng/mL TGFβ3 (**IC**). Brightfield images at week 1 (**Top Row**) show the difference in aggregate size in which the aggregates in the IC medium was the biggest. Alcian Blue staining at week 2 and 3 (**Row 2–4**) shows maturation of the cartilage extracellular matrix; aggregates in the IC medium were stained most intensely and uniformly. Hypertrophic cells can be found at both week 2 and week 3 in the IM, BC and IC medium.

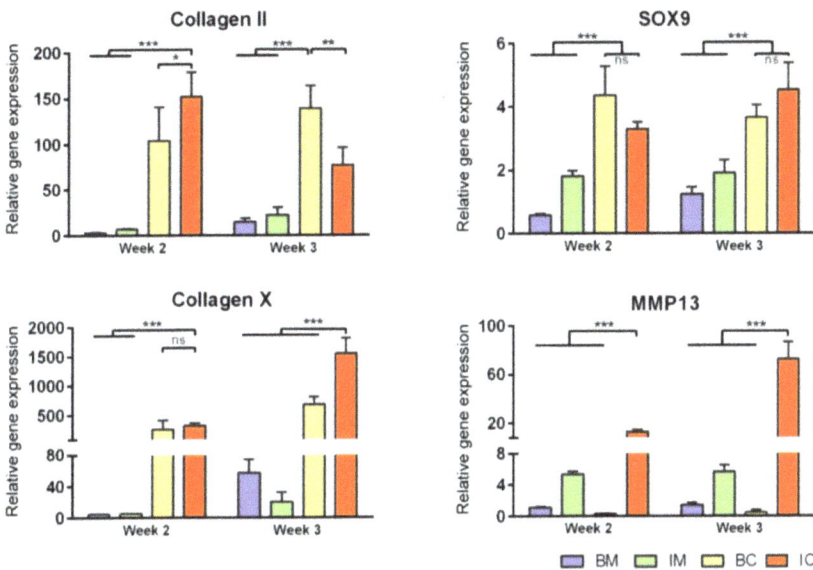

Figure 3. Effect of different media on MiTEC gene expression. Gene expression analysis of aggregates cultured in basic medium (BM—blue bar), BM + ITS (IM—green bar), BM + TGFβ + Dex (BC—yellow bar), and BM + ITS + TGFβ + Dex (IC—red bar) at week 2–3. Error bars represent standard deviation (n = 3). (*) denotes $p < 0.05$, (**) denotes $p < 0.01$, (***) denotes $p < 0.001$, and ns denotes non-significant.

3.3. Induction of MiTEC Mineralization with Beta-Glycerophosphate

Just prior to endochondral ossification, end stage hypertrophic chondrocytes direct the formation of mineralized matrix, which becomes a scaffold for osteoprogenitor cells to interact with and secrete osteoid [31]. Pre-mineralizing the hypertrophic cartilage construct in vivo may improve and accelerate bone formation upon in vivo implantation. In this experiment, we induced in vivo mineralization of MiTECs with beta-glycerophosphate (bGP). MiTECs were cultured for 2 or 3 weeks in IC medium, followed by 1 week in mineralization medium with 10 mM bGP. MiTECs were collected at week 3 (2 weeks in IC medium plus 1 week in mineralization medium) and week 4 (3 weeks in IC medium plus 1 week in mineralization medium) for analysis. Calcium analysis showed a significant increase in the calcium content of MiTECs cultured in the mineralization medium (Figure 4A). Hydroxyproline content (estimated organic content of the extracellular matrix) increased from week 3–4 but was not affected by the bGP treatment. Histological analysis with Alizarin Red staining showed intense red nodules in the bGP condition (Figure 4B). Gene expression analysis was performed for the hypertrophic markers HIF2α, ALP, VEGF, collagen 10 and MMP13 (Figure S2A). Interestingly, the addition of bGP increased HIF2α, VEGF, collagen X and MMP13 expression at week 4 but not at week 3 of the culture. Expression of ALP after 1 week in mineralization medium either decreased (week 3) or was unchanged (week 4). Overall, the in vivo mineralization of MiTEC could be efficiently achieved with the bGP treatment, which may add an edge to the in vivo performance of the material.

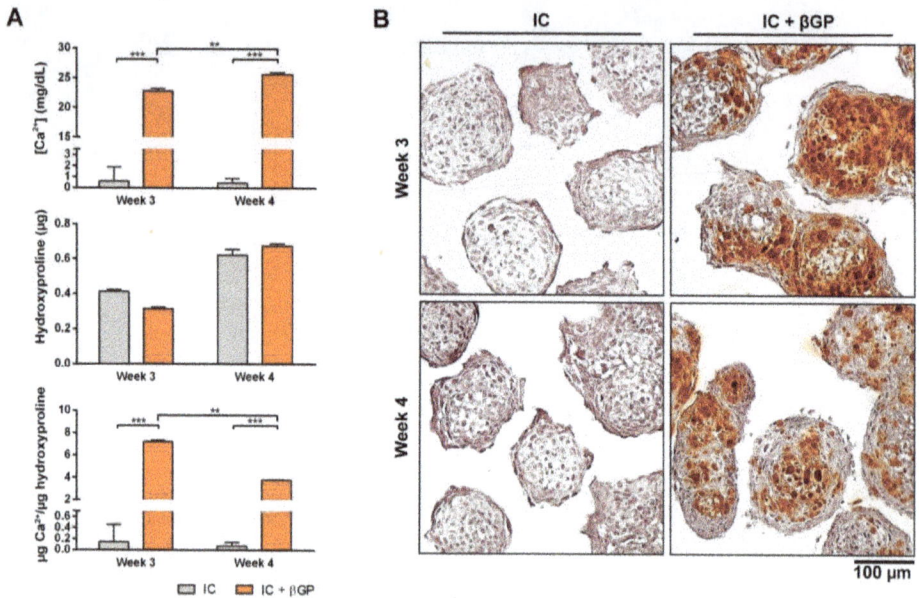

Figure 4. Induction of MiTEC mineralization with beta-glycerophosphate. Calcium content, hydroxyproline content and calcium content per μg of hydroxyproline of aggregates cultured in IC medium for 2 or 3 weeks, plus 1 week treatment with beta-glycerophosphate (bGP) (**A**). Error bars represent the standard deviation (n = 3). (******) denotes $p < 0.01$, and (*******) denotes $p < 0.001$. Alizarin Red staining of aggregates cultured in IC medium for 2 or 3 weeks, plus 1 week treatment with bGP; red nodules can be seen homogeneously inside the aggregates (**B**).

3.4. Boosting Vascular Endothelial Growth Factor (VEGF) Secretion from MiTEC Using the Hypoxia Mimetic Phenanthroline

Vascular invasion of the hypertrophic cartilage is a crucial event in endochondral bone formation and VEGF plays a critical role in it [32,33]. Enriching the extracellular matrix with VEGF may improve MiTEC performance. Previously, using high throughput screening, we identified phenanthroline as a hypoxia mimicking molecule capable of inducing VEGF expression and secretion in hMSCs [30]. Preliminary experiments were done to verify that phenanthroline can also stimulate VEGF expression and secretion of ATDC5 cells cultured in a monolayer (data not shown). In the aggregate culture, VEGF expression was highest in the IM medium (Figure S1B), but VEGF secretion as detected in the medium was highest in the IC medium at about 2000 pg/mL (Figure 5, top graph). To test the effect of phenanthroline on MiTEC, we cultured the aggregates for 2 or 3 weeks in IC medium, followed by a 2, 3 or 6 day exposure to 50 μM phenanthroline. Phenanthroline induced a 7-fold induction of VEGF expression after a 2 day exposure at week 2 of the culture (Fig 5, bottom graph). However, this expression reduced if the exposure was prolonged to 3 days and 6 days. Exposing MiTEC with phenanthroline for 2 days at week 3 of the culture also resulted in an 8-fold increase in the mRNA level. The VEGF secretion baseline at 2000 pg/mL in the IC medium was more than doubled when phenanthroline was added for 2 days at week 2 of the culture (Figure 5, middle graph). However, when phenanthroline treatment was extended to 6 days, the secretion reduced to about 3000 pg/mL. A 2-day stimulation in week 3 resulted in the same secretion level as in week 2. Thus, using phenanthroline, we could efficiently boost VEGF expression and secretion from MiTEC.

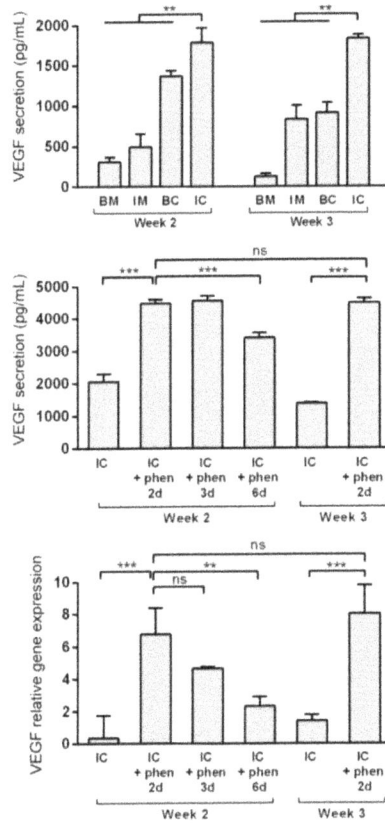

Figure 5. Boosting vascular endothelial growth factor (VEGF) expression and secretion from MiTEC using the hypoxia mimetic phenanthroline. VEGF secretion of aggregates cultured in BM (blue bar), IM (green bar), BC (yellow bar) and IC (red bar) medium at week 2–3 (top graph). VEGF secretion (middle graph) and expression (bottom graph) of aggregates cultured in IC medium for 2 or 3 weeks followed by phenanthroline treatment for 2, 3 or 6 days. Error bars represent standard deviation (n = 3). (**) denotes $p < 0.01$, (***) denotes $p < 0.001$, and ns denotes non-significant.

3.5. Devitalization and Decellularization of MiTEC

To make MiTEC an off-the-shelf product, devitalization/decellularization is necessary in order to reduce the immunogenicity of the material. We devitalized MiTEC by liquid nitrogen (LN2) freeze-thawing and decellularized MiTEC by SDS processing following established protocols. Devitalized/decellularized MiTECs were tested for cell survival by a metabolism assay where no metabolic activity was found (data not shown). The amount of MiTECs harvested from one 12-well plate, decellularized with SDS and air dried is shown in Fig S2B. The average diameter of an aggregate after a 3-week culture in IC medium was 300 μm (Figure 6). Assuming each aggregate is a sphere; its volume is $\frac{4}{3}\pi \times 150^3 = 14,137,167$ μm^3 or 0.014 mm^3. Each well of the 12-well plate containing 1585 aggregates yielded 22.4 mm^3, and one 12-well plate yielded 268.9 mm^3 of tissue. Four culture plates would be needed to make 1CC of tissue. Histological analysis with Alcian Blue and immunostaining for collagen type 2 and type X is shown in Figure 6. No cell nuclei were visible in the histological images of the decellularized MiTEC. Alcian Blue staining was reduced significantly in the decellularized samples, however collagen type 2 and X staining were similar to that of the devitalized samples. Collagen type

2 staining was more eminent at the periphery of the aggregates, while collagen type 10 was distributed more uniformly.

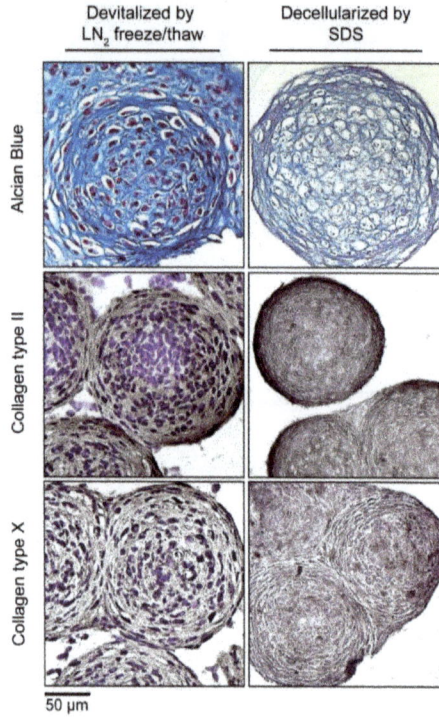

Figure 6. Devitalization and decellularization of MiTEC. Aggregates were cultured for 2 weeks in IC medium, and then were either devitalized by repeated liquid nitrogen (LN2) freeze/thaw or decellularized by SDS. Picture panel shows Alcian Blue staining (**Top Row**); collagen type 2 staining (**Middle Row**); and collagen type 10 staining (**Bottom Row**).

3.6. DCM Influences Chondrogenic Differentiation of hMSCs

To test the biological properties of our DCM, devitalized/decellularized MiTECs were mixed with hMSCs and pellet-cultured for 4 weeks in either basic medium or chondrogenic differentiation medium. Pellets of hMSCs mixed with LN2-devitalized MiTEC are referred to as LN2-pellets, and pellets of hMSCs mixed with SDS-decellularized MiTEC are referred to as SDS-pellets. As a control, hMSCs were cultured in a pellet of 250,000 cells which is the same number of cells used in the mix-culture with MiTEC. After 4 weeks, the LN2-pellets and SDS-pellets cultured in chondrogenic medium developed a glassy appearance and felt very firm (Figure S2C). Gene expression analysis was performed for early chondrogenesis makers collagen type 2, aggrecan and SOX9 (Figure 7A). Relative to hMSC pellets, expression of these markers increased significantly in the SDS-pellet in chondrogenic medium. Even in basic medium, aggrecan expression increased 20-fold in the SDS-pellet compared to the hMSCs pellet. Expression of the 3 markers in the LN2-pellet was also higher than hMSC alone control, but lower than the SDS-pellets. Alcian Blue staining showed that the devitalized/decellularized MiTECs were still visible and embedded inside the cell pellets (Figure 7B). No cell was found inside the SDS treated MiTECs. In basic medium, beside the intense blue stain of the devitalized MiTEC aggregates, the rest of the pellet was weakly stained. In chondrogenic differentiation medium, the hMSCs alone control developed some blue stains only in some parts of the pellets. However, when hMSCs were co-cultured with either LN2 or SDS treated MiTEC, Alcian Blue was intensely stained throughout the pellets. The MiTEC appeared to be shrunken inside the pellets under the chondrogenic medium condition, with a big gap between MiTEC and the human cells. With this experiment, we showed that devitalized/decellularized MiTEC has chondro-inductive potential in vivo.

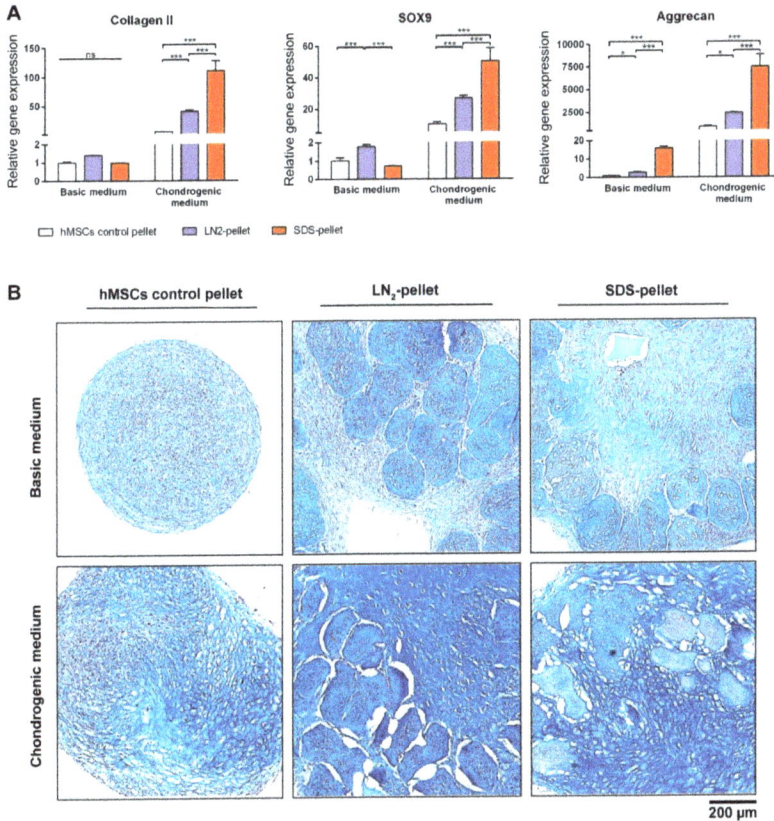

Figure 7. MiTEC affects chondrogenic differentiation of human mesenchymal stem cells (hMSCs). Gene expression analysis of hMSCs co-cultured with devitalized or decellularized MiTEC in basic medium or chondrogenic medium (**A**). Error bars represent standard deviation (n = 3). (*) denotes $p < 0.05$, (**) denotes $p < 0.01$, (***) denotes $p < 0.001$, and ns denotes non-significant. Alcian Blue staining of hMSCs co-cultured with devitalized or decellularized MiTEC in basic medium (top row) or chondrogenic medium (bottom row) (**B**).

4. Discussion

Although autologous bone is considered as the most superior grafting material for bone regeneration [34], other bone graft substitutes are increasingly preferred not only for the convenience of the surgeons but also for the good of the patients [35]. In nature, bone healing occurs through both endochondral and intramembranous ossification [36]. While intramembranous ossification is the fastest route of building bone matrix, it can only handle small and mechanically stable defects [36,37]. Endochondral ossification, while it is slow and requires a lot more energy, is the predominant route of bone healing in fractures. During the process, mesenchymal progenitor cells differentiate into chondrocytes which deposit cartilaginous matrix called the soft callus. In animal models, the soft callus formation peaks at 7-9 days post trauma with a peak in collagen type 2 and proteoglycan such as aggrecan [38]. The chondrocytes of the soft callus undergo maturation towards hypertrophy, becoming enlarged in size, and secreting alkaline phosphatase which mineralizes the extracellular matrix. The fate of the hypertrophic chondrocytes remains controversial. Classically, the hypertrophic chondrocytes undergo apoptosis and the osteoprogenitor cells invade the callus and replace the cartilage with bone. Alternatively, studies have shown that a proportion of hypertrophic chondrocytes do not undergo apoptosis and instead transdifferentiate into osteoblasts [12,39]. In the classical model, the role of hypertrophic chondrocytes is less important after its accomplishment of synthesizing the necessary growth factors. This suggests that a hypertrophic cartilage matrix void of cells but high in endogenous growth factors can continue its route to be transformed into bone in vivo. To date, no clinical case using hypertrophic cartilage for bone regeneration has been reported. Despite abundant proof-of-principle studies, no available method can yet produce sufficient hypertrophic cartilage for clinical use. Here we demonstrated that by using the cell line ATDC5 cultured in micro-aggregates, it was feasible to produce hypertrophic cartilage in unlimited amounts. According to the FDA's guideline for clinical issues concerning the use of xenotransplantation products in humans [40], "cell lines from animals may be established and used in the production of xenotransplantation products". Compared to primary cells, cell lines are easier to maintain and more consistent in quality. Since cell lines are carcinogenic, devitalization of the hypertrophic cartilage is necessary to reduce immunogenic concerns. Whether or not the devitalized MiTEC is still capable of inducing endochondral ossification in vivo needs further experiments. Bourgine et al. demonstrated that apoptosis-induced devitalized hypertrophic cartilage constructs could form bone in vivo while freeze-thawed devitalized constructs could not [18]. They attributed this to the significant loss of glycosaminoglycans, mineral content, and ECM-bound cytokines during the freeze-thaw cycles. We also observed a loss of glycosaminoglycans, as indicated by Alcian Blue staining, in the SDS decellularized MiTEC, but not in the freeze-thaw devitalized MiTEC. Apparently, the bioactivity of the hypertrophic cartilage ECM may be lost when a sub-optimal devitalization/decellularization process is used. Hence, the balance of removing immunogenicity and retaining osteoinductivity needs to be fine-tuned, for which many devitalization/decellularization methods have been reported [41–43]. Our model can potentially be adapted into a high throughput screening platforms in vivo and in vivo, allowing the devitalization/decellularization protocol to be empirically optimized.

Vascularization is a critical factor for the successful integration of large grafts. Hypertrophic cartilage has an intrinsic property of produce angiogenic growth factors, which play a crucial role in endochondral ossification and many studies have shown the positive effect of adding VEGF in bone regeneration [33,44]. It has been shown that the lack of vascularization in the DCM constructs could be attributed to the loss of VEGF during the devitalization process [18]. Vascularization in the case of endochondral bone formation is essential for the recruitment of the host cells in order to remodel the cartilage template and subsequent ossification. We showed that stimulating MiTEC with the hypoxia mimicking molecule phenanthroline boosted VEGF secretion to double its basal level, although the VEGF content which remained in the decellularized MiTEC has not been analyzed. Since vascularization is paramount to the success of this model, it may be necessary to further optimize it for instance by combining it with current vascularization strategies, i.e., VEGF impregnation [45]. Similarly, pre-mineralization of MiTEC in vivo may be beneficial for bone formation in vivo. Calcium phosphate ceramics have a positive effect on osteogenesis [46] and even soluble calcium ions have a positive effect on the osteogenic differentiation of hMSCs [47]. The degree of mineralization is another aspect which can be optimized for bone formation in vivo.

The inductive potential of decellularized ECM on stem cells [48,49] has been reported. It was hypothesized that the acellular ECM of a tissue possessed the instructive cues that drive the differentiation of stem cells into this particular tissue type [50,51]. The instructive cues are the soluble factors and the macromolecules that regulate cell fate. To date, no study has demonstrated the inductive potential of hypertrophic cartilage matrix in vivo. In this paper, we show that

Bioengineering **2017**, *4*, 35

devitalized/decellularized MiTEC, especially in combination with chondrogenic medium, enhanced the chondrogenic differentiation of hMSCs in vivo. From histological images it appeared that the MiTEC ECM remained intact and hMSCs were not able to enter the cartilage matrix. Thus, it's arguable that the inductive potential of devitalized/decellularized MiTEC is caused by the soluble factors released from it, although the surface chemistry and topography of the tissue might also play a role. Interestingly, SDS decellularized MiTEC appeared to be more potent than the freeze-thaw devitalized aggregates. This may be similar to the biological activity of bone versus demineralized bone, where the removal of bone mineral makes the osteogenic molecules available for interaction with the cells [52].

Unlike natural products harvested from cadavers where donor variation is inevitable, hypertrophic cartilage culture in vivo is a totally controllable process. There are many concerns over the variation in quality among allogenic bone grafts produced by different companies or even from different batches of product from the same company [53,54]. Moreover, some products such as DBM and platelet gels containing "autologous growth factors" are not subjected to high level of regulatory scrutiny [55]. In contrast, MiTEC can be cultured and tested for both safety and efficacy following stringent good manufacturing practice (GMP) protocols. Here, we demonstrated how MiTEC can be manipulated in a number of ways to modify its extracellular matrix composition. The well plate format of this system allows for high throughput screening to be used in drug discovery and, using a different cell source or cell sources, one can even switch this model to the production of a totally different type of tissue, for instance to produce liver tissue or to study tumor cell biology. In conclusion, we have shown a method to produce clinically relevant-sized hypertrophic cartilage for bone regeneration by endochondral ossification. We decellularized the hypertrophic tissue and showed that the remaining ECM had inductive potential on chondrogenic differentiation of hMSCs in vivo. The logical next phase of this work is the pre-clinical evaluation of MiTEC in orthotopic models.

5. Conclusions

The results of this study demonstrate the feasibility of producing in large amounts and to readily vary the chemical composition of hypertrophic cartilage tissue in vivo using the ATDC5 cell line cultured in micro-aggregates (MiTEC). Moreover, under appropriate culturing and devitalizing conditions, the devitalized MiTEC can enhance chondrogenic differentiation of hMSCs, suggesting that devitalized MiTEC represents a promising advance for clinical applications in bone regeneration.

Supplementary Materials: The supplementary materials are available online at http://www.mdpi.com/2306-5354/4/2/35/s1.

Acknowledgments: We thank Marcel Karperien for providing the ATDC5 cell line, Nicolas Rivron and Erik Vrij for providing the stamps and PDMS molds for the spheroid culture system, and Ana Barradas for optimizing the micro-aggregate culture system. J.d.B. and C.v.B. acknowledge the financial support of the Dutch province of Limburg, and B.Q.L. acknowledges the financial support of Pieken in de Delta Osst Nederland (PIDON) grant 91014.

Author Contributions: Bach Quang Le—Project design and implementation, data collection, analysis and manuscript drafting. Clemens van Blitterswijk and Jan de Boer—Funding and project conception, staff supervision and project implementation, data interpretation and manuscript drafting and editing.

Conflicts of Interest: The authors declare no conflict of interest.

References

1. Ferguson, C.; Alpern, E.; Miclau, T.; Helms, J.A. Does adult fracture repair recapitulate embryonic skeletal formation? *Mech. Dev.* **1999**, *87*, 57–66. [CrossRef]
2. Einhorn, T.A.; Gerstenfeld, L.C. Fracture healing: Mechanisms and interventions. *Nat. Rev. Rheumatol.* **2015**, *11*, 45–54. [CrossRef] [PubMed]
3. Gerstenfeld, L.C.; Cullinane, D.M.; Barnes, G.L.; Graves, D.T.; Einhorn, T.A. Fracture healing as a post-natal developmental process: Molecular, spatial, and temporal aspects of its regulation. *J. Cell. Biochem.* **2003**, *88*, 873–884. [CrossRef] [PubMed]

4. Durao, S.F.; Gomes, P.S.; Silva-Marques, J.M.; Fonseca, H.R.; Carvalho, J.F.; Duarte, J.A.; Fernandes, M.H. Bone regeneration in osteoporotic conditions: Healing of subcritical-size calvarial defects in the ovariectomized rat. *Int. J. Oral Maxillofac. Implants* **2012**, *27*, 1400–1408. [PubMed]
5. Dinopoulos, H.; Dimitriou, R.; Giannoudis, P.V. Bone graft substitutes: What are the options? *Surg. J. R. Coll. Surg. Edinb. Irel.* **2012**, *10*, 230–239.
6. Jukes, J.M.; Both, S.K.; Leusink, A.; Sterk, L.M.; van Blitterswijk, C.A.; de Boer, J. Endochondral bone tissue engineering using embryonic stem cells. *Proc. Natl. Acad. Sci. USA* **2008**, *105*, 6840–6845. [CrossRef] [PubMed]
7. Scotti, C.; Tonnarelli, B.; Papadimitropoulos, A.; Scherberich, A.; Schaeren, S.; Schauerte, A.; Lopez-Rios, J.; Zeller, R.; Barbero, A.; Martin, I. Recapitulation of endochondral bone formation using human adult mesenchymal stem cells as a paradigm for developmental engineering. *Proc. Natl. Acad. Sci. USA* **2010**, *107*, 7251–7256. [CrossRef] [PubMed]
8. Weiss, H.E.; Roberts, S.J.; Schrooten, J.; Luyten, F.P. A semi-autonomous model of endochondral ossification for developmental tissue engineering. *Tissue Eng. Part A* **2012**, *18*, 1334–1343. [CrossRef] [PubMed]
9. Farrell, E.; Both, S.K.; Odorfer, K.I.; Koevoet, W.; Kops, N.; O'Brien, F.J.; Baatenburg de Jong, R.J.; Verhaar, J.A.; Cuijpers, V.; Jansen, J.; et al. In-vivo generation of bone via endochondral ossification by in-vitro chondrogenic priming of adult human and rat mesenchymal stem cells. *BMC Musculoskelet. Disord.* **2011**, *12*, 31. [CrossRef] [PubMed]
10. Gawlitta, D.; Farrell, E.; Malda, J.; Creemers, L.B.; Alblas, J.; Dhert, W.J. Modulating endochondral ossification of multipotent stromal cells for bone regeneration. *Tissue Eng. Part B Rev.* **2010**, *16*, 385–395. [CrossRef] [PubMed]
11. Scotti, C.; Piccinini, E.; Takizawa, H.; Todorov, A.; Bourgine, P.; Papadimitropoulos, A.; Barbero, A.; Manz, M.G.; Martin, I. Engineering of a functional bone organ through endochondral ossification. *Proc. Natl. Acad. Sci. USA* **2013**, *110*, 3997–4002. [CrossRef] [PubMed]
12. Bahney, C.S.; Hu, D.P.; Taylor, A.J.; Ferro, F.; Britz, H.M.; Hallgrimsson, B.; Johnstone, B.; Miclau, T.; Marcucio, R.S. Stem cell-derived endochondral cartilage stimulates bone healing by tissue transformation. *J. Bone Miner. Res.* **2014**, *29*, 1269–1282. [CrossRef] [PubMed]
13. Urist, M.R. Bone: Formation by autoinduction. *Science* **1965**, *150*, 893–899. [CrossRef] [PubMed]
14. Bridges, J.B.; Pritchard, J.J. Bone and cartilage induction in the rabbit. *J. Anat.* **1958**, *92*, 28–38. [PubMed]
15. Urist, M.R.; Mc, L.F. Osteogenetic potency and new-bone formation by induction in transplants to the anterior chamber of the eye. *J. Bone Jt. Surg. Am.* **1952**, *34-A*, 443–476. [CrossRef]
16. Urist, M.R.; Wallace, T.H.; Adams, T. The function of fibrocartilaginous fracture callus. Observations on transplants labelled with tritiated thymidine. *J. Bone Jt. Surg. Br.* **1965**, *47*, 304–318.
17. Urist, M.R.; Adams, T. Cartilage or bone induction by articular cartilage. Observations with radioisotope labelling techniques. *J. Bone Jt. Surg. Br.* **1968**, *50*, 198–215.
18. Bourgine, P.E.; Scotti, C.; Pigeot, S.; Tchang, L.A.; Todorov, A.; Martin, I. Osteoinductivity of engineered cartilaginous templates devitalized by inducible apoptosis. *Proc. Natl. Acad. Sci. USA* **2014**, *111*, 17426–17431. [CrossRef] [PubMed]
19. Cunniffe, G.M.; Vinardell, T.; Murphy, J.M.; Thompson, E.M.; Matsiko, A.; O'Brien, F.J.; Kelly, D.J. Porous decellularized tissue engineered hypertrophic cartilage as a scaffold for large bone defect healing. *Acta Biomater.* **2015**, *23*, 82–90. [CrossRef] [PubMed]
20. Jukes, J.M.; Moroni, L.; van Blitterswijk, C.A.; de Boer, J. Critical steps toward a tissue-engineered cartilage implant using embryonic stem cells. *Tissue Eng. Part A* **2008**, *14*, 135–147. [CrossRef] [PubMed]
21. Siddappa, R.; Licht, R.; van Blitterswijk, C.; de Boer, J. Donor variation and loss of multipotency during in vivo expansion of human mesenchymal stem cells for bone tissue engineering. *J. Orthop. Res.* **2007**, *25*, 1029–1041. [CrossRef] [PubMed]
22. Yao, Y.; Wang, Y. Atdc5: An excellent in vivo model cell line for skeletal development. *J. Cell. Biochem.* **2013**, *114*, 1223–1229. [CrossRef] [PubMed]
23. Altaf, F.M.; Hering, T.M.; Kazmi, N.H.; Yoo, J.U.; Johnstone, B. Ascorbate-enhanced chondrogenesis of atdc5 cells. *Eur. Cells Mater.* **2006**, *12*, 64–69; discussion 69–70. [CrossRef]
24. Caron, M.M.; Emans, P.J.; Cremers, A.; Surtel, D.A.; Coolsen, M.M.; van Rhijn, L.W.; Welting, T.J. Hypertrophic differentiation during chondrogenic differentiation of progenitor cells is stimulated by bmp-2 but suppressed by bmp-7. *Osteoarthr. Cartil.* **2013**, *21*, 604–613. [CrossRef] [PubMed]

25. Rivron, N.C.; Vrij, E.J.; Rouwkema, J.; Le Gac, S.; van den Berg, A.; Truckenmuller, R.K.; van Blitterswijk, C.A. Tissue deformation spatially modulates vegf signaling and angiogenesis. *Proc. Natl. Acad. Sci. USA* **2012**, *109*, 6886–6891. [CrossRef] [PubMed]

26. Fennema, E.; Rivron, N.; Rouwkema, J.; van Blitterswijk, C.; de Boer, J. Spheroid culture as a tool for creating 3d complex tissues. *Trends Biotechnol.* **2013**, *31*, 108–115. [CrossRef] [PubMed]

27. Alves, H.; Mentink, A.; Le, B.; van Blitterswijk, C.A.; de Boer, J. Effect of antioxidant supplementation on the total yield, oxidative stress levels, and multipotency of bone marrow-derived human mesenchymal stromal cells. *Tissue Eng. Part A* **2013**, *19*, 928–937. [CrossRef] [PubMed]

28. Mackay, A.M.; Beck, S.C.; Murphy, J.M.; Barry, F.P.; Chichester, C.O.; Pittenger, M.F. Chondrogenic differentiation of cultured human mesenchymal stem cells from marrow. *Tissue Eng.* **1998**, *4*, 415–428. [CrossRef] [PubMed]

29. Kheir, E.; Stapleton, T.; Shaw, D.; Jin, Z.; Fisher, J.; Ingham, E. Development and characterization of an acellular porcine cartilage bone matrix for use in tissue engineering. *J. Biomed. Mater. Res. Part A* **2011**, *99*, 283–294. [CrossRef] [PubMed]

30. Doorn, J.; Fernandes, H.A.; Le, B.Q.; van de Peppel, J.; van Leeuwen, J.P.; De Vries, M.R.; Aref, Z.; Quax, P.H.; Myklebost, O.; Saris, D.B.; et al. A small molecule approach to engineering vascularized tissue. *Biomaterials* **2013**, *34*, 3053–3063. [CrossRef] [PubMed]

31. Kronenberg, H.M. Developmental regulation of the growth plate. *Nature* **2003**, *423*, 332–336. [CrossRef] [PubMed]

32. Dai, J.; Rabie, A.B. Vegf: An essential mediator of both angiogenesis and endochondral ossification. *J. Dent. Res.* **2007**, *86*, 937–950. [CrossRef] [PubMed]

33. Yang, Y.Q.; Tan, Y.Y.; Wong, R.; Wenden, A.; Zhang, L.K.; Rabie, A.B. The role of vascular endothelial growth factor in ossification. *Int. J. Oral Sci.* **2012**, *4*, 64–68. [CrossRef] [PubMed]

34. Pape, H.C.; Evans, A.; Kobbe, P. Autologous bone graft: Properties and techniques. *J. Orthop. Trauma* **2010**, *24* (Suppl. 1), S36–S40. [CrossRef] [PubMed]

35. Parikh, S.N. Bone graft substitutes: Past, present, future. *J. Postgrad. Med.* **2002**, *48*, 142–148. [PubMed]

36. Marsell, R.; Einhorn, T.A. The biology of fracture healing. *Injury* **2011**, *42*, 551–555. [CrossRef] [PubMed]

37. Shapiro, F. Bone development and its relation to fracture repair. The role of mesenchymal osteoblasts and surface osteoblasts. *Eur. Cells Mater.* **2008**, *15*, 53–76. [CrossRef]

38. Einhorn, T.A. The cell and molecular biology of fracture healing. *Clin. Orthop. Relat. Res.* **1998**, *355*, S7–S21. [CrossRef]

39. Hu, D.P.; Ferro, F.; Yang, F.; Taylor, A.J.; Chang, W.; Miclau, T.; Marcucio, R.S.; Bahney, C.S. Cartilage to bone transformation during fracture healing is coordinated by the invading vasculature and induction of the core pluripotency genes. *Development* **2017**, *144*, 221–234. [CrossRef] [PubMed]

40. Food and Drug Administration. *Guidance for Industry: Source animal, Product, Preclinical, and Clinical Issues Concerning the Use of Xenotransplantation Products in Humans*; Food and Drug Administration: Rockville, MD, USA, 2011.

41. Lu, H.; Hoshiba, T.; Kawazoe, N.; Chen, G. Comparison of decellularization techniques for preparation of extracellular matrix scaffolds derived from three-dimensional cell culture. *J. Biomed. Mater. Res. Part A* **2012**, *100*, 2507–2516. [CrossRef] [PubMed]

42. Crapo, P.M.; Gilbert, T.W.; Badylak, S.F. An overview of tissue and whole organ decellularization processes. *Biomaterials* **2011**, *32*, 3233–3243. [CrossRef] [PubMed]

43. Dong, J.; Mo, X.; Li, Y.; Chen, D. [recent research progress of decellularization of native tissues]. *Sheng Wu Yi Xue Gong Cheng Xue Za Zhi* **2012**, *29*, 1007–1013. [PubMed]

44. Aryal, R.; Chen, X.P.; Fang, C.; Hu, Y.C. Bone morphogenetic protein-2 and vascular endothelial growth factor in bone tissue regeneration: New insight and perspectives. *Orthop. Surg.* **2014**, *6*, 171–178. [CrossRef] [PubMed]

45. Krishnan, L.; Willett, N.J.; Guldberg, R.E. Vascularization strategies for bone regeneration. *Ann. Biomed. Eng.* **2014**, *42*, 432–444. [CrossRef] [PubMed]

46. Zhang, J.; Luo, X.; Barbieri, D.; Barradas, A.M.; de Bruijn, J.D.; van Blitterswijk, C.A.; Yuan, H. The size of surface microstructures as an osteogenic factor in calcium phosphate ceramics. *Acta Biomater.* **2014**, *10*, 3254–3263. [CrossRef] [PubMed]

47. Barradas, A.M.; Fernandes, H.A.; Groen, N.; Chai, Y.C.; Schrooten, J.; van de Peppel, J.; van Leeuwen, J.P.; van Blitterswijk, C.A.; de Boer, J. A calcium-induced signaling cascade leading to osteogenic differentiation of human bone marrow-derived mesenchymal stromal cells. *Biomaterials* **2012**, *33*, 3205–3215. [CrossRef] [PubMed]

48. Hoganson, D.M.; Meppelink, A.M.; Hinkel, C.J.; Goldman, S.M.; Liu, X.H.; Nunley, R.M.; Gaut, J.P.; Vacanti, J.P. Differentiation of human bone marrow mesenchymal stem cells on decellularized extracellular matrix materials. *J. Biomed. Mater. Res. Part A* **2014**, *102*, 2875–2883. [CrossRef] [PubMed]

49. Guo, Y.; Zeng, Q.; Yan, Y.; Shen, L.; Liu, L.; Li, R.; Zhang, X.; Wu, J.; Guan, J.; Huang, S. Proliferative effect and osteoinductive potential of extracellular matrix coated on cell culture plates. *SpringerPlus* **2013**, *2*, 303. [CrossRef] [PubMed]

50. Brown, B.N.; Badylak, S.F. Extracellular matrix as an inductive scaffold for functional tissue reconstruction. *Transl. Res.* **2014**, *163*, 268–285. [CrossRef] [PubMed]

51. Reilly, G.C.; Engler, A.J. Intrinsic extracellular matrix properties regulate stem cell differentiation. *J. Biomech.* **2010**, *43*, 55–62. [CrossRef] [PubMed]

52. Zhang, M.; Powers, R.M., Jr.; Wolfinbarger, L., Jr. A quantitative assessment of osteoinductivity of human demineralized bone matrix. *J. Periodontol.* **1997**, *68*, 1076–1084. [CrossRef] [PubMed]

53. Aghdasi, B.; Montgomery, S.R.; Daubs, M.D.; Wang, J.C. A review of demineralized bone matrices for spinal fusion: The evidence for efficacy. *Surg. J. R. Coll. Surg. Edinb. Irel.* **2013**, *11*, 39–48. [CrossRef] [PubMed]

54. Bae, H.W.; Zhao, L.; Kanim, L.E.; Wong, P.; Delamarter, R.B.; Dawson, E.G. Intervariability and intravariability of bone morphogenetic proteins in commercially available demineralized bone matrix products. *Spine* **2006**, *31*, 1299–1306. [CrossRef] [PubMed]

55. Greenwald, A.S.; Boden, S.D.; Goldberg, V.M.; Khan, Y.; Laurencin, C.T.; Rosier, R.N. Bone-graft substitutes: Facts, fictions, and applications. *J. Bone Jt. Surg. Am.* **2001**, *83-A* (Suppl. 2 Pt 2), 98–103. [CrossRef]

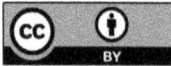

bioengineering

MDPI

Article

Development of Self-Assembled Nanoribbon Bound Peptide-Polyaniline Composite Scaffolds and Their Interactions with Neural Cortical Cells

Andrew M. Smith, Harrison T. Pajovich and Ipsita A. Banerjee *

Department of Chemistry, Fordham University, 441 East Fordham Road, Bronx, New York, NY 10458, USA; asmith169@fordham.edu (A.M.S.); hpajovich@fordham.edu (H.T.P.)
* Correspondence: banerjee@fordham.edu; Tel.: +1-718-817-4445

Academic Editor: Gary Chinga Carrasco
Received: 4 November 2017; Accepted: 8 January 2018; Published: 13 January 2018

Abstract: Degenerative neurological disorders and traumatic brain injuries cause significant damage to quality of life and often impact survival. As a result, novel treatments are necessary that can allow for the regeneration of neural tissue. In this work, a new biomimetic scaffold was designed with potential for applications in neural tissue regeneration. To develop the scaffold, we first prepared a new bolaamphiphile that was capable of undergoing self-assembly into nanoribbons at pH 7. Those nanoribbons were then utilized as templates for conjugation with specific proteins known to play a critical role in neural tissue growth. The template (Ile-TMG-Ile) was prepared by conjugating tetramethyleneglutaric acid with isoleucine and the ability of the bolaamphiphile to self-assemble was probed at a pH range of 4 through 9. The nanoribbons formed under neutral conditions were then functionalized step-wise with the basement membrane protein laminin, the neurotropic factor artemin and Type IV collagen. The conductive polymer polyaniline (PANI) was then incorporated through electrostatic and π–π stacking interactions to the scaffold to impart electrical properties. Distinct morphology changes were observed upon conjugation with each layer, which was also accompanied by an increase in Young's Modulus as well as surface roughness. The Young's Modulus of the dried PANI-bound biocomposite scaffolds was found to be 5.5 GPa, indicating the mechanical strength of the scaffold. Thermal phase changes studied indicated broad endothermic peaks upon incorporation of the proteins which were diminished upon binding with PANI. The scaffolds also exhibited in vitro biodegradable behavior over a period of three weeks. Furthermore, we observed cell proliferation and short neurite outgrowths in the presence of rat neural cortical cells, confirming that the scaffolds may be applicable in neural tissue regeneration. The electrochemical properties of the scaffolds were also studied by generating I-V curves by conducting cyclic voltammetry. Thus, we have developed a new biomimetic composite scaffold that may have potential applications in neural tissue regeneration.

Keywords: self-assembly; templates; tissue regeneration; peptide amphiphiles

---

1. Introduction

The nervous system consists of a network of interconnected cells that play a critical role in the reception and transmission of electrical signals throughout the body [1,2]. However, damage to the nervous system caused by brain injuries or neurodegenerative disorders such as, Alzheimer's, Parkinson's, epilepsy, multiple sclerosis, or chronic traumatic encephalopathy, can lead to severe impairment in daily function and quality of life [3,4]. The slow growth and fragility of nervous tissue poses a unique challenge for treatment interventions. Current treatments are limited to nerve autographing and the use of nerve conduits [5], as well as development of novel antagonists [6]. These methods are challenged by the lack of donors, tissue rejection, scar tissue growth, implantation decay and lack of sufficient structural and biochemical information at the biomolecular level [7]. Tissue Engineering (TE) poses an alternative treatment option to conventional methods. TE seeks to repair, restore and replace damaged tissues and harbor growth of healthy tissue [8]. This is accomplished by creating a biomimetic three-dimensional matrix that exemplifies properties of the extracellular matrix (ECM), which can eventually aid in re-growing tissue [9]. These scaffolds are tailored to specific tissues to ensure compatibility and alleviate immune response and scar tissue growth and support new tissue by proper adhesion and integration [10,11].

Since the inception of TE, a multitude of materials, both natural and synthetic, have been discovered to promote neural tissue growth [12]. For example, functionalized carbon nanotubes and graphene nanotubes have been successful in promoting cell differentiation and migration, while efficiently maintaining conductive properties within the tissue [13–15]. Polymers [16] such as polyethylene glycol (PEG), poly ε-caprolactone (PCL), poly(lactic-co-glycolic acid) (PLGA) and poly-lactic acid (PLA) are some of the most widely used synthetic polymers [17]. Specifically, they have been used to create neural guidance conduits and cylindrical porous electrospun composites to promote axonal growth and to bridge neural ending defects [18]. For instance, it was reported that composites of poly ε-caprolactone electrospun membranes and gelatin improved cell adhesion, proliferation and differentiation of PC-12 nerve cells and supported neurite outgrowth [19]. In a recent study, it was shown that irradiation of graphitic carbon nitride integrated with graphene oxide (GO) that was bound to electrospun PCL/gelatin fibers resulted in neural stimulation upon irradiation with visible-light and thereby supported neuronal differentiation [20]. Amongst the naturally occurring proteoglycans, hyaluronic acid, chitosan, chondrotin sulfate and heparin sulfate have gained significant prominence [21] in the preparation of composite materials for neural TE. For example, in one study, chondroitin-6-sulfate and neural growth factor (NGF) were fused into PEG gels and promoted neurite extension and viability of cortical cells [22,23]. In a separate study, heparin-mimicking polymers—prepared by combining glucosamine-like 2-methacrylamido glucopyranose monomers with three separate sulfonated units—showed higher cytocompatibility and promoted differentiation of embryonic stem cells to neuronal cells as compared to natural heparin [24]. Forsythe and co-workers developed three-dimensional graphene-heparin-poly-L-lysine polyelectrolytes that promoted neuron cell adhesion, proliferation and neurite outgrowth [25]. It has also been shown that hyaluronic acid bound electrospun PCL scaffolds as well as agarose-chitosan blends enhance mechanical properties and increased proliferation of neural cells [26,27].

In addition to the aforementioned biomaterials, peptide amphiphiles have gained prominence in numerous biomedical applications due to their facile self-assembling properties, biocompatibility and relative ease of functionalization [28]. For example, when peptide nanofibers formed by self-assembly of amphiphilic (palmitoyl-GGGAAAKRK) were utilized for siRNA delivery into the brain, they showed higher intra-cellular uptake after being delivered intra-cranially [29]. Stupp and co-workers recently showed that hybrid DNA-peptide nanotubes that had been prepared by altering the sequence of the DNA strands and incorporating the cell-adhesion motif RGDS displayed selectivity and enhanced cell adhesion and differentiation of neural stem cells into neurons but not astrocytes [30]. Scaffolds formed by utilizing the self-assembling peptide RADA16-I have demonstrated potential in closing neural gaps and regenerating axons and healing spinal cord injuries [31]. Researchers have also developed hybrid matrices by combining Type I collagen and peptide amphiphile based nanofibrous scaffolds functionalized with IKVAV or YIGSR that showed specific responses to cerebellar cortex Granule cells and Purkinje cells. Specifically, the IKVAV hybrid scaffolds showed an increase in granule cell density and growth of Purkinje cell dendrite and axons in the presence of peptide nanofibers over specific concentration ranges compared to collagen [32].

In this work, we have developed a new biomimetic scaffold with potential for neural tissue engineering. We conjugated 3,3-tetramethylene glutaric acid (TMG) with isoleucine (Ile) to form a new bolaamphiphile, wherein TMG was the inner head group while the two isoleucine groups formed the tail groups at each end. The self-assembling ability of the Ile-TMG-Ile conjugate was probed at a pH range of 4–9. We observed that under neutral conditions, the conjugate self-assembled into nanoribbons, which were then utilized as templates for developing the scaffold. TMG has been shown to be biocompatible and is a well-known aldose-reductase inhibitor in vitro. It was once touted for its potential in inhibiting diabetic angiopathy and cataract formation by preventing the formation of sorbitol [33]. However, it was found to be relatively inactive as an aldose-reductase inhibitor in vivo, as significant amounts of TMG were unable to reach the retina or lens. We utilized TMG due to its unique structure containing the glutaric acid back bone functionalized with a cyclopentyl ring system. We conjugated it with isoleucine, as it is a key factor known to enhance the activity of alanine-serine-cysteine transporter (Asc-1), which mediates the release of Gly and Ser from neurons and modulates N-methyl-D-aspartate receptor (NMDAR) synaptic activity [34]. The nanoribbons formed upon self-assembly were utilized as templates for preparing tailored scaffolds for neural tissue regeneration. The template Ile-TMG-Ile nanoribbons were first conjugated with laminin, a major component of the extracellular matrix of vascular tissue in the brain. Laminin has been shown to increase the binding abilities of nanoscaffolds as well as to promote cell migration in newly formed cells [35,36]. A recent study conducted using a laminin functionalized PCl-chitosan scaffold showed increased mechanical properties, cell attachment and proliferation [37]. Another study found that laminin based scaffolds vastly improved neuronal survival in the injured brains of mice, which led to greater performance on spatial learning tasks [38].

We then conjugated the laminin bound assemblies with Artemin, which is a glial cell line derived neurotropic factor. Artemin is known to support signaling and increase growth in both peripheral and central nervous tissue by binding to GFR alpha3–RET, an artemin specific receptor in the MAP kinase pathway [39]. It has also been shown to attenuate neuropathic pain in individuals with spinal cord injuries and plays a protective role against deteriorating motor neurons in ALS patients [40,41]. To form the biocomposite, we then conjugated the laminin-artemin-bound templates with Type IV Collagen. It is well known that Type IV Collagen is a component of the basement membrane of vascular tissues in brain and forms mesh-like structures with advantageous mechanical properties. Furthermore, Type IV collagen promotes cell adhesion and stability [42].

Finally, emeraldine base polyaniline (PANI)—a conductive polymer—was incorporated to impart electric properties to the scaffold. PANI consists of repeat units of benzene rings which are separated by secondary amine groups and a quinoid ring system attached to imine groups [43]. The protonated form of emeraldine is conductive as it can form a semiquinone radical cation [44]. In a study where emeraldine polyaniline was blended with gelatin and then electrospun into nanofibers, the scaffold showed a marked increase in conductivity after incorporation of PANI [45]. Thus, we have created a new composite scaffold that consists of self-assembled nanoribbons, conjugated with key proteinaceous components to enhance growth and proliferation of neuronal cells as well as a conductive polymer, polyaniline to impart electrical properties. The formed scaffold demonstrated biodegradability, enhanced mechanical properties as well as promoted growth and proliferation of cortical cells and promoted axonal outgrowth Thus, these newly formed scaffolds may have potential applications in neural tissue engineering.

2. Materials and Methods

Amino acid isoleucine and 3,3-tetramethylene glutaric acid, dimethylformamide (DMF), N-Hydroxy Succinimide (NHS), 1-ethyl-3-(3-dimethylaminopropyl) carbodiimide (EDAC) and triethylamine (TEA), Bradford reagent, Bovine serum albumin (BSA) were purchased from Sigma Aldrich. Buffer solutions of various pH values were purchased from Fisher Scientific. Mouse laminin (sc-29012) and laminin alpha-2 antibody (B-4) were purchased from Santa Cruz Biotechnology. NHS-rhodamine was purchased from Thermo Scientific. Anti-collagen Type IV (rabbit) antibody was purchased from Rockland. Human artemin (category 4515-20, lot P70215) was purchased from Bio Vision. Type IV collagen (AG 19502) was purchased from Neuromics. Rat cortical cells (E18) and cell culture media (NbActiv4) were purchased from BrainBits. Neuroblast cell culture media and Glutamax were purchased from Gibco. Polyaniline was purchased from Ark Pharmaceuticals. Solvent *N*-methyl-2-Pyrrolidine was purchased from VWR. The digital multimeter model M-1000D was purchased from Elenco and a 1.62 mm diameter platinum electrode was purchased from Bioanalytical Systems Incorporated.

2.1. Synthesis of Ile-TMG-Ile

To TMG (1M) were added NHS (0.1M) and EDAC (0.1M) in DMF for activating the carboxylic acid groups of TMG. The mixture was stirred for one hour at 4 °C followed by the addition of Ile (2M). Two drops of TEA were added and the reaction mixture was stirred at 4 °C for 24 h. After 24 h, the solution was rotary evaporated to remove the solvent. The product obtained was found to be a white solid. The ESI-MS obtained by HPLC-MS (Agilent 6100 series, Santa Clara, CA, USA) showed a very weak M+ peak at m/z 411.2; peaks were also observed at m/z 952.4 and at m/z 805.5 due to the formation of oligmers. The strongest peak was seen at m/z 393.2 due to loss of hydroxyl radical. The product most likely undergoes McLafferty rearrangement, as expected for amides. Smaller fragments were observed at m/z = 360.2; 230.7, 361.2 and 115.0. Thus, in addition to Ile-TMG-Ile, side products that included oligomers were also formed. The product was recrystallized using methanol and dried under vacuum before further analysis. The yield of the product was found to 57.2%. The formation of the product was confirmed by ^{1}H NMR spectroscopy using a Bruker 400 MHz NMR (Billerica, MA, USA) in deuterated DMSO with TMS as a solvent. ^{1}H NMR (DMSO-d6) spectrum showed peaks at δ 0.9 (t, 6H); δ 1.2 (d, 6H); δ 1.4 (t, 2H); δ 1.7 (m, 4H); δ 2.3 (d, 2H); δ 2.7 (s, 4H); δ 2.9 (s, 4H); 3.4 (s, 4H); δ 8.1 (s, 2H); δ 12.2 (s, 2H). ^{13}C NMR (DMSO-d6) showed peaks at δ 17.3; δ 22.2; 25.3; δ 29.6; δ 33.4; δ 39.5 δ 42.7; δ 45.9 and δ 174.2.

2.2. Self-Assembly of Ile-TMG-Ile Template

The synthesized product was allowed to self-assemble in buffer solutions of varying pH values. In general, the product (45 mM) was allowed to assemble under acidic (pH 4, potassium acid phthalate buffer); neutral (pH 7, potassium phosphate monobasic-sodium hydroxide buffer) and basic (pH 9, boric acid, potassium chloride, sodium hydroxide buffer) conditions over a period of three to four weeks at room temperature. The growth of assemblies was monitored by dynamic light scattering periodically. After four weeks of growth, the assemblies were centrifuged and washed thrice with deionized water to remove the buffer and left in deionized water for further analysis.

2.3. Preparation of Scaffold

The washed Ile-TMG-Ile assemblies grown at pH 7 were utilized for preparation of scaffolds. An aqueous solution of the fibrillar assemblies (2 mM) was treated with EDAC (1 mM) and NHS (1 mM) for one hour at 4 °C to activate the free carboxylic groups in Ile-TMG-Ile. Mouse laminin (0.1 mg/ mL, 200 µL) was then added to the activated template. The mixture was stirred at 4 °C for 24 h to allow for adhesion of laminin. The laminin bound templates were then washed and centrifuged thrice with deionized water to remove any unbound laminin followed by addition of EDAC (1 mM) and NHS (1 mM) for one hour at 4 °C. To the laminin bound templates, artemin (0.1 mg/mL, 200 µL) was then added and shaken at 4 °C for 24 h and washed and centrifuged thrice to remove unbound artemin. The laminin and artemin functionalized construct was once again allowed to react with EDAC (1 mM) and NHS (1 mM) for one hour at 4 °C followed by the addition of Type IV collagen (0.1 mg/mL, 100 µL) and was shaken at 4 °C for 24 h. The biocomposite was washed and centrifuged to remove unbound collagen. The formed biocomposite scaffold was then vacuum dried. To the dried scaffold, polyaniline (PANI) (0.1 mg/mL) in *N*-methyl-2-Pyrrolidine (5 mL) was added and the mixture was shaken at 4 °C for 24 h and then centrifuged for three hours to remove unbound PANI.

2.4. Binding Efficiency of Laminin, Artemin and Type IV Collagen on the Assemblies

The efficiency of binding of each of the protein components was examined by UV-Vis spectroscopy which was monitored at 272 nm and the absorbance before and after binding to each of the proteins was measured. The absorbance of laminin (0.1 mg/mL, 200 μL) was compared, with that of washed laminin bound assemblies which were prepared as described above. The volumes of the solutions were kept constant. Our results indicated 84.6% binding of laminin to the assemblies. Subsequently the protein concentration of laminin bound assemblies was determined using the Bradford method, based on a standard curve obtained for BSA (1 mg/mL). The concentration of laminin on the assemblies was found to be 2.5 μM. Similarly, upon binding with artemin, the binding efficiency was found to be 92.3% and the protein concentration was found to be 3.19 μM. Finally, for Type IV collagen, the binding efficiency was found to be 88.3% and the protein concentration after binding to Type IV Collagen was found to be 3.65 μM.

2.5. In Vitro Biodegradability Studies

To examine the biodegradability of the formed scaffold, 45 mg of the scaffold was weighed in a petri dish to which 10 mL of simulated body fluid buffer (SBF) was added. The weight of the scaffold was measured every 10 h over a period of 22 days. In general, at each time point, the scaffold was rinsed with deionized water and air dried at room temperature before measurement of weight. The SBF was replaced as necessary each time with the same volume (10 mL). Studies were carried out in triplicate. The results were then analyzed as a function of time. The SBF was prepared according to previously established methods [46]. Briefly, to prepare the simulated body fluid (SBF) for biodegradability studies, 750 mL of distilled water was first brought to a constant temperature of 36.5 °C. The solution was constantly stirred while adding 7.996 g of NaCl, 0.350 g NaHCO$_3$, 0.224 g KCl, 0.228 g K$_2$HPO$_4$ 3H$_2$O, 0.305 g MgCl$_2$ 6H$_2$O, 40 mL HCl (1 M), 0.278 g CaCl$_2$, 0.071 g Na$_2$SO$_4$ and 6.057 g (CH$_2$OH)$_3$CNH$_2$. The pH was adjusted to 7.4 with dropwise addition of 1 M HCl. The total volume was then brought to 1 L using distilled water and then the solution was stored at 4 °C before use.

2.6. Cell Studies

To examine cell viability, rat cortical cells (E18, lot, BrainBits) were cultured in NbActiv4 media (BrainBits) containing 1% 10,000 g/mL amphotericin and 100 units/mL penicillin and streptomycin. The cells were grown to confluence and kept in a humidified atmosphere of 5% CO$_2$ at 37 °C. To examine the effects of the scaffold, cells were plated in 12-well Falcon polystyrene tissue culture plates at a density of 1×10^3 cells per well. After allowing the cells to adhere to the well plates for two hours, scaffolds were added at varying concentration (6 μM, 10 μM and 13 μM). The scaffolds were allowed to interact with the cells for 24, 48 and 72 h. These studies were carried out in triplicate. After each allotted period of time, cell viability and growth was examined by via trypan blue method. Cortical cells in media alone were used as a control for this study. Once stained with trypan blue, live and dead cells were counted using a hemocytometer and averaged. The percent viability was then calculated as follows: (living cortical cells)/(living cortical cells + dead cortical cells) × 100. To observe the interactions of the cortical cells with the scaffolds, cells were plated and allowed to interact with scaffolds as before. The media was changed every 48 h. Images were taken using an AmScope IN200TA-P Inverted Tissue Culture Microscope (Irvine, CA, USA) with a USB camera at various magnifications every 24 h over a period of seven days.

2.7. Electrochemical Studies

We first examined the resistance of control PANI, PANI-bound scaffolds and the biocomposite scaffold in the absence of PANI and determined the conductivity. The resistance of the scaffolds was tested in HCl (1M). A digital multimeter, model M-1000D, from Elenco (Philadelphia, PA, USA) was then used to determine the resistance. To examine the electrochemical properties of the scaffold, we conducted cyclic voltammetry in the presence of PANI, PANI-bound scaffolds and the biocomposite scaffold before it was bound to PANI as control. To obtain I-V curves, the solutions were dried directly onto the 2.01 mm^2 electrode using a vacuum pump for a period of 24 h, adding an addition layer every 6 h. A voltage cell was created using this working electrode, a platinum counter electrode, an Ag/AgCl reference electrode and 1M HCl. Prior to electrochemical measurements, nitrogen was bubbled into the cell for 20 min to remove dissolved oxygen from the solution. PowerSuite by Princeton Applied Research and a Princeton Applied Research potentiostat model 263A (Oakridge, TN, USA) were used to obtain I-V curves from a potential of -0.2 V to 0.9 V at 10 mV/s.

2.8. Characterization

2.8.1. Fourier Transform Infrared (FTIR) Spectroscopy

FTIR spectroscopy was conducted using a Thermo Scientific Nicolet IS50 FTIR (Waltham, MA, USA) with OMNIC software. In general, samples were run at a range of 400 cm^{-1} to 4000 cm^{-1} with 100 scans per sample and the data obtained was averaged.

2.8.2. Scanning Electron Microscopy (SEM)

To examine the morphologies of the assemblies as well as the incorporation of each layer after conjugation, samples were air-dried on to carbon double stick tape and carbon coated to prevent charging. Samples were imaged at various magnifications between of 2 kV to 10 kV utilizing a Zeiss EVO MA10 scanning electron microscope (Thornwood, NY, USA).

2.8.3. Transmission Electron Microscopy (TEM)

In order to further elucidate the morphologies of the assemblies we also conducted TEM analysis using JEOL 1200 EX transmission electron microscope (Peabody, MA, USA). Samples were air-dried on to formvar/carbon 200 mesh copper grids overnight before analysis. Samples were imaged at various magnifications at 80 KeV.

2.8.4. Dynamic Light Scattering (DLS)

To monitor the growth of the assemblies, we conducted DLS using a NICOMP 380 ZLS sizer (Willow Grove, PA, USA). Samples were diluted to appropriate concentrations and each sample was run at least three times and the data obtained was averaged.

2.8.5. Atomic Force Microscopy (AFM)

We examined the nanoscale morphology of the assemblies after conjugation with each layer using a Bruker Multimode 8 AFM (Santa Barbara, CA, USA). Furthermore, the mechanical properties of the scaffolds were also determined by conducting Peak Force Microscopy. The tip was moved to various points (at least five points per sample) on each sample and the values obtained were averaged. Young's Modulus was determined by fitting the data into a Hertzian Model. In general, we used RTESPA-175 Antimony (n) doped Si tip with a spring constant of 40 N/m.

2.8.6. Differential Scanning Calorimetry (DSC)

To explore the thermal phase changes of the scaffolds, we conducted DSC analysis. For each analysis, 0.1 mg samples were dried under vacuum and weighed. We examined the phase changes for each layer of the scaffold using a TA instruments, model Q200 instrument (New Castle, DE, USA) at a temperature range of 0 °C to 250 °C at scanning rate of 10 °C per minute.

2.8.7. Fluorescence Microscopy

Fluorescence microscopy was carried out to examine the interactions of FITC labeled laminin -2 antibody (B-4) with laminin bound assemblies and rhodamine labeled Type IV collagen with the biocomposites using a Phase Contrast Amscope Fluorescence Inverted Microscope (Irvine, CA, USA). To prepare samples for binding with laminin antibody, the laminin bound assemblies were washed and centrifuged with deionized water followed by the addition of BSA Blocker solution (1% BSA) in tris buffered saline to prevent non-specific binding. The sample was vortexed for two minutes and allowed to incubate at room temperature for 4 h. The sample was then centrifuged and washed once with TBS followed by washing with deionized water. To the sample, we then added FITC labeled laminin -2 antibody (B-4) (50 μg/mL). The sample was incubated overnight at 4 °C. Samples were then washed and centrifuged with deionized water and imaged on poly-L-lysine coated glass slides which was covered by a coverslip. Samples were then excited at 450 nm. A similar protocol was followed for examining the interactions of rhodamine labeled collagen IV antibody, where in the collagen IV-artemin-laminin-bound Ile-TMG-Ile assemblies were first washed and centrifuged, followed by the addition of 1% BSA blocking agent before incubation with the antibody. Finally samples were transferred to glass-slides covered with coverslips and imaged at 588 nm excitation.

2.8.8. UV-Vis Spectroscopy

To determine the binding efficiency and protein concentrations of the biocomposite assemblies after each layer of protein (laminin, artemin and Type IV collagen) was added, we carried out UV-Vis spectroscopy using a Nanodrop 2000 spectrophotometer (Waltham, MA, USA).

2.9. Statistical Analysis

We used two-tailed Student's t-test for carrying out statistical analysis. Studies were carried out in triplicate (n = 3). Data are presented as the mean value ± standard deviation (SD) of each sample group.

3. Results and Discussion

3.1. Self-Assembly of Ile-TMG-Ile

Molecular self-assembly of biomolecules transpires through weak, non-covalent interactions that include electrostatic, hydrophobic interactions, hydrogen bonds, van der Waals interactions and π–π stacking forces that result in the formation of stable and functional supramolecular structures [47]. Self-assembling peptides, in particular form unique supramolecular assemblies and offer several advantages. Thus, such materials pose a plethora of applications in tissue engineering as they are highly biocompatible and modifiable [48].

In this work, we designed a new bolaamphiphile by conjugating the amino acid Ile with the dicarboxylic acid 3,3 tetramethylene glutaric acid (TMG) resulting the in the formation of (2S,2′S,3S,3′S)-2,2′-((2,2′-(cyclopentane-1,1-diyl)bis(acetyl))bis(azanediyl))bis(3-methylpentanoic cid), abbreviated as Ile-TMG-Ile (Figure 1). In previous work, peptide based bolaamphiphiles containing amino acid moieties such as glycine, conjugated with dicarboxylic acids such as azelaic acid have been shown to self-assemble into nano and microtubes with closed ends or single layered sheets [49]. In an earlier study, we have shown that when phenylalanine was conjugated with dicarboxylic acids of different chain lengths, supramolecular assemblies of a variety of morphologies were formed depending upon the growth conditions used [50]. It has also been shown that peptide amphiphiles containing N-terminus palmitoylated groups such as CH_3-$(CH_2)_{14}CO$-NH-X-Ala_3-Glu_4-CO-NH_2, where in the amino acid X was varied between Ile, Phe or Val, self-assembled into micelles, nanoribbons or nanofibers depending upon the pH of the growth conditions [51].

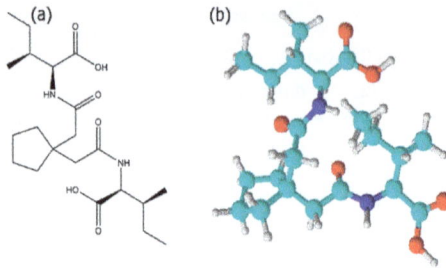

Figure 1. (a) Chemical structure of Ile-TMG-Ile; (b) ball and stick model.

Herein, we examined the self-assembly of Ile-TMG-Ile at pH values of 4 through 9 for a period of four weeks. To examine the morphologies of the formed assemblies, we conducted SEM and TEM microscopy. Figure 2 shows the SEM and TEM images of assemblies formed at varying pH. SEM analysis at pH 4 (Figure 2a) indicates the formation of short, thick nanofibers in the diameter range of 500 nm to 1 μm, while at pH 7 (Figure 2b) we observed the formation of long, multilayered nanoribbons several micrometers in length, with an average diameter of 500 nm to 1 μm. Figure 2c shows the structures of the assemblies formed under basic conditions (pH 9). Results indicated that under basic conditions, structures of a variety of shapes and sizes (spherical micelles, microtubes and fibers) in the range of 2 μm to 5 μm in diameter were formed. Corresponding TEM images, also indicated similar morphologies as shown in Figure 2d–f which correspond to assemblies formed at pH 4, 7 and 9 respectively. The sizes obtained by the TEM analysis, indicate that the average diameter of the nanofibers formed at pH 4 was found to be 20 nm, while those grown at pH 7 were in the size range of 500 nm to 1μm. The assemblies formed at pH 9 were found to be in the range of 200 nm to 500 nm. The size differences between TEM and SEM are attributed to the fact that the assemblies are intrinsically multiscale in nature and, vary in sizes. The TEM images display higher resolution and smaller sample sizes are most likely revealed by TEM analysis. Overall, self-assembly of Ile-TMG-Ile was found to be pH dependent.

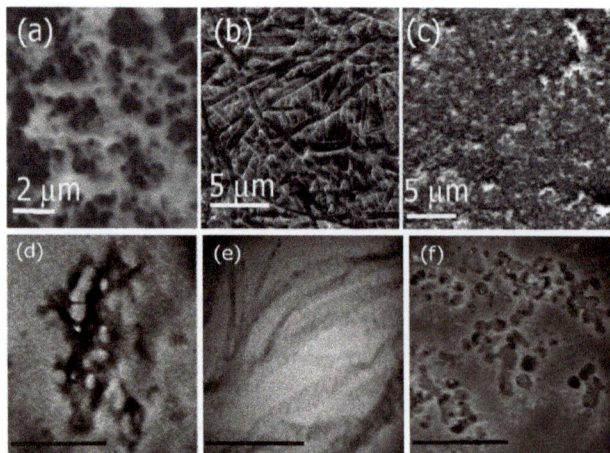

Figure 2. SEM images of Ile-TMG-Ile assemblies formed at (a) pH 4; (b) pH 7 and at (c) pH 9. TEM images of the assemblies are shown at (d) pH 4 (scale bar = 500 nm); (e) pH 7 (scale bar = 2 μm) and (f) pH 9 (scale bar = 1 μm nm).

The formation of short, thick nanofibers under acidic conditions is attributed to higher H-bonding interactions under acidic conditions as the carboxylic groups of the side chain isoleucines are likely to be protonated under those conditions. Additionally, assembly formation is promoted due to intermolecular H-bonding interactions between the –NH and O=C groups of the amide groups of the bolaamphiphile. Studies conducted previously with peptide amphiphiles such as bis(*N*-α-amido-glycylglycine)-1,7-heptane dicarboxylate have shown that at a pH range of 4 to 5, the formation of nanotubes is promoted due to higher H-bonding interactions and beta-sheet formation [52]. In the case of Ile-TMG-Ile, it is likely that beta-sheet formation is promoted, particularly due to the hydrophobicity of the Ile moieties which have been known to induce nanofiber formation [53]. Under neutral conditions, there appears to be a transition between beta-sheet structures to random coil due to changes in H-bonding interactions as the carboxyl groups are progressively deprotonated, resulting in the formation of uniform nanoribbons. Similar phenomena have been observed in the case of bola-glycolipids where changes in morphologies of supramolecular structures were observed, resulting in nanoribbon formation under neutral conditions. This was primarily attributed to a combination of hydrophobic interactions, chirality as well as well as changes in pH [54]. Under basic conditions, we observed a mixture of nanostructures as under those conditions the Ile-TMG-Ile bolaamphiphle is completely deprotonated and H-bonding is significantly diminished. Although C=O–NH amide H-bonding still exists under basic conditions, the carboxylate groups are negatively charged under those conditions and may result in repulsion between the negatively charged carboxylate groups. Thus, a variety of structures including micelles and few fibrillar structures are formed due to a combination of hydrophobic interactions, as well as amide-amide H-bonding and uniform assemblies are not formed.

We also monitored the growth of assemblies periodically using dynamic light scattering in all cases and over time. Results obtained after two weeks of growth are shown in Figure 3. As seen in the figure, the assemblies obtained were polydisperse. This is most likely because the assemblies are not uniform. They are mostly fibrillar, or ribbon shaped (in the case of assemblies grown at pH 4 and pH 7) or display a variety of morphologies as seen in the case of assemblies grown at pH 9. It is likely that aggregates of the assemblies at different stages of growth are observed. Overall, due to the formation of ribbon like structures under neutral conditions, we selected those assemblies for preparation of the scaffold.

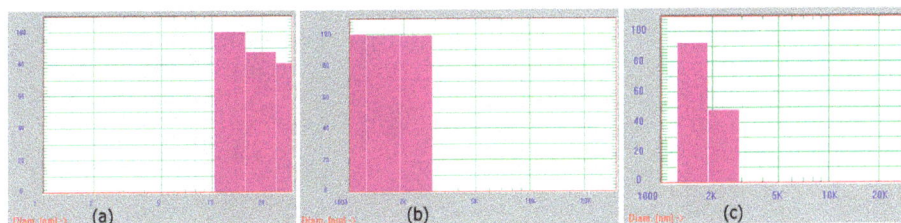

Figure 3. Dynamic light scattering analyses of assemblies formed at (**a**) pH 4; (**b**) pH 7 and (**c**) pH 9.

3.2. Functionalization of Ile-TMG-Ile and Preparation of Scaffold

To prepare the scaffolds that can be tailored for potential neural TE applications, we incorporated protein constituents that may aid in neural tissue regeneration due to their specific functional properties. The conjugation of each component was examined by SEM and TEM imaging as shown in Figure 4. We first conjugated the washed nanoribbons with laminin, a major component of the ECM of neural tissue. Upon incorporation of laminin, changes in morphology were observed (Figure 4a). The SEM image of laminin bound assemblies showed a relatively rough, gelatinous coating on the nanoribbons compared to the smooth surfaces in the absence of laminin as seen in Figure 2b. The corresponding TEM image (Figure 4e) showed a fibrous mesh like network upon conjugation with laminin. In general, laminin consists of both globular and rod-shaped domains and forms alpha-helical coiled coil structures [55]. Upon conjugation with the nanoribbons, laminin binds to nanoribbons, forming a gelatinous network intertwined with the nanoribbons. In general, laminin has been known to polymerize and form laminin networks, in cells due to interactions between the α-short arms of the amino terminal domain and β and γ-short arms of laminin [56]. It is likely that it wraps around Ile-TMG-Ile nanoribbon assemblies upon conjugation resulting in the mesh like networks.

Upon conjugation with artemin, further morphology changes were observed. In the SEM image (Figure 4b), we observed the incorporation of globular, rosette like structures throughout the gelatinous matrix. Similar structures were observed in the in the corresponding TEM image (Figure 4f). Previous studies have revealed that artemin monomers tend to self-assemble into rosette-like oligomers [57] and it is also known to be an exceptionally stable neurotrophic factor that can induce changes in the folding process of proteins as it functions as a molecular chaperone [58]. Thus, the morphology changes observed on the surfaces of the laminin bound nanoribbons further confirm the successful conjugation of artemin. We then conjugated the composite nanoribbons with Type IV collagen (Figure 4c,g). SEM and TEM images confirmed morphological changes after incorporation of Type IV collagen as the formation of large fibrillar mesh like structures were observed, integrated with rosette structures of artemin. In several studies, it has been shown that collagens tend to form long fibrillar structures, due to the formation of triple-helices and impart structural integrity to scaffolds [59]. Thus, our results confirm the formation of the biocomposite nanoribbons integrated with laminin, artemin and Type IV collagen. To impart electrical properties, essential for developing scaffolds for neural TE, we then incubated the conductive polymer polyaniline (PANI) with the biocomposite scaffolds. Previous studies have shown that PANI in the presence of dopants can self-assemble into nanostructures [60]. The presence of the amine groups of PANI, allow for electrostatic and H-bonding interactions between the carbonyl groups of the protein bound nanoribbons and PANI. Additionally, stacking interactions with the aromatic ring systems of PANI are also promoted between the proline and hydroxyproline moieties of Type IV Collagen. Distinct changes in morphology were observed upon incorporation of PANI into the biocomposite (Figure 4d,h) showing the formation of aggregates of PANI on the scaffold indicating its successful assimilation.

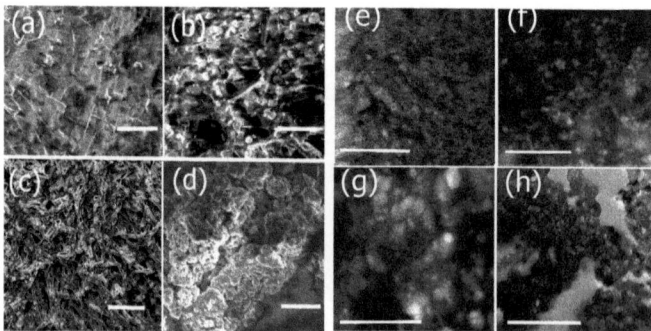

Figure 4. SEM and TEM images showing morphology changes after functionalization with each component. (**a**) SEM image of nanoribbons functionalized with laminin (scale bar = 2 μm); (**b**) SEM image showing subsequent conjugation with Artemin (scale bar = 2 μm); (**c**) SEM image after incorporation of Type IV collagen to laminin-artemin-bound nanoribbons (scale bar = 5 μm); (**d**) SEM image after incorporation of PANI to the functionalized biocomposite (scale bar = 5 μm). (**e**) TEM image of nanoribbons functionalized with laminin (scale bar = 2 μm); (**f**) TEM image showing subsequent conjugation with Artemin (scale bar = 2 μm); (**g**) TEM image after incorporation of Type IV collagen to laminin-artemin-bound nanoribbons (scale bar = 3 μm); (**h**) TEM image after incorporation of PANI to the functionalized biocomposite (scale bar = 3 μm).

3.3. FTIR Spectroscopy

To further confirm the formation of the scaffold, we conducted FTIR spectroscopy (Figure 5). As shown in Figure 5a, the self-assembled template nanoribbons showed characteristic peaks in the amide I region at 1658 cm^{-1} and at 1650 cm^{-1} with a shoulder at 1634 cm^{-1} along with peaks at 1450 cm^{-1} and 1413 cm^{-1} in the amide II region. These peaks are indicative of formation of a mix of random coil, alpha helical and beta-sheet structures [61] that resulted in the formation of nanoribbons. Previous studies using protein analogs with C terminus isoleucine are consistent with these findings of mostly alpha helical and random coil structures [62]. Additionally, a strong peak was observed at 1286 cm^{-1} and at 1075 cm^{-1}, attributed to C–O and C–H stretching respectively. Upon conjugation with laminin (Figure 5b), the amide I peaks were observed at 1656 cm^{-1} and at 1628 cm^{-1} indicating increased beta-sheet formation along with the presence of alpha helices. The amide II peaks were observed at 1550 cm^{-1} and at 1519 cm^{-1} while the C–O and C–H stretching peaks were seen at 1295 cm^{-1} and at 1059 cm^{-1} respectively [63]. It has been reported that laminins generally tend to polymerize into sheet like structures [64], which is consistent with our results. Furthermore, similar shifts were also seen after incorporation of laminin onto a poly(l-lactide-co- glycolide) scaffold, indicating successful conjugation of laminin with the nanoribbons [65]. After conjugation with artemin (Figure 5c), further shifts were observed. The amide I band was shifted to 1632 cm^{-1} with a shoulder at 1662 cm^{-1} while the amide II peaks shifted to 1535 cm^{-1} and 1514 cm^{-1}. The C–O and C–H stretching peaks were observed at 1299 cm^{-1} and at 1064 cm^{-1} with a shoulder at 1054 cm^{-1} respectively. These peaks are indicative of increase in beta-sheets along with the appearance of beta-turn structure.

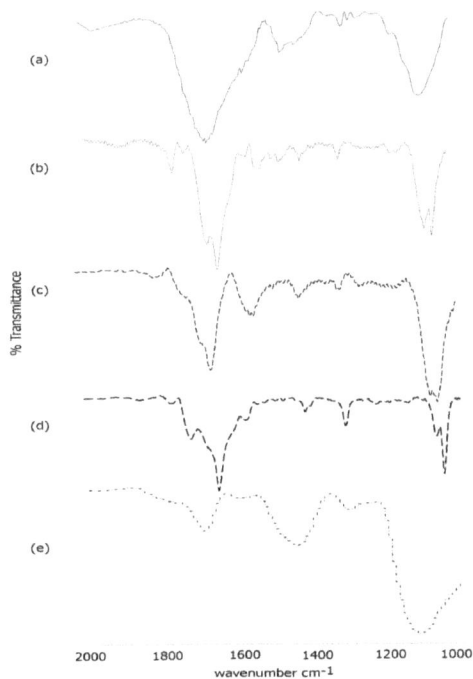

Figure 5. FTIR spectra of (**a**) self-assembled Ile-TMG-Ile nanoribbons; (**b**) Nanoribbons bound to laminin; (**c**) Artemin conjugated with laminin bound nanoribbons; (**d**) Type IV collagen conjugated with artemin-laminin bound nanoribbons; (**e**) PANI bound to Type IV collagen-artemin-laminin bound nanoribbons.

Upon incorporation of Type IV collagen (Figure 5d), the FTIR spectra showed peaks in the amide I region at 1629 cm^{-1} with a shoulder at 1652 cm^{-1} and a peak at 1699 cm^{-1}. The amide II peak was found to be at 1558 cm^{-1} while the C-O and C-H stretching peaks were observed at 1293 cm^{-1} and at 1035 cm^{-1} respectively. These changes confirm the incorporation of Type IV collagen. Furthermore, the secondary structure reveals the presence of alpha-helical content along with beta-strands and β and γ-turns [66] due to blending of Type IV collagen with artemin-laminin bound nanoribbons. Distinct changes were observed upon incorporation of PANI. As seen in Figure 4e, peaks were found at 1680 cm^{-1}, 1560 cm^{-1} and at 1430cm^{-1}, 1280 cm^{-1} and at 1112 cm^{-1}. The peaks at 1630 cm^{-1} at 1450 cm^{-1} are indicative of vibrations from quinoid rings and benzenoid ring systems as seen in PANI bound polystyrene nanocomposites [67]. These results further confirm the formation of the composite scaffold.

3.4. Fluorescence Microscopy

In order to confirm that the proteins retained biological activity after conjugation with the assemblies, we examined the binding affinity of the laminin bound assemblies as well as the Type IV collagen bound biocomposites with corresponding antibodies. We used FITC labeled laminin -2 antibody (B-4) for laminin bound assemblies and rhodamine labeled anti-collagen (Type IV) antibody for Type IV collagen bound biocomposites respectively and examined the interactions using fluorescence microscopy. In previous work, it has been shown that conjugation of different biological moieties including specific peptide sequences such as RGD, TAT peptides, or proteins such as transferrin, antibodies with nanomaterials not only increases the stability of the proteins but also enhances the applications of the nanomaterials themselves [68]. Furthermore, such conjugations allow for interactions with cell receptors or biological membranes, thereby promoting the use of such materials for a variety of biomedical applications. As shown in Figure 6, FITC conjugated anti-laminin bound antibodies efficiently bound to the laminin bound assemblies, (Figure 6a) and rhodamine conjugated anti-collagen IV antibodies bound to the biocomposite (Figure 6b). These results confirmed that laminin and Collagen IV retained their biological activity upon binding with the assemblies.

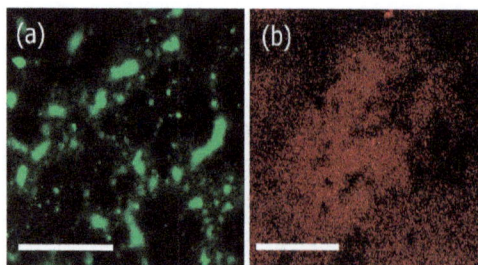

Figure 6. Fluorescence microscopy images of (**a**) FITC labeled laminin α-2 antibody bound to laminin bound assemblies; (**b**) Rhodamine labeled collagen IV antibody bound to biocomposite assemblies (collagen IV-artemin-laminin bound Ile-TMG-Ile). Scale bars = 20 μm.

3.5. Differential Scanning Calorimetry

In order to explore the thermal properties, we examined phase changes of the assemblies before and after conjugation with each component utilized in the formation of the scaffold (Figure 7). Short endothermic peaks were observed in the case of the Ile-TMG-Ile assemblies (Figure 7a) at 14.9 °C and at 36.7 °C followed by another endothermic peak at 99.6 °C, due to loss of loosely bound water. After functionalization with laminin, (Figure 7b) a large, broad endothermic peak was observed in the temperature range of 50 °C to 100 °C, followed by shallow endothermic peaks at 172.4 °C and at 232.1 °C. The significantly broad endothermic peak at the lower temperature is indicative loss of free water, due to the presence of hydrophilic amino acids in the protein. This is primarily due to the fact that hydrophilic groups can cause significant hydration and upon heating, changes in H-bonding interactions and consequently conformation changes in the laminin bound nanoribbons occur. This is a common occurrence in self-assembled peptides and proteins due to the rearrangement of components because of changes in inter and intra-molecular interactions [69]. The short peak at 171.4 °C is likely due to thermal melting, followed by crystallization at a higher temperature (232.1 °C). After further functionalization with artemin (Figure 7c) a similar broad endothermic peak was observed in the temperature range of 50 °C to 100 °C, (though the intensity was lower). Slight shifts were observed in the higher temperature range, with the thermal melting appearing at 172.6 °C and the subsequent short crystallization peak was observed at 242.1 °C. Upon binding with Type IV collagen, (Figure 7d) the composite once again showed a broad endothermic peak, between 50 °C to 100 °C, though the intensity of the peak was lesser than the previous layer, due to higher cross-linking in the presence of collagen and notably, peaks at higher temperature were diminished.

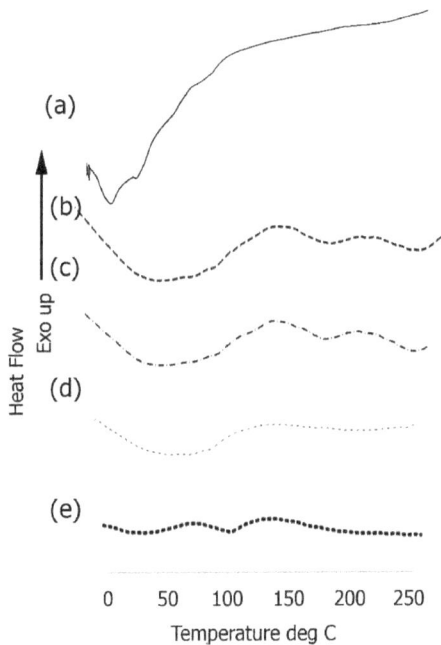

Figure 7. DSC thermograms of (**a**) self-assembled Ile-TMG-Ile nanoribbons; (**b**) Nanoribbons bound to laminin; (**c**) Artemin conjugated with laminin bound nanoribbons; (**d**) Type IV collagen conjugated with artemin-laminin bound nanoribbons; (**e**) PANI bound to Type IV collagen-artemin-laminin bound nanoribbons.

However, a significant change was observed upon incorporation of PANI (Figure 7e), where in the intensity of the broad endothermic peaks seen in the protein bound scaffold was significantly reduced. Relatively short endothermic peaks are observed at 52 °C and at 102 °C due loss of loosely bound water and no other significant peaks are observed. PANI is significantly hydrophobic compared to the proteinaceous components, resulting in shallow peaks due to loss of free unbound water. These results further confirm the integration of PANI.

3.6. Mechanical and Surface Properties

It is paramount that the designed scaffolds should be able to bear force loads in order to adequately support seeded cells and potentially boost the formation of new tissue. We utilized peak force microscopy to determine the mechanical properties of the scaffold. In general, nanoindentation was carried out using AFM to examine the changes in attractive and repulsive forces and the depth of indentation as the tip of the cantilever contacts the sample and is deformed. At least three to five points were selected for each sample to obtain force vs. separation curves and the data obtained was fit into Hertzian model to obtain the Young's modulus. The results obtained for average Young's Modulus values after incorporation of each of the components of the scaffold are shown in Table 1.

Table 1. Youngs Modulus values of constructs after consecutive incorporation of each layer.

Construct	Young's Modulus (GPa)
Self-Assembled nanoribbons	0.757
Nanoribbons bound to Laminin	1.805
Nanoribbons bound to Laminin-Artemin-Collagen	2.985
Nanoribbons bound to Laminin-Artemin-Collagen-PANI	5.522

These results indicate that as each protein layer was conjugated with the nanoribbons, the Young's Modulus (YM) was found to increase, demonstrating that each protein component consecutively increased the stiffness and mechanical strength of the scaffold. The YM values obtained were for dried scaffolds alone and are most likely higher than those one would expect for wet scaffolds, under in vivo or in vitro conditions. Previous nanoindentation studies have shown that native single collagen fibrils have an YM value in the range of 1 to 2 GPa [70]. It has also been reported that protein structures and self-assembled collagen based constructs designed to have properties to mimic the extracellular matrix display Young's Moduli averaging 1.2 GPa [71]. We also determined the Young's Modulus of control Type IV collagen by nanoindentation and the YM was found to be 532.2 ± 3 MPa, while control PANI films were found to have a YM of 1.52 ± 5 GPa. Thus, our results indicate that for the protein functionalized nanoribbon biocomposite, the overall mechanical strength of the scaffold increases due to the multi-component nature of the scaffold. Furthermore, it was found that the highest YM value was obtained after incorporation of PANI. A comparison of AFM images of scaffolds before and after incorporation of PANI and the corresponding force curves are shown in Figure 8.

AFM topography images indicate that the surface of the bicomposite before binding to PANI (Figure 8a) shows a more fibrillar structure, due to top layer of the scaffold being Type IV collagen, while after binding to PANI, more globular structures were observed to be deposited on the scaffold (Figure 8b). These results indicate changes in surface roughness and morphology of the scaffold after incorporation of PANI. Additionally, the force-curves also showed significant changes upon binding with PANI (Figure 8c,d). These results are consistent with previous nanoindentation studies, where it has been demonstrated that when PANI was deposited on vertical arrays of carbon nanotubes (CNTs), the Young's Modulus value dramatically increased due to strong electrostatic and π–π stacking interactions with CNTs [72]. It is expected that similar interactions occur between the biocomposite and PANI that leads to a higher YM. In general, the Young's Modulus values of pyrrolidinone and polyaniline films have been reported to be in the range of 200 MPa–5 GPa [73]. Thus, our results after incorporation of PANI with the biocomposite scaffold are within the values reported previously in the literature.

We also probed the changes in the surface roughness of the scaffold before and after incorporation of PANI. In general, it is known that surface roughness plays a key role in cell adhesion of scaffolds [74] For instance, it has been shown that silk fibroin bound PLA fibers with higher surface roughness promoted increased growth and adhesion of osteoblast cells [75]. For the biocomposite scaffold before incorporation of PANI, the average surface roughness (Ra) was found to be 154 nm, while the maximum roughness (Rmax) was determined to be 209 nm. We found that incorporation of PANI resulted in a significant increase in the surface roughness. The Ra was found to be 377 nm and the Rmax was found to be 2065 nm, further confirming the formation of the composite.

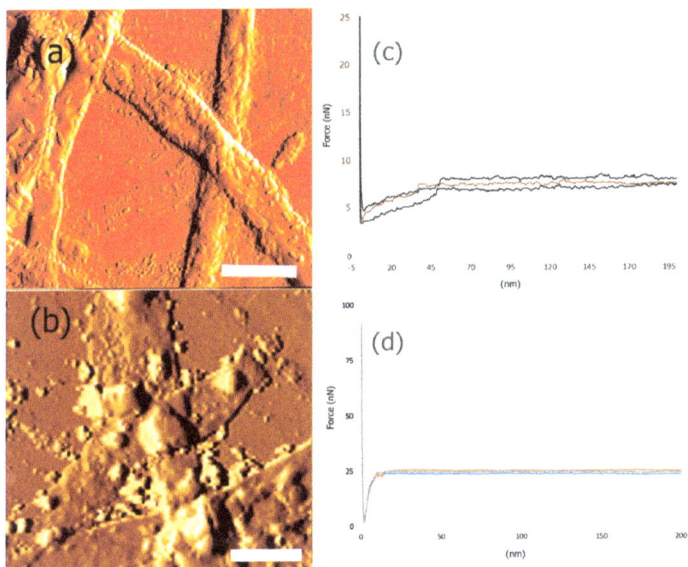

Figure 8. AFM amplitude image of (**a**) biocomposite nanoribbons bound to laminin, artemin and collagen. Scale Bar = 10 μm; (**b**) nanoribbons bound to laminin, artemin and collagen and PANI. Scale Bar = 5 μm. (**c**) Force curves obtained for biocomposite nanoribbons bound to laminin, artemin and collagen; (**d**) Force curves obtained for nanoribbons bound to laminin, artemin and collagen and PANI.

3.7. In Vitro Biodegradability Studies

When developing a scaffold for tissue engineering, the biodegradability of a scaffold plays a vital role. It has been reported that biodegradability promotes growth and proliferation of cells, as well as production of native ECM [76]. In comparison to non-biodegradable scaffolds, biodegradable composites are able to aid in the growth of new tissues at a highly expedited rate due to the increased proliferation and lack of hindrance for cell growth [77]. We examined the biodegradability of the formed scaffold in simulated body fluid buffer in order to mimic in vivo conditions. Figure 9 shows the results obtained over a period of three weeks in simulated body fluid. The scaffold shows a mass loss of 48.7% after 22 days. Overall, the scaffold showed degradation at a moderate rate, which is preferential to highly vascular nervous tissue [78]. This result is consistent with other polymer and basement membrane mimicking scaffolds for tissue engineering; such as, poly(3-hydroxybutyric acid) with chitin and chitosan which demonstrated biodegradability from 45–70% and collagen, hyaluronic acid and gelatin scaffolds which demonstrated 45% biodegradability [79].

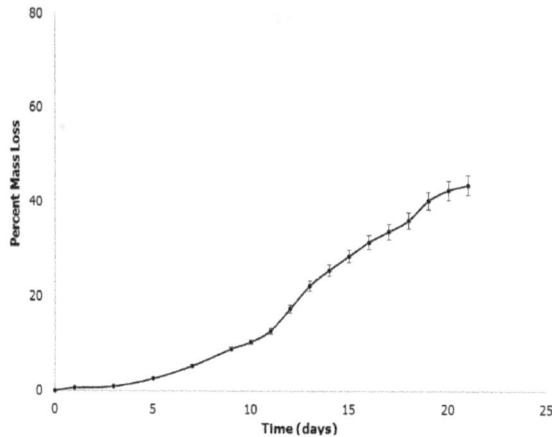

Figure 9. Biodegradation studies of the scaffolds showing mass loss over a period of 20 days.

3.8. Cell Studies

To examine if the formed scaffolds would be suitable for applications in neural TE, we conducted cell viability studies with rat neural cortical cells. We examined the effects of scaffolds before and after incorporation of PANI as shown in Figure 10. The data shown are representative of results obtained in the presence of 10 μM scaffolds in comparison with control untreated cells. Our results indicate that the cells continued to proliferate over a period of 72 h in the presence of scaffolds. Although cell proliferation continued over time, the rate of cell growth for the PANI bound construct was lower compared to the controls due to the known cytotoxicity of PANI [80]. This is most likely that proliferation continued due to the synergistic effects of the protein components of the scaffolds, which play a role in enhancing biocompatibility of the PANI bound scaffold. Previous studies have shown that laminin bound nanofibers significantly increased the attachment and neurite extension of cells in vitro [81] while artemin promotes axonal growth in damaged neural tissue, as well as regeneration of sensory neurons [82]. Other research has shown that after damage, artemin increases survivability of injured neurons [83]. The incorporation of Type IV collagen increases the influx of nutrients to growing and damaged neural tissue, increasing new growth and proliferation. We also studied the growth and proliferation in the presence of 6 μM and 13 μM scaffolds which showed similar trends of cell viability (data not shown). In general, no significant differences were observed in the proliferation at varying concentrations of the scaffold. These results indicated growth and proliferation of cortical cells continued and were comparative to the control throughout various time periods and concentrations of the construct.

To further investigate the cell proliferation of neural cortical cells and morphologies in the presence and absence of PANI bound scaffolds, we conducted phase contrast optical microscopy studies. The results obtained are shown in Figure 11. As seen in the figure, there was a major difference in the morphologies of the cells grown in the presence of PANI bound scaffolds over a period of seven days in comparison to those after 48 h. As shown in Figure 11a,b, in the absence of scaffold, cells continued to proliferate over time. However, we did not observe cluster formation or axonal outgrowths. Upon incubation with PANI bound scaffolds. After 48 h (Figure 11c), the cells appeared to relatively more elongated compared to controls However after seven days, we observed cluster formation and axonal outgrowth (Figure 11d). These results indicated that the cells efficiently continued to proliferate in the presence of the PANI bound scaffolds and enhanced neural cell growth as well as cell-cell adhesion, further confirming that the scaffolds were conducive to forming cell-scaffold matrices and provide an environment for the growth and support of neural cortical cells.

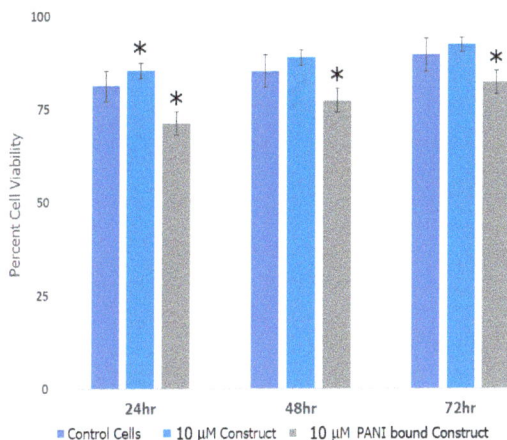

Figure 10. Cortical cell viability in the presence of scaffold constructs before and after incorporation of PANI. (* = p < 0.05 was determined to be statistically significant).

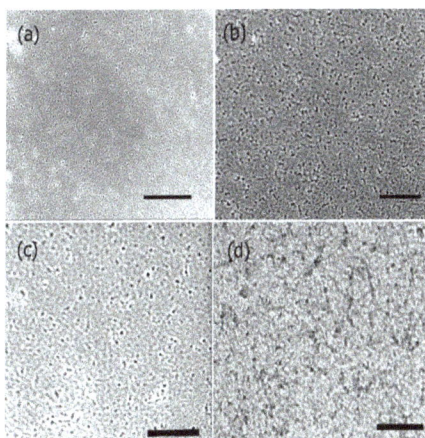

Figure 11. Phase contrast microscopy images showing the growth of neural cortical cells (**a**) control cells after 24 h; (**b**) control cells after 72 h; (**c**) cells with PANI bound scaffolds after 48 h and (**d**) cells with PANI bound scaffolds after 7 days. Scale bars: (**a**) 50 μm; (**b**) 50 μm; (**c**) 30 μm; (**d**) 50 μm.

3.9. Cyclic Voltammetry

To examine the electrochemical properties of the PANI bound scaffold, cyclic voltammetry was conducted. Prior to performing the experiment, the control PANI or the scaffold bound PANI were dried onto the platinum electrodes in vacuum overnight. After connecting the electrodes to the potentiostat, nitrogen was bubbled into the HCl cell solution to remove oxygen from the solution. Potential between -0.2 V to 0.9 V was applied at 10 mV/s to obtain I-V curves. At a voltage of 0.1 mV, an anodic oxidation peak was observed of approximately 2.6×10^{-7} Amps current, with a corresponding cathodic reduction peak at 0.27 mV of approximately -2.85×10^{-7} Amps current in the case of the control PANI. Cyclic voltammetry was then conducted with scaffold bound PANI. Our results indicated that oxidation peaks were observed at 0.213 mV at 1.13×10^{-5} amps current and at 0.56 mV at 1.12×10^{-5} Amps which correspond to the lecuoemeraldine-emeraldine and emeraldine-pernigraniline oxidation processes [84]. The reduction peaks were observed at cathodic currents of -1.39×10^{-5} Amps and at -1.54×10^{-5} Amps at 0.67 mV and at 0.32 mV respectively. These results are shown in Figure 12. Similar cyclic voltagrams have been observed for electrospun polycaprolactone and polyaniline fibers used in skeletal tissue engineering [85].

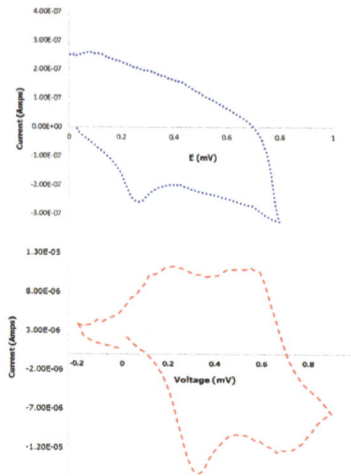

Figure 12. Comparison of cyclic voltagrams of control PANI (top) and PANI bound scaffold (bottom).

Cyclic voltammetry of polyaniline-carbon nanotubes also yielded similar voltammograms [86]. We also compared the cyclic voltagrams with scaffolds formed before incorporation of PANI which did not show any peaks (data not shown). To further examine the electrical properties of the scaffolds, we measured the resistance of the scaffolds to determine the conductivity. Our results showed that the PANI bound scaffolds displayed a conductance of 1.5×10^{-3} S/cm; while the scaffolds in the absence of PANI displayed zero conductivity. Control PANI displayed a conductivity of 2.0×10^{-3} S/cm, which was higher than the PANI bound scaffolds. Overall, these results are indicative that upon binding to PANI the scaffolds display electrical properties, compared to absence of PANI, which is essential for scaffolds for neural tissue regeneration.

4. Conclusions

In this work, 3,3 tetramethyleneglutaric acid and isoleucine were coupled and allowed to self-assemble into a nanoribbon matrix. The nanoribbons were then functionalized with laminin, a primary component in the neural cell basement membrane, along with artemin a glial cell line derived neurotropic factor and Type IV collagen another key component of the ECM of neural tissues. To impart electrical properties, we then incorporated polyaniline a conductive polymer into the scaffold matrix. Peak force microscopy studies revealed that the scaffolds had high mechanical strength and the Young's Modulus increased with conjugation with each protein layer. The scaffolds also displayed biodegradability. Furthermore, the scaffolds were found to promote cell proliferation and encouraged neurite outgrowths. Although cell proliferation was relatively lower for the PANI bound scaffolds, compared to scaffolds without PANI, our results indicated that the biological components of the scaffold overall aided in cell growth. Additionally, cyclic voltammetry conducted showed that PANI bound scaffolds displayed electrochemical properties. Thus, we have created supramolecular composite scaffolds that may be have applications in neural tissue engineering.

Acknowledgments: Andrew M. Smith and Harrison T. Pajovich would like to thank Fordham University Research Grants for financial support of this work. Ipsita A. Banerjee thanks NSF MRI Grant No. 1626378 for support of this work. The authors would also like to thank McMahon for his suggestions and help with the conductivity studies and Fath at the Queens College core facility for Imaging, Cellular and Molecular Biology for the use of the transmission electron microscope

Author Contributions: Andrew M. Smith synthesized the scaffolds, performed experiments and worked on data acquisition for the various studies conducted. Andrew M. Smith was also involved in writing the initial drafts. Harrison T. Pajovich performed some of the analytical experiments. Ipsita A. Banerjee conceived and designed the experiments, analyzed the data and wrote the paper.

Conflicts of Interest: The authors declare no conflict of interest. The founding sponsors had no role in the design of the study; in the collection, analyses, or interpretation of data; in the writing of the manuscript and in the decision to publish the results.

References

1. Saaty, T. Neurons the decision makers, Part I: The firing function of a single neuron. *Neural Netw.* **2017**, *86*, 102–114. [CrossRef] [PubMed]
2. Hammond, C.; Cayre, M.; Panatier, A.; Avignone, E. Neuron-glial cell cooperation. In *Cellular and Molecular Neurophysiology*, 4th ed.; Academic Press: Cambridge, MA, USA, 2015; pp. 25–37. ISBN 9780123970329.
3. Katsu-Jiménez, Y.; Alves, R.M.P.; Giménez-Cassina, A. Food for thought: Impact of metabolism on neuronal excitability. *Exp. Cell Res.* **2017**, *36*, 41–46. [CrossRef] [PubMed]
4. Gupta, M.K.; Jayaram, S.; Madugundu, A.K.; Chavan, S.; Advani, J.; Pandey, A.; Thongboonkerd, V.; Sirdeshmukh, R. Chromosome-centric human proteome project: Deciphering proteins associated with glioma and neurodegenerative disorders on chromosome 12. *J. Proteome Res.* **2014**, *13*, 3178–3190. [CrossRef] [PubMed]
5. Yu, X.; Bellamkonda, R.V. Tissue-Engineered scaffolds are Effective alternatives to autografts for bridging peripheral nerve gaps. *Tissue Eng.* **2003**, *9*, 421–430. [CrossRef] [PubMed]
6. Otto, R.; Penzis, R.; Gaube, F.; Adolph, O.; Föhr, K.J.; Warncke, P.; Robaa, D.; Appenroth, D.; Fleck, C.; Enzensperger, C.; et al. Evaluation of homobivalent carbolines as designed multiple ligands for the treatment of neurodegenerative disorders. *J. Med. Chem.* **2015**, *58*, 6710–6715. [CrossRef] [PubMed]
7. Carriel, V.; Alaminos, M.; Garzón, I.; Campos, A.; Cornelissen, M. Tissue engineering of the peripheral nervous system. *Expert Rev. Neurother.* **2014**, *14*, 301–318. [CrossRef] [PubMed]
8. Williams, D. Benefit and risk in tissue engineering. *Mater. Today* **2004**, *7*, 24–29. [CrossRef]
9. Evans, N.D.; Gentleman, E.; Polak, J.M. Scaffolds for stem cells. *Mater. Today* **2006**, *9*, 26–33. [CrossRef]
10. Gu, X.; Ding, F.; Williams, D.F. Neural tissue engineering options for peripheral nerve regeneration. *Biomaterials* **2014**, *35*, 6143–6156. [CrossRef] [PubMed]
11. Koss, K.M.; Unsworth, L.D. Neural tissue engineering: Bioresponsive nanoscaffolds using engineered self-assembling peptides. *Acta Biomater.* **2016**, *44*, 2–15. [CrossRef] [PubMed]
12. Skop, N.B.; Calderon, F.; Cho, C.H.; Gandhi, C.D.; Levison, S.W. Improvements in biomaterial matrices for neural precursor cell transplantation. *Mol. Cell. Ther.* **2014**, *2*, 19. [CrossRef] [PubMed]
13. Tanaka, M.; Sato, Y.; Haniu, H.; Nomura, H.; Kobayashi, S.; Takanashi, S.; Okamoto, M.; Takizawa, T.; Aoki, K.; Usui, Y.; et al. A three-dimensional block structure consisting exclusively of carbon nanotubes serving as bone regeneration scaffold and as bone defect filler. *PLoS ONE* **2017**, *12*, e0172601. [CrossRef] [PubMed]
14. Perkins, B.L.; Naderi, N. Carbon nanostructures in bone tissue engineering. *Open Orthop. J.* **2016**, *10*, 877–899. [CrossRef] [PubMed]
15. Palejwala, A.H.; Fridley, J.S.; Mata, J.A.; Samuel, E.L.G.; Luerssen, T.G.; Perlaky, L.; Kent, T.A.; Tour, J.M.; Jea, A. Biocompatibility of reduced graphene oxide nanoscaffolds following acute spinal cord injury in rats. *Surg. Neurol. Int.* **2016**, *7*, 75. [CrossRef] [PubMed]
16. Kohane, D.S.; Langer, R. Polymeric biomaterials in tissue engineering. *Pediatr. Res.* **2008**, *63*, 487–491. [CrossRef] [PubMed]
17. Chen, G.; Ushida, T.; Tateishi, T. Scaffold design for tissue engineering. *Macromol. Biosci.* **2002**, *2*, 67–77. [CrossRef]

18. Fukunishi, T.; Shoji, T.; Shinoka, T. Nanofiber composites in vascular tissue engineering. In *Nanofiber Composites for Biomedical Applications*; Woodhead Publishing: Cambridge, UK, 2017; pp. 455–481. ISBN 9780081001738.

19. Alvarez-Perez, M.A.; Guarino, V.; Cirillo, V.; Ambrosio, L. Influence of gelatin cues in PCL electrospun membranes on nerve outgrowth. *Biomacromolecules* **2010**, *11*, 2238–2246. [CrossRef] [PubMed]

20. Zhang, Z.; Xu, R.; Wang, Z.; Dong, M.; Cui, B.; Chen, M. Visible-Light neural stimulation on graphitic-carbon nitride/graphene photocatalytic fibers. *ACS Appl. Mater. Interfaces* **2017**, *9*, 34736–34743. [CrossRef] [PubMed]

21. Hemshekhar, M.; Thushara, R.M.; Chandranayaka, S.; Sherman, L.S.; Kemparaju, K.; Girish, K.S. Emerging roles of hyaluronic acid bioscaffolds in tissue engineering and regenerative medicine. *Int. J. Biol. Macromol.* **2016**, *86*, 917–928. [CrossRef] [PubMed]

22. Butterfield, K.C.; Conovaloff, A.W.; Panitch, A. Development of affinity-based delivery of NGF from a chondroitin sulfate biomaterial. *Biomatter* **2011**, *1*, 174–181. [CrossRef] [PubMed]

23. Weyers, A.; Linhardt, R.J. Neoproteoglycans in tissue engineering. *FEBS J.* **2013**, *280*, 2511–2522. [CrossRef] [PubMed]

24. Lei, J.; Yuan, Y.; Lyu, Z.; Wang, M.; Liu, Q.; Wang, H.; Yuan, L.; Chen, H. Deciphering the role of sulfonated unit in heparin-mimicking polymer to promote neural differentiation of embryonic stem cells. *ACS Appl. Mater. Interfaces* **2017**, *9*, 28209–28221. [CrossRef] [PubMed]

25. Zhou, K.; Thouas, G.A.; Bernard, C.C.; Nisbet, D.R.; Finkelstein, D.I.; Li, D.; Forsythe, J.S. Method to impart electro- and biofunctionality to neural scaffolds using graphene-polyelectrolyte multilayers. *ACS Appl. Mater. Interfaces* **2012**, *4*, 4524–4531. [CrossRef] [PubMed]

26. Cao, Z.; Gilbert, R.J.; He, W. Simple agarose-chitosan gel composite system for enhanced neuronal growth in three dimensions. *Biomacromolecules* **2009**, *10*, 2954–2959. [CrossRef] [PubMed]

27. Entekhabi, E.; Haghbin Nazarpak, M.; Moztarzadeh, F.; Sadeghi, A. Design and manufacture of neural tissue engineering scaffolds using hyaluronic acid and polycaprolactone nanofibers with controlled porosity. *Mater. Sci. Eng. C* **2016**, *69*, 380–387. [CrossRef] [PubMed]

28. Rad-Malekshahi, M.; Lempsink, L.; Amidi, M.; Hennink, W.E.; Mastrobattista, E. Biomedical Applications of Self-Assembling Peptides. *Bioconjug. Chem.* **2016**, *27*, 3–18. [CrossRef] [PubMed]

29. Mazza, M.; Hadjidemetriou, M.; De Lázaro, I.; Bussy, C.; Kostarelos, K. Peptide nanofiber complexes with siRNA for deep brain gene silencing by stereotactic neurosurgery. *ACS Nano* **2015**, *9*, 1137–1149. [CrossRef] [PubMed]

30. Stephanopoulos, N.; Freeman, R.; North, H.A.; Sur, S.; Jeong, S.J.; Tantakitti, F.; Kessler, J.A.; Stupp, S.I. Bioactive DNA-peptide nanotubes enhance the differentiation of neural stem cells into neurons. *Nano Lett.* **2015**, *15*, 603–609. [CrossRef] [PubMed]

31. Ellis-Behnke, R.G.; Liang, Y.-X.; You, S.-W.; Tay, D.K.C.; Zhang, S.; So, K.-F.; Schneider, G.E. Nano neuro knitting: peptide nanofiber scaffold for brain repair and axon regeneration with functional return of vision. *Proc. Natl. Acad. Sci. USA* **2006**, *103*, 5054–5059. [CrossRef] [PubMed]

32. Sur, S.; Pashuck, E.T.; Guler, M.O.; Ito, M.; Stupp, S.I.; Launey, T. A hybrid nanofiber matrix to control the survival and maturation of brain neurons. *Biomaterials* **2012**, *33*, 545–555. [CrossRef] [PubMed]

33. Hutton, J.C.; Schofield, P.J.; Williams, J.F.; Hollows, F.C. The failure of aldose reductase inhibitor 3,3'-tetramethylene glutaric acid to inhibit in vivo sorbitol accumulation in lens and retina in diabetes. *Biochem. Pharmacol.* **1974**, *23*, 2991–2998. [CrossRef]

34. Rosenberyg, D.; Artoul, S.; Segal, A.C.; Kolodney, G.; Radzishevsky, I.; Dikpoltsev, E.; Foltyn, V.N.; Inoue, R.; Mori, H.; Billard, J.-M.; et al. Neuronal D-Serine and Glycine Release Via the Asc-1 Transporter Regulates NMDA Receptor-Dependent Synaptic Activity. *J. Neurosci.* **2013**, *33*, 3533–3544. [CrossRef] [PubMed]

35. Arulmoli, J.; Pathak, M.M.; McDonnell, L.P.; Nourse, J.L.; Tombola, F.; Earthman, J.C.; Flanagan, L.A. Static stretch affects neural stem cell differentiation in an extracellular matrix-dependent manner. *Sci. Rep.* **2015**, *5*, 8499. [CrossRef] [PubMed]

36. Joo, S.; Yeon Kim, J.; Lee, E.; Hong, N.; Sun, W.; Nam, Y. Effects of ECM protein micropatterns on the migration and differentiation of adult neural stem cells. *Sci. Rep.* **2015**, *5*, 13043. [CrossRef] [PubMed]

37. Junka, R.; Valmikinathan, C.M.; Kalyon, D.M.; Yu, X. Laminin functionalized biomimetic nanofibers for nerve tissue engineering. *J. Biomater. Tissue Eng.* **2013**, *3*, 494–502. [CrossRef] [PubMed]

38. Tate, C.C.; Shear, D.A.; Tate, M.C.; Archer, D.R.; Stein, D.G.; LaPlaca, M.C. Laminin and fibronectin scaffolds enhance neural stem cell transplantation into the injured brain. *J. Tissue Eng. Regen. Med.* **2009**, *3*, 208–217. [CrossRef] [PubMed]

39. Baloh, R.H.; Tansey, M.G.; Lampe, P.A.; Fahrner, T.J.; Enomoto, H.; Simburger, K.S.; Leitner, M.L.; Araki, T.; Johnson, E.M.; Milbrandt, J. Artemin, a novel member of the GDNF ligand family, supports peripheral and central neurons and signals through the GFRα3-RET receptor complex. *Neuron* **1998**, *21*, 1291–1302. [CrossRef]

40. Detloff, M.R.; Smith, E.J.; Quiros Molina, D.; Ganzer, P.D.; Houlé, J.D. Acute exercise prevents the development of neuropathic pain and the sprouting of non-peptidergic (GDNF- and artemin-responsive) c-fibers after spinal cord injury. *Exp. Neurol.* **2014**, *255*, 38–48. [CrossRef] [PubMed]

41. Allen, S.J.; Watson, J.J.; Shoemark, D.K.; Barua, N.U.; Patel, N.K. GDNF, NGF and BDNF as therapeutic options for neurodegeneration. *Pharmacol. Ther.* **2013**, *138*, 155–175. [CrossRef] [PubMed]

42. Timpl, R.; Wiedmann, H.; van Delden, V.; Furthmayr, H.; Kühn, K. A network model for the organization of type IV collagen molecules in basement membranes. *Eur. J. Biochem.* **1981**, *120*, 203–211. [CrossRef] [PubMed]

43. Boeva, Z.A.; Sergeyev, V.G. Polyaniline: Synthesis, properties and application. *Polym. Sci. Ser. C* **2014**, *56*, 144–153. [CrossRef]

44. Magnuson, M.; Guo, J.-H.; Butorin, S.M.; Agui, A.; Sathe, C.; Nordgren, J. The electronic structure of polyaniline and doped phases studied by soft X-ray absorption and emission spectroscopies. *J. Chem. Phys.* **1999**, *111*, 4756–4763. [CrossRef]

45. Li, M.; Guo, Y.; Wei, Y.; MacDiarmid, A.G.; Lelkes, P.I. Electrospinning polyaniline-contained gelatin nanofibers for tissue engineering applications. *Biomaterials* **2006**, *27*, 2705–2715. [CrossRef] [PubMed]

46. He, Q.; Shi, J.; Zhu, M.; Chen, Y.; Chen, F. The three-stage in vitro degradation behavior of mesoporous silica in simulated body fluid. *Microporous Mesoporous Mater.* **2010**, *131*, 314–320. [CrossRef]

47. Sun, L.; Zheng, C.; Webster, T.J. Self-assembled peptide nanomaterials for biomedical applications: Promises and pitfalls. *Int. J. Nanomed.* **2017**, 73–86. [CrossRef] [PubMed]

48. Wan, S.; Borland, S.; Richardson, S.M.; Merry, C.L.R.; Saiani, A.; Gough, J.E. Self-assembling peptide hydrogel for intervertebral disc tissue engineering. *Acta Biomater.* **2016**, *46*, 29–40. [CrossRef] [PubMed]

49. Kogiso, M.; Ohnishi, S.; Yase, K.; Masuda, M.; Shimizu, T. Dicarboxylic oligopeptide bolaamphiphiles: Proton-triggered self-assembly of microtubes with loose solid surfaces. *Langmuir* **1998**, *14*, 4978–4986. [CrossRef]

50. Menzenski, M.Z.; Banerjee, I.A. Self-assembly of supramolecular nanostructures from phenylalanine derived bolaamphiphiles. *New J. Chem.* **2007**, *31*, 1674. [CrossRef]

51. Cote, Y.; Fu, I.W.; Dobson, E.T.; Goldberger, J.E.; Nguyen, H.D.; Shen, J.K. Mechanism of the pH-controlled self-assembly of nanofibers from peptide amphiphiles. *J. Phys. Chem. C* **2014**, *118*, 16272–16278. [CrossRef] [PubMed]

52. Matsui, H.; Gologan, B. Crystalline glycylglycine bolaamphiphile tubules and their pH-sensitive structural transformation. *J. Phys. Chem. B* **2000**, *104*, 3383–3386. [CrossRef]

53. Loo, Y.; Zhang, S.; Hauser, C.A.E. From short peptides to nanofibers to macromolecular assemblies in biomedicine. *Biotechnol. Adv.* **2012**, *30*, 593–603. [CrossRef] [PubMed]

54. Cuvier, A.-S.; Berton, J.; Stevens, C.V.; Fadda, G.C.; Babonneau, F.; Van Bogaert, I.N.A.; Soetaert, W.; Pehau-Arnaudet, G.; Baccile, N. pH-triggered formation of nanoribbons from yeast-derived glycolipid biosurfactants. *Soft Matter* **2014**, *10*, 3950–3959. [CrossRef] [PubMed]

55. Macdonald, P.R.; Lustig, A.; Steinmetz, M.O.; Kammerer, R.A. Laminin chain assembly is regulated by specific coiled-coil interactions. *J. Struct. Biol.* **2010**, *170*, 398–405. [CrossRef] [PubMed]

56. Hussain, S.-A.; Carafoli, F.; Hohenester, E. Determinants of laminin polymerization revealed by the structure of the α5 chain amino-terminal region. *EMBO Rep.* **2011**, *12*, 276–282. [CrossRef] [PubMed]

57. De Graaf, J.; Amons, R.; Möller, W. The primary structure of artemin from Artemia cysts. *Eur. J. Biochem.* **1990**, *193*, 737–741. [CrossRef] [PubMed]

58. Hassani, L.; Sajedi, R.H. Effect of artemin on structural transition of lactoglobulin. *Spectrochim. Acta A Mol. Biomol. Spectrosc.* **2013**, *105*, 24–28. [CrossRef] [PubMed]

59. Liu, G.Y.; Agarwal, R.; Ko, K.R.; Ruthven, M.; Sarhan, H.T.; Frampton, J.P. Templated assembly of collagen fibers directs cell growth in 2D and 3D. *Sci. Rep.* **2017**, *7*, 9628. [CrossRef] [PubMed]

60. Huang, K.; Wan, M. Self-assembled polyaniline nanostructures with photoisomerization function. *Chem. Mater.* **2002**, *14*, 3486–3492. [CrossRef]

61. Kong, J.; Yu, S. Fourier transform infrared spectroscopic analysis of protein secondary structures. *Acta Biochim. Biophys. Sin. (Shanghai)* **2007**, *39*, 549–559. [CrossRef] [PubMed]

62. Almlén, A.; Vandenbussche, G.; Linderholm, B.; Haegerstrand-Björkman, M.; Johansson, J.; Curstedt, T. Alterations of the C-terminal end do not affect in vitro or in vivo activity of surfactant protein C analogs. *Biochim. Biophys. Acta. Biomembr.* **2012**, *1818*, 27–32. [CrossRef] [PubMed]

63. Langham, A.A.; Waring, A.J.; Kaznessis, Y.N. Comparison of interactions between beta-hairpin decapeptides and SDS/DPC micelles from experimental and simulation data. *BMC Biochem.* **2007**, *8*, 11. [CrossRef] [PubMed]

64. Baker, B.R.; Garrell, R.L. g-Factor analysis of protein secondary structure in solutions and thin films. *Faraday Discuss.* **2004**, *126*, 209. [CrossRef] [PubMed]

65. Wen, X.; Wang, Y.; Guo, Z.; Meng, H.; Huang, J.; Zhang, L.; Zhao, B.; Zhao, Q.; Zheng, Y.; Peng, J. Cauda equina-derived extracellular matrix for fabrication of nanostructured hybrid scaffolds applied to neural tissue engineering. *Tissue Eng. Part A* **2015**, *21*, 1095–1105. [CrossRef] [PubMed]

66. Vass, E.; Hollósi, M.; Besson, F.; Buchet, R. Vibrational spectroscopic detection of beta- and gamma-turns in synthetic and natural peptides and proteins. *Chem. Rev.* **2003**, *103*, 1917–1954. [CrossRef] [PubMed]

67. Pud, A.A.; Nikolayeva, O.A.; Vretik, L.O.; Noskov, Y.V.; Ogurtsov, N.A.; Kruglyak, O.S.; Fedorenko, E.A. New nanocomposites of polystyrene with polyaniline doped with lauryl sulfuric acid. *Nanoscale Res. Lett.* **2017**, *12*, 493. [CrossRef] [PubMed]

68. Arruebo, M.; Valladares, M.; Gonzalez-Fernandez, A. Antibody conjugated nanoparticles for biomedical applications. *J. Nanomaterials* **2009**, *2009*, 37. [CrossRef]

69. Gröschel, A.H.; Müller, A.H.E. Self-assembly concepts for multicompartment nanostructures. *Nanoscale* **2015**, *7*, 11841–11876. [CrossRef] [PubMed]

70. Heim, A.J.; Matthews, W.G.; Koob, T.J. Determination of the elastic modulus of native collagen fibrils via radial indentation. *Appl. Phys. Lett.* **2006**, *89*. [CrossRef]

71. Muiznieks, L.D.; Keeley, F.W. Molecular assembly and mechanical properties of the extracellular matrix: A fibrous protein perspective. *Biochim. Biophys. Acta* **2012**, *1832*, 866–875. [CrossRef] [PubMed]

72. Ding, J.; Li, X.; Wang, X.; Zhang, J.; Yu, D.; Qiu, B. Fabrication of vertical array CNTs/polyaniline composite membranes by microwave-assisted in situ polymerization. *Nanoscale Res. Lett.* **2015**, *10*, 493. [CrossRef] [PubMed]

73. Wei, Y.; Jang, G.W.; Hsueh, K.F.; Scherr, E.M.; MacDiarmid, A.G.; Epstein, A.J. Thermal transitions and mechanical properties of films of chemically prepared polyaniline. *Polymer (Guildf)* **1992**, *33*, 314–322. [CrossRef]

74. Xu, C.; Yang, F.; Wang, S.; Ramakrishna, S. In vitro study of human vascular endothelial cell function on materials with various surface roughness. *J. Biomed. Mater. Res. A* **2004**, *71*, 154–161. [CrossRef] [PubMed]

75. Chen, B.-Q.; Kankala, R.K.; Chen, A.-Z.; Yang, D.-Z.; Cheng, X.-X.; Jiang, N.-N.; Zhu, K.; Wang, S.-B. Investigation of silk fibroin nanoparticle-decorated poly(l-lactic acid) composite scaffolds for osteoblast growth and differentiation. *Int. J. Nanomed.* **2017**, *12*, 1877–1890. [CrossRef] [PubMed]

76. Nguyen, K.T.; West, J.L. Photopolymerizable hydrogels for tissue engineering applications. *Biomaterials* **2002**, *23*, 4307–4314. [CrossRef]

77. Sheikh, Z.; Najeeb, S.; Khurshid, Z.; Verma, V.; Rashid, H.; Glogauer, M. Biodegradable materials for bone repair and tissue engineering applications. *Materials (Basel)* **2015**, *8*, 5744–5794. [CrossRef] [PubMed]

78. Serbo, J.V.; Gerecht, S. Vascular tissue engineering: biodegradable scaffold platforms to promote angiogenesis. *Stem Cell Res. Ther.* **2013**, *4*, 8. [CrossRef] [PubMed]

79. Ikejima, T.; Inoue, Y. Crystallization behavior and environmental biodegradability of the blend films of poly(3-hydroxybutyric acid) with chitin and chitosan. *Carbohydr. Polym.* **2000**, *41*, 351–356. [CrossRef]

80. Bober, P.; Humpolíček, P.; Pacherník, J.; Stejskal, J.; Lindfors, T. Conducting polyaniline based cell culture substrate for embryonic stem cells and embryoid bodies. *RSC Adv.* **2015**, *5*, 50328–50335. [CrossRef]

81. Neal, R.A.; Lenz, S.M.; Wang, T.; Abebayehu, D.; Brooks, B.P.C.; Ogle, R.C.; Botchwey, E.A. Laminin- and basement membranepolycaprolactone blend nanofibers as a scaffold for regenerative medicine. *Nanomater. Environ.* **2014**, *2*, 1–12. [CrossRef] [PubMed]

82. Wong, L.E.; Gibson, M.E.; Arnold, H.M.; Pepinsky, B.; Frank, E. Artemin promotes functional long-distance axonal regeneration to the brainstem after dorsal root crush. *Proc. Natl. Acad. Sci. USA* **2015**, *112*, 6170–6175. [CrossRef] [PubMed]

83. Önger, M.E.; Delibaş, B.; Türkmen, A.P.; Erener, E.; Altunkaynak, B.Z.; Kaplan, S. The role of growth factors in nerve regeneration. *Drug Discov. Ther.* **2016**, *3*, 285–291. [CrossRef] [PubMed]

Bioengineering **2018**, *5*, 6

84. Shin, Y.J.; Kim, S.H.; Yang, D.H.; Kwon, H.; Shin, J.S. Amperometric glucose biosensor by means of electrostatic layer-by-layer adsorption onto polyaniline-coated polyester films. *J. Ind. Eng. Chem.* **2010**, *16*, 380–384. [CrossRef]

85. Ku, S.H.; Lee, S.H.; Park, C.B. Synergic effects of nanofiber alignment and electroactivity on myoblast differentiation. *Biomaterials* **2012**, *33*, 6098–6104. [CrossRef] [PubMed]

86. Gajendran, P.; Saraswathi, R. Polyaniline-carbon nanotube composites. *Pure Appl. Chem.* **2008**, *80*, 2377–2395. [CrossRef]

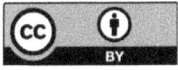

bioengineering

MDPI

Article

Effects of Heterologous tRNA Modifications on the Production of Proteins Containing Noncanonical Amino Acids

Ana Crnković [1,†], Oscar Vargas-Rodriguez [1,†], Anna Merkuryev [2] and Dieter Söll [1,2,*]

[1] Department of Molecular Biophysics and Biochemistry, Yale University, New Haven, CT 06520, USA; ana.crnkovic@yale.edu (A.C.); oscar.vargas@yale.edu (O.V.-R.)

[2] Department of Chemistry, Yale University, New Haven, CT 06520, USA; anna.merkuryev@yale.edu

* Correspondence: dieter.soll@yale.edu; Tel.: +1-203-432-6200

† These authors contributed equally to this work.

Academic Editor: Gary Chinga Carrasco
Received: 19 December 2017; Accepted: 31 January 2018; Published: 2 February 2018

Abstract: Synthesis of proteins with noncanonical amino acids (ncAAs) enables the creation of protein-based biomaterials with diverse new chemical properties that may be attractive for material science. Current methods for large-scale production of ncAA-containing proteins, frequently carried out in *Escherichia coli*, involve the use of orthogonal aminoacyl-tRNA synthetases (o-aaRSs) and tRNAs (o-tRNAs). Although o-tRNAs are designed to be orthogonal to endogenous aaRSs, their orthogonality to the components of the *E. coli* metabolism remains largely unexplored. We systematically investigated how the *E. coli* tRNA modification machinery affects the efficiency and orthogonality of o-tRNA^{Sep} used for production of proteins with the ncAA *O*-phosphoserine (Sep). The incorporation of Sep into a green fluorescent protein (GFP) in 42 *E. coli* strains carrying deletions of single tRNA modification genes identified several genes that affect the o-tRNA activity. Deletion of cysteine desulfurase (*iscS*) increased the yield of Sep-containing GFP more than eightfold, while overexpression of dimethylallyltransferase MiaA and pseudouridine synthase TruB improved the specificity of Sep incorporation. These results highlight the importance of tRNA modifications for the biosynthesis of proteins containing ncAAs, and provide a novel framework for optimization of o-tRNAs.

Keywords: noncanonical amino acids; genetic code expansion; protein translation; tRNA; aminoacyl-tRNA synthetases; posttranscriptional modifications; phosphoserine

1. Introduction

Our increasing understanding of protein structure and function, together with the ease of robust recombinant protein expression systems, facilitates the design of protein-based biomaterials. These biopolymers are of great interest in the field of materials science due to their mechanical and biological properties that are, in many cases, superior to those of synthetic biomaterials. Protein-based materials have become particularly important in the development of medical devices and drug discovery because of their chemical flexibility, biocompatibility, and biodegradability [1]. A disadvantage in the design and fabrication of proteinogenic materials has been the small number of building blocks with reactive handles available through the twenty canonical amino acids. However, recent methodological advances to genetically incorporate noncanonical amino acids (ncAAs) into proteins have expanded the chemical functionalities of natural proteins and allowed the design of more sophisticated polypeptides [2]. Over 150 chemically and structurally diverse ncAAs have been genetically incorporated into proteins, which have enabled a variety of applications across different disciplines [3]. Photoactive [4], fluorinated [5], unsaturated [6], and β-amino acids [7] have been incorporated to facilitate processes such as photopatterning [8], to enhance protein stability [6], or to create proteins with unique properties [9]. However, incorporation of each ncAA requires a devoted aminoacyl-tRNA synthetase (aaRS), which first needs to be created by directed evolution [10]. This can be bypassed, in part, by genetic incorporation of the ncAA *O*-phosphoserine (Sep), whose phosphate group can be converted to a myriad of functional groups by a recently reported method [11].

Robust production of ncAA-containing proteins requires altered translational components. Primary is an engineered aminoacyl-tRNA synthetase (aaRS)•tRNA pair specific for the desired ncAA. This orthogonal translation system (OTS) must operate in a host cell being agnostic of the endogenous aaRSs and tRNAs, while interacting normally with the host translation machinery (e.g., elongation factor and ribosome, [12]). For these reasons, most OTSs are obtained from organisms of a different domain of life; thus, the OTSs used in *Escherichia coli* are usually of archaeal or eukaryotic origin [3,12]. In addition, site-specific ncAA incorporation needs codon reassignment. The major strategies are based on stop codon (UAG) suppression to minimize errors in sense codon decoding during protein synthesis. Collectively, this process is known as genetic code expansion. The current challenges are low orthogonality and polyspecificity which affect the yield and purity of the synthesized protein [13]. Lack of orthogonality may result from anticodons in orthogonal tRNAs (o-tRNAs) that are recognized by host aaRSs causing formation of the wrong aa-tRNA and leading to incorporation of an undesired amino acid [14]. Installation of antideterminants against the offending host aaRSs will prevent misacylation. However, improving OTS specificity will require a labor-intensive redesign of the orthogonal aaRS (o-aaRS) [10]. Yet, for some exotic ncAAs, engineering of other cellular components is sometimes necessary (e.g., the elongation factor Tu (EF-Tu) [15], the ribosome [7], or amino acid transporters [16]).

Although substantial progress has been made in tackling the issues described above, further improvement of OTSs will require consideration of other cellular factors that may influence ncAA translation. For instance, little is known about how the post-transcriptional modification system of the host interacts with and affects the activity of o-tRNAs. In *E. coli*, many different tRNA modifications [17] are responsible for accurate tRNA aminoacylation and codon/anticodon pairing on the ribosome. Thus, heterologous modifications of o-tRNAs may significantly influence their activity. Because most OTSs used in *E. coli* include foreign tRNAs, it is difficult to predict whether their modification pattern is similar to that of endogenous *E. coli* tRNAs. To investigate this, we employed a translation system for site-specific Sep incorporation (Sep-OTS) in *E. coli*. Using single-gene knockout strains of tRNA modification genes [18], and a green fluorescent protein (GFP) reporter system [19], we identified *E. coli* enzymes whose absence influences homogeneity of Sep-containing proteins. Unexpectedly, we found that the deletion of cysteine desulfurase gene (*iscS*) increases the total yield of GFP sixfold, while preserving the relative ratio of phosphorylated protein in the mixture. Taken together, these results underscore the essential role of tRNA modifications in genetic code expansion studies.

2. Materials and Methods

2.1. Strains and Plasmid Constructions

Oligonucleotide synthesis, DNA sequencing, and LC-MS/MS were performed by the Keck Foundation Biotechnology Resource Laboratory at Yale University. *O*-phospho-L-serine (Sep) was purchased from Sigma-Aldrich (Milwaukee, WI USA). *E. coli* TOP10 cells were used for general cloning. *E. coli* BL21(DE3), BW25113, and selected Keio knockout strains (Supplementary Table S1, [18]) were used for super-folder GFP (sfGFP) production. The reporter-containing plasmids (pET-sfGFP-sepT and all derivatives) (Supplementary Table S2) were adapted from a previously developed pET-sfGFP-pylT plasmid [19]. The plasmid pET-sfGFP-sepT-Trm5 was generated by introducing the gene encoding Trm5 from *Methanococcus maripaludis* under the *lpp* promoter and the *rrnC* terminator.

A codon-optimized version of the SepRS gene was placed under an *lpp* promoter in a modified pCDF2 vector. For the experiments involving archaeal Trm5, an engineered variant of SepRS was used (SepRS9), encoded in the same manner in the pCDF2 plasmid. Plasmids pCDF-lpp.SepRS-Para.MiaA and pCDF-lpp.SepRS-Para.TruB were created by introducing *araC* and the arabinose promoter into a pCDF2 backbone (Supplementary Figure S1).

2.2. Growth Media

All *E. coli* strains were grown in Luria-Bertani (LB) medium, supplemented with 5 mM Sep where indicated, and sfGFP production was induced by adding 1 mM isopropyl β-D-1-thiogalactopyranoside (IPTG). MiaA and TruB expression from the corresponding pCDF vectors was induced by 1 mM arabinose.

2.3. SfGFP-Based Activity Assays

High-throughput sfGFP stop codon read-through assays were carried out in 96-well plates as previously described with minor modifications [20]. Briefly, *E. coli* strains were either transformed with pET-sfGFP-sepT or co-transformed with pET-sfGFP-sepT and pCDF2-SepRS. Individual colonies were grown in 1.5 mL LB medium supplemented with 50 μg/mL spectinomycin and 100 μg/mL ampicillin at 37 °C. Keio collection knockout strains were grown in 12.5 μg/mL kanamycin. Overnight cultures were diluted 1:100 in 100 μL LB medium (with or without Sep and IPTG) and transferred to a 96-well assay plate (CORNING). Growth and fluorescence (excitation wavelength 485/20 nm; emission wavelength 528/20 nm) were monitored for 24 h at 37 °C in a Synergy HT plate reader (BioTek). To quantify the amount of GFP synthesized, values obtained for relative fluorescence units (RFU) and OD_{600} in blank wells were subtracted from corresponding values collected in wells containing cells of interest. Then, the corrected fluorescence units were divided by the corrected OD_{600}. The mean and standard deviations correspond to the average of at least three distinct colonies, each measured with two technical replicates.

2.4. SfGFP Purification and Phos-Tag Analysis

A single colony containing pET-sfGFP-2TAG-sepT(G37A) and pCDF2-SepRS or pCDF-lpp.SepRS-Para.MiaA and pCDF-lpp.SepRS-Para.TruB was inoculated into 1.5 mL LB medium and grown overnight. The overnight culture was diluted 1:200 in 25 mL LB medium with 5 mM Sep. Cells were grown to an OD_{600} of 0.5, after which the protein expression was induced. Cells were grown for 12 h after induction. Cells were lysed using BugBuster (EMD Millipore, Billerica, MA, USA) and buffer A (50 mM Tris, pH 7.5, 300 mM NaCl, 10 mM imidazole, pH 7.6 and 10% (*v/v*) glycerol). Lysed cells were centrifuged at 11,000× *g* for 30 min at 4 °C, and the supernatant was loaded on a pre-equilibrated Ni-NA slurry (200 μL). The resin was washed with buffers A and B (same as A but with 35 mM imidazole). Finally, the protein was eluted with buffer C (300 mM imidazole, pH 7.6, 200 mM NaCl, 5% (*v/v*) glycerol). Eluted protein was then concentrated to ~A_{280} = 1 and stored at −20 °C.

For the Phos-tag™ mobility shift and Western blot analysis of sfGFP, 2 μg of isolated sfGFP was loaded onto a 10% or 12% polyacrylamide gel containing 50 μM Mn^{2+}-Phos-tag™ acrylamide (Wako Pure Chemical Industries, Ltd., Osaka, Japan). After electrophoresis, the gel was washed in transfer buffer with 1 mM EDTA to remove the Mn^{2+} ions and then in an EDTA-free transfer buffer (25 mM Tris, 191 mM Gly, 20% (*v/v*) ethanol). PVDF membrane was soaked in methanol and then equilibrated in the transfer buffer. Transfer was executed at 65 mA for 30 min. The membrane was blotted with 1:1000 anti-GFP (rabbit IgG fraction, conjugated to horseradish peroxidase, Life Technologies, Grand Island, NY USA). The chemiluminescent signal was detected and captured on a ChemiDoc MP camera (Bio-Rad, Hercules, CA, USA). Recorded signals were quantified by ImageJ (developer Wayne Rasband, Research Services Branch of NIH, Research Triangle Park, NC, USA) [21].

3. Results and Discussion

3.1. Implications of Post-Transcriptional Modifications in Orthogonal tRNAs

Because of their pivotal role in translation of the genetic code, tRNAs are tightly regulated through an intricate metabolic cycle which includes a myriad of post-transcriptional chemical modifications across the tRNA structure. Over 100 currently identified modifications perform versatile tasks in tRNA processing, stability, and functionality [17,22,23]. tRNAs are more comprehensively modified in the anticodon region, especially at positions 34 (first base of the anticodon) and 37 (base following the anticodon) [24]. These particular modifications are critical for faithful translation of the genetic code as they ensure proper amino acid pairing with cognate tRNAs and correct matching of the codon/anticodon at the ribosome [25,26]. However, bacterial, archaeal, and eukaryal enzymes devoted to their formation sometimes differ and tRNAs from different kingdoms may bear different nucleotide determinants (e.g., [27]). Despite their essential role in protein synthesis, and the fact that o-tRNAs might be undermodified or improperly modified within the host, tRNA modifications have been mostly overlooked in the development or optimization of OTSs.

Here we explored the influence of *E. coli*-specific post-transcriptional modifications on the performance of Sep-OTS. tRNA$^{Sep}_{CUA}$ was originally created by introducing three base substitutions in the archaeal *Methanocaldococcus jannaschii* tRNA^{Cys} [15]. *M. maripaludis* phosphoseryl-tRNA synthetase (SepRS) aminoacylates tRNA$^{Sep}_{CUA}$ with phosphoserine, thereby enabling site-specific incorporation of Sep in response to a UAG stop codon (Figure 1a). The Sep-OTS has been of particular interest since it simplifies the preparation of Sep-containing proteins and enables precise placement of Sep within a protein. Naturally present in proteins as a reversible post-translational modification, Sep is fundamental in the regulation of protein activity in all organisms. While Sep-OTS has already aided mechanistic studies of serine phosphorylation/dephosphorylation (e.g., [28]), the overall efficiency and specificity of the system has presented complications that compromise sample yields and purity. To overcome these issues, most efforts so far have focused on improving aminoacylation efficiency by engineering of tRNA^{Sep} [29,30], SepRS [30,31], and elongation factor Tu (EF-Tu, [15,31]). In the case of tRNA^{Sep}, optimization has involved the evolution of more efficient tRNA^{Sep} mutants [30] and/or the improvement of tRNA expression levels [29], with no consideration to the potential role of heterologous modifications on tRNA^{Sep}.

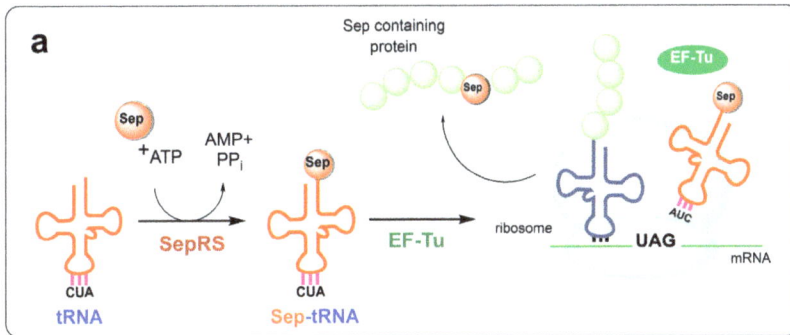

Figure 1. *Cont.*

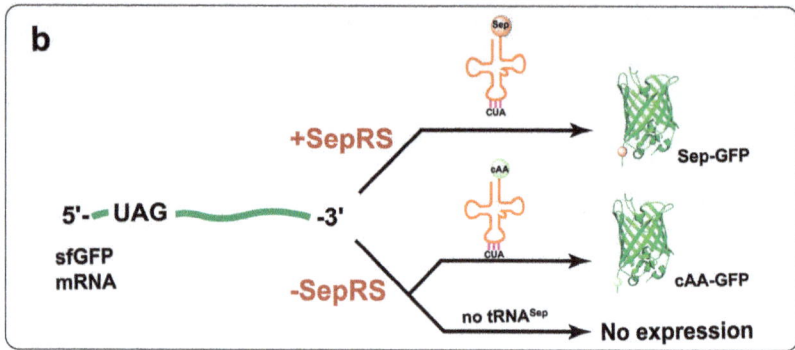

Figure 1. (**a**) Schematic representation of stop codon suppression with noncanonical amino acids (ncAAs). An orthogonal aminoacyl-tRNA synthetase (aaRS) (represented by SepRS) aminoacylates an orthogonal suppressor tRNA (anticodon CUA, shown in orange) with a noncognate amino acid (Sep). Sep-tRNA^{Sep}$_{CUA}$ is delivered to the ribosome by the modified version of the host elongation factor EF-Tu. At the ribosome, the Sep-tRNA^{Sep}$_{CUA}$ decodes an internal stop codon (UAG) and the ncAA is incorporated in the nascent protein. (**b**) Schematic depiction of a stop codon read-through assay using super-folder green fluorescent protein (sfGFP)-2TAG. A stop codon containing mRNA can be translated only in the presence of suppressor tRNA (here, tRNA^{Sep}$_{CUA}$). In the presence of SepRS, tRNA^{Sep}$_{CUA}$ is aminoacylated with phosphoserine, which is subsequently incorporated into sfGFP. In the absence of SepRS, an endogenous aaRS may misacylate tRNA^{Sep}$_{CUA}$ with a canonical amino acid, which then becomes incorporated into sfGFP.

To gain insights into whether modifications influence o-tRNA activity in the host organism, we began our investigation using the first generation of tRNA^{Sep}, which contains G at position 37 (Figure 2a). In *M. jannaschii*, the parental tRNA^{Cys} is methylated at G37 by the methyltransferase Trm5 [27]. Because this modification substantially increases aminoacylation efficiency by SepRS [32], G37 methylation of tRNA^{Sep} in *E. coli* might increase the overall efficiency of the Sep-OTS. However, it is unknown whether the essential *E. coli* methyltransferase TrmD—an evolutionarily divergent homolog of Trm5—can catalyze the methylation of tRNA^{Sep} G37 [18]. We were unable to assess the influence of TrmD on tRNA^{Sep}, as the *trmD* deletion strain is not part of the Keio collection. Therefore, to test whether methylation of tRNA^{Sep} G37 can increase aminoacylation by SepRS, and, consequently, Sep incorporation, we co-expressed archaeal Trm5 with tRNA^{Sep} in *E. coli*. We tested this system in the absence and presence of a SepRS mutant (SepRS9) that was previously engineered to improve the aminoacylation of tRNA^{Sep} by altering its anticodon binding domain [31]. The effect of Trm5 on tRNA^{Sep} was monitored by using a super-folder GFP (sfGFP) reporter gene [33] with an amber UAG codon replacing a Ser codon at position 2 (sfGFP-2TAG, [19]). In this assay, suppression (read-through) of the amber stop codon by tRNA^{Sep} leads to synthesis of sfGFP (Figure 1b). Using this platform, we found that the orthogonality of tRNA^{Sep} in the absence of SepRS appears to be compromised by host aaRSs (previously, Gln incorporation has been reported, [15]). However, in the presence of SepRS9, sfGFP synthesis was reduced, which is the result of tRNA^{Sep} sequestration by SepRS that prevents misacylation of tRNA^{Sep} by host aaRSs and reduces read-through. Interestingly, co-expression of Trm5 improved tRNA^{Sep} orthogonality almost sixfold. This result suggests that methylation of G37 can significantly prevent aminoacylation of tRNA^{Sep} by *E. coli* aaRSs (Figure 2b). Low sfGFP yields in cells co-expressing Trm5 and wild-type SepRS suggest that the G37 methylation does not improve the aminoacylation activity of wild-type SepRS for tRNA^{Sep} (Figure 2b). On the other hand, expression of SepRS9 with Trm5 increased the GFP yields approximately twofold, indicating that the anticodon binding domain of SepRS9 is more accommodating for the CUA anticodon with the adjacent G37 methyl group. However, the Phos-tag^{TM} analysis indicates that a significant amount of misincorporation still occurs in the presence of Trm5 and SepRS9 (Figure 2b).

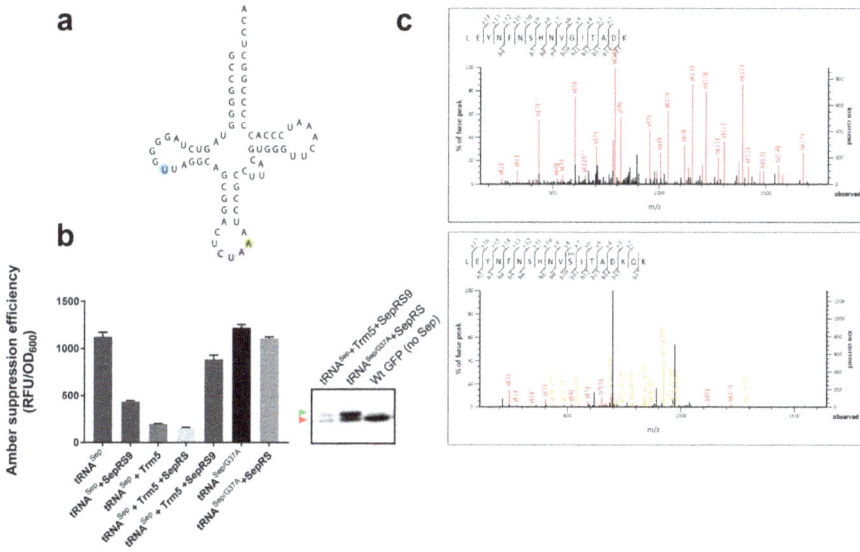

Figure 2. (**a**) Secondary structure of tRNA$^{Sep/G37A}$. Anticodon bases are highlighted and the G37A mutation is indicated. (**b**) The effect of *M. maripaludis* Trm5 on the stop codon read-through with original tRNA^{Sep} and tRNA$^{Sep/G37A}$ in the presence or absence of wild-type SepRS or SepRS9 variant. sfGFP-2TAG expression was monitored by fluorescence in a BL21(DE3) strain grown in Luria-Bertani (LB) medium supplemented with 5 mM Sep. Responses were taken at 20 h. The amber suppression efficiency is measured relative to the cell density (OD$_{600}$). Phos-tag^{TM} mobility shift analysis of GFP-2TAG isolated from the strains harboring tRNA^{Sep}, SepRS9, and Trm5 and tRNA$^{Sep/G37A}$ variant and wild-type SepRS. OTS components are indicated above the wells. Proteins were detected by Western blot using anti-GFP antibodies. The green arrow indicates the position of the Sep-containing GFP, while the red one points to the position of cAA-containing GFP. (**c**) Endogenous GlyRS likely charges MjtRNA^{Sep} with Gly. LC-MS/MS analyses of sfGFP-151TAG demonstrate that in the presence of Sep-OTS (tRNA$^{Sep}_{CUA}$^{G37A} system), both Sep and Gly incorporation occur. The tandem mass spectrum of the peptides (residues 141–156) LEYNFNSHNVGITADK (ion score 116.5) and LEYNFNSHNVSepITADK (ion score 52.9) from purified sfGFP with one amber codon at position 151 from *E. coli* BL21 (DE3), using the tRNA$^{Sep}_{CUA}$^{G37A}-containing Sep-OTS. Cells were grown without additional Sep in the medium.

Because OTS optimization entails establishing a platform that maintains the o-aaRS aminoacylation efficiency, retains or increases o-tRNA orthogonality, and maximizes EF-Tu acceptance and o-tRNA decoding capacity, we decided to test a tRNA^{Sep} variant with a G37-to-A mutation (tRNA$^{Sep/G37A}$) that was previously shown to enhance the suppression activity of the tRNA [29]. Because G37 [34] and its methylated counterpart [32] act as determinants for SepRS aminoacylation, the success of o-tRNA$^{Sep/G37A}$ most likely originates from its improved decoding ability [26]. In fact, adenosine at position 37 is common in strong natural and artificial UAG suppressors [3,35], suggesting that A37 improves the tRNA suppression activity. It is well known that the stabilizing modifications such as ct^{6}Aand ms^{2}i^{6}A accompany weak A1-U36 or U1-A36 codon–anticodon base pairs in *E. coli* (the same base pairing pattern occurs in the decoding of amber stop codons). Indeed, co-expression of SepRS and tRNA$^{Sep/G37A}$ yielded a similar suppression efficiency as that of tRNA$^{Sep/G37A}$ alone, and a 2.5× increase in comparison to G37-containing tRNA^{Sep}. Although G73A did not improve tRNA orthogonality, it improved the suppression efficiency without decreasing the percentage of specific Sep incorporation (Figure 2b). In addition to Phos-tag^{TM} analysis, we confirmed Sep incorporation in a purified recombinant sfGFP using tandem mass spectrometry (LC-MS/MS) (Figure 2c). In addition to Sep, Gly was detected. This can result from misacylation of tRNA$^{Sep/G37A}$, which shares sequence elements with *E. coli* tRNA^{Gly}, with Gly by *E. coli* glycyl-tRNA synthetase [34,36].

3.2. Sep-OTS Activity in the Absence of Individual Post-transcriptional Modification Enzymes

In *E. coli*, an archaeal o-tRNA can be challenged by endogenous tRNA modification enzymes that (a) may introduce bacteria-specific modifications (only half of archaeal modifications are found in bacterial milieu) and (b) can act on the o-tRNA in a sequence-specific manner characteristic of bacterial tRNAs [23,37]. On the other hand, archaeal o-tRNAs can also be challenged by the absence of native archaeal modifications. For example, specific modifications that contribute to tRNA folding and stabilization might be missing in bacteria [38,39].

To determine if heterologous tRNA modifications play a role in the activity of Sep-OTS in *E. coli*, we used the sfGFP2-TAG reporter assay in a series of *E. coli* single-gene knockout strains from Keio collection [18]. These strains are suitable for stop codon read-through assays, because they do not possess genomic copies of tRNA suppressors, and, as indicated by the sfGFP-2TAG synthesis in tRNA$^{Sep/G37A}$ absence (Supplementary Figure S2), show very low levels (<1%) of near cognate suppression. Therefore, the observed sfGFP-2TAG production is exclusively based on the activity of tRNA$^{Sep/G37A}$. We tested 42 strains in which a single gene encoding a nonessential enzyme involved in post-transcriptional tRNA modification was deleted (a full list of strains is given in Supplementary Table S1). Although only a few of these enzymes operate independently, we decided to investigate all enzymes participating in the biosynthesis of post-transcriptional modifications because of their mutual interactions and their connection to other metabolic processes [40–42].

We observed significant variations in the efficiency of the Sep-OTS in the absence of particular modification enzymes (Figure 3a, Supplementary Figures S3 and S4, Tables S3 and S4). For example, in the strains lacking GluQRS, MiaA, ThiI, or TruB, sfGFP expression was decreased. Enzymes MiaA, ThiI, and TruB are involved in the i^{6}A37, s^{4}U8, and Ψ55 modifications, respectively, suggesting that these modifications may be important for the activity of the Sep-OTS. How the absence of GluQRS impairs sfGFP synthesis is unclear since this enzyme operates on U34, which is missing in tRNA$^{Sep/G37A}$ (Supplementary Table S1). Synthesis of wild-type sfGFP in ΔthiI and ΔtruB strains demonstrates that in these strains the overall translation is somewhat diminished (Supplementary Figure S5 and Table S5), thereby indicating that their absence might affect the activities of endogenous tRNAs, not only tRNA$^{Sep/G37A}$. In contrast, the yield of WT sfGFP in the ΔmiaA strain is comparable to the yield in the wild-type BW25113 strain (Supplementary Figure S5 and Table S5), implying that the lack of i^{6}A37 modification directly affects tRNA$^{Sep/G37A}$ (and therefore Sep-OTS).

3.3. Effects of Post-transcriptional Modifications on the Orthogonality of tRNA$^{Sep/G37A}$

We also analyzed the role of modifications on the orthogonality of tRNA$^{Sep/G37A}$ by expressing this tRNA in the absence of SepRS (Figure 3b, Supplementary Figure S4). In this context, a decrease in sfGFP expression signal can be interpreted as an increase in tRNA$^{Sep/G37A}$ orthogonality, which may be related to the absence of modifications that improve mischarging of tRNA$^{Sep/G37A}$ by endogenous aaRSs. Mischarging with canonical amino acids (cAAs) results in the cAA-tRNA$^{Sep/G37A}$ formation which can seemingly increase the sfGFP-2TAG synthesis, mask the true Sep incorporation efficacy, and reduce Sep incorporation by competing for the binding to the UAG codons (discussed in Sections 3.4 and 3.5).

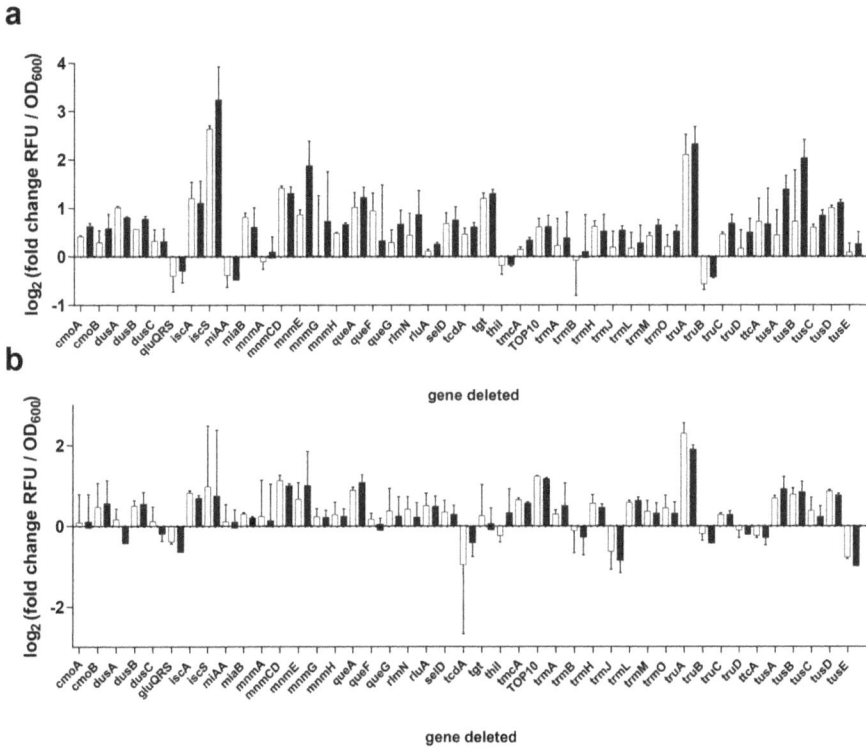

Figure 3. Stop codon read-through assays with sfGFP-2TAG in 42 selected Keio collection strains with full Sep-OTS (**a**) and with suppressor tRNA$^{Sep}_{CUA}$^{G37A} only (**b**). First column (white) corresponds to the signal recorded in the media without, and the second (black) with 5 mM Sep. Fold change values were derived from 4–8 (**a**) and 3–6 biological replicates (**b**).

Some of the strains allow for minor improvements in tRNA$^{Sep/G37A}$ orthogonality (1.4–1.8-fold) according to the mean decrease in sfGFP synthesis. Corresponding decreases were recorded in strains lacking GluQRS, TrmJ, and TusE (Figure 3b, Supplementary Table S4). Strains lacking DusA, TcdA, TruB, TtcA offer a marginal improvement of 1.2–1.4-fold. Among these enzymes, DusA, TcdA, TrmJ, TruB, and TtcA can theoretically operate on tRNA$^{Sep/G37A}$ (Supplementary Table S1). TrmJ and TtcA modify base C32, thereby influencing the conformation of the anticodon stem-loop. The corresponding modifications Cm and s^{2}C reduce the RNA conformational flexibility, thereby making this tRNA part rigid [26]. Because anticodon stem-loop modifications directly influence its conformation, the lack of these modifications may result in mirrored effects in screens with or without SepRS; in other words, the lack of modifications placed in the tRNA anticodon will, most likely, reflect the changes in the tRNAs' decoding capacity. DusA catalyzes dihydrouridine formation on U20, which influences D-loop flexibility and tRNA folding [22]. TcdA acts on premodified base A37, which is not likely to form in the context of tRNA$^{Sep/G37A}$ [43]. Because wild-type GFP translation is decreased in both Δ*tcdA* and Δ*ttcA*, these enzymes may affect overall translation (Supplementary Figure S5 and Table S5), whereas DusA and TrmJ may actually introduce modifications in tRNA$^{Sep/G37A}$ that influence its orthogonality. In contrast, deletion of *truB* decreases sfGFP-2TAG synthesis in the absence and presence of SepRS; thus, it is likely that the corresponding modification influences tRNA$^{Sep/G37A}$ stability overall, and not the interaction of tRNA$^{Sep/G37A}$ with endogenous aaRSs.

The highest increase in sfGFP synthesis occurs in *E. coli* strains lacking IscS, MnmCD, MnmE, TGT, TruA, TusA, or TusB enzymes (Figure 3a, Supplementary Table S3). However, this effect is accompanied by a decrease in orthogonality (Figure 3b, Supplementary Table S4). In comparison with the wild-type strain, a significant decrease in orthogonality also occurs in the ∆queA strain. MnmCD, MnmE, QueA, and TGT should not act on $tRNA^{Sep/G37A}$, as this tRNA does not possess the necessary nucleotide sequence for their recognition (Supplementary Table S1). It is possible that the lack of modifications on the *E. coli* tRNAs reduces the affinity of their corresponding aaRSs, resulting in improved misacylation of $tRNA^{Sep/G37A}$. IscS, TusA, and TusB participate in the sulfur transfer required for the biosynthesis of sulfur-containing post-transcriptional modifications [44] and have no tRNA substrates as such. Curiously, sfGFP-2TAG synthesis is approximately twofold higher in *E. coli* TOP10 cells containing $tRNA^{Sep/G37A}$, indicating that the BW25113 genetic background might be more appropriate for Sep-OTS-assisted stop codon suppression and production of Sep-containing proteins.

3.4. Deletion of iscS Leads to a Significant Increase of Sep-Containing sfGFP

Efficiency of site-specific incorporation of ncAAs via nonsense suppression depends on the catalytic prowess of the OTS [3], the availability of ncAA (depending on the ncAA intake and its participation in the cellular metabolism, [45]), the suitability of ncAA-o-tRNA for EF-Tu binding [12], and the capacity of ncAA-o-tRNA to decode the stop codon of interest [26] and outcompete the release factor for binding to the same site [46]. Because each of these processes is usually less efficient than for endogenous translation systems, yields of ncAA-containing proteins are typically low. Prompted by the fact that some of the deletion strains tested in this study show markedly increased yields of GFP-2TAG (Figure 3a), we decided to quantitatively explore the efficiency of Sep incorporation in these strains. We isolated GFP-2TAG synthesized in the presence of Sep-OTS in these select strains and analyzed the level of Sep incorporation by Phos-tag^{TM} technology [47].

We chose strains with medium (∆dusA, ∆dusB, ∆iscA, ∆trmJ, and ∆tusD) and high (∆iscS, ∆mnmCD, ∆mnmE, ∆truA, ∆tusA, and ∆tusB) increases in GFP-2TAG synthesis relative to the wild-type (parental BW25113) strain. GFP isolated from these strains was subjected to Phos-tag^{TM} analysis—a mobility shift assay using an alkoxide-bridged dinuclear metal complex that can be employed to monitor stoichiometric incorporation of Sep [47]. Because phosphoserine residues form complexes with Mn^{2+}-ions immobilized within the gel via chelating agent Phos-tag^{TM}, the fraction with Sep-containing GFP is decelerated in the gel and separates from the cAA-containing GFP. Using anti-GFP antibodies, these fractions can be quantified and relative amounts of Sep-GFP in the total mixture calculated (Figure 4a,b).

The result of Phos-tag^{TM} analysis is shown in Figure 4a. Densitometric quantification of the slower, Sep-containing fraction shows that in the wild-type strain, Sep-GFP accounts for 65% of the total protein. This ratio is preserved in ∆dusB, ∆iscS, ∆trmJ, and ∆tusA strains (57%, 54%, 58%, and 53% of Sep-GFP, respectively). In strains ∆dusA, ∆mnmCD, ∆mnmE, and ∆truA, it is considerably lower (33%, 37%, 37%, and 39%, respectively). The mean increase in GFP production, as monitored by the fluorescence (Figure 3a), multiplied by the fraction of Sep-containing GFP, as determined by Phos-tag^{TM} analysis (Figure 4b), allows us to establish factual increases in Sep-GFP production (Figure 4c). These values demonstrate that deletion strains lacking TruA, TusB, and MnmE, while showing more than fourfold increase in total GFP synthesis, provide a less than threefold improvement in Sep-GFP production. While this is still an improvement, ∆dusA and ∆trmJ—strains with moderate (less than twofold) increases in GFP-2TAG production (Figure 3a, Supplementary Figure S3 and Table S3)—actually produce less Sep-GFP than the wild-type (Figure 4c). In conclusion, only the *iscS* deletion strain offers a substantial improvement in Sep-GFP synthesis (Figure 4c).

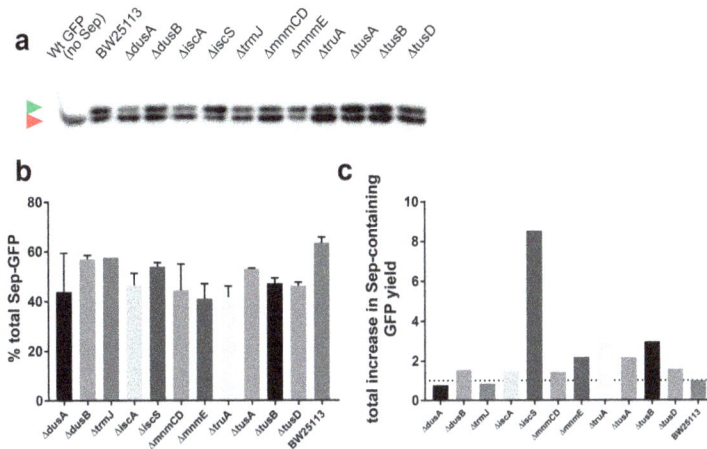

Figure 4. Some of the deletion strains showing increased GFP-2TAG synthesis while preserving the relative Sep-GFP to cAA-GFP ratio. (**a**) Phos-tag™ mobility shift analysis of GFP-2TAG isolated from the corresponding knockout strains. Strain names are indicated above the wells. Proteins were analyzed by the Phos-tag method and detected by Western blot using anti-GFP antibodies. The green arrow shows the position of the Sep-containing GFP, while the red one points to the position of nonphosphorylated, cAA-containing GFP. Wild-type GFP controls are also shown. (**b**) Quantification of the shifted bands allows the estimation of Sep incorporation efficiency. Percentages of Sep-modified GFP in the corresponding isolate are shown. Values are presented as mean ± S.D. derived from two biological replicates. (**c**) Mean increase in total GFP-2TAG synthesis (Figure 3, Supplementary Figure S3 and Table S3) multiplied by the mean percentage of Sep-containing GFP in the matching strain shows the factual increase in Sep-GFP production.

3.5. Overexpression of MiaA and TruB Leads to a Higher Purity of Sep-Containing sfGFP

The analysis of the Sep-OTS-facilitated production of GFP-2TAG in the deletion strains (Figure 3a, Supplementary Table S3) suggested that the modifications i^6A37, s^4U8, and $\Psi55$ influence Sep-OTS performance. Because natural tRNA suppressors lacking i^6A are significantly less active [35,48], we decided to test whether overexpression of dimethylallyltransferase MiaA can increase production of Sep-GFP. The i^6A37 modification in the anticodon loop prevents unwanted hydrogen bond formation between the C32 and A38, as well as the A37 and U33, thereby ensuring productive conformation of this element [26]. The A36-A37-A38 motif (present in tRNA$^{Sep/G37A}$, Figure 2a) serves as an identity element for the *E. coli* MiaA enzyme [49]. In addition to MiaA, we examined pseudouridine synthase TruB, which not only catalyzes pseudouridine formation but also acts as a general RNA chaperone [50]. We reasoned that the overexpression of MiaA and TruB may increase the fraction of tRNA$^{Sep/G37A}$ with i^6A37 and $\Psi55$, respectively, while TruB may also facilitate folding of this o-tRNA.

Genes encoding MiaA and TruB were separately introduced into a pCDF-derived plasmid containing a copy of the *SepRS* gene. We decided to place the *miaA* and *truB* genes under the control of the arabinose promoter to enable tight control of their expression, while *SepRS* expression was driven by the constitutive *lpp* promoter. This experimental design allows us to compare Sep-OTS assisted sfGFP-2TAG production with natural and artificially increased levels of MiaA and TruB.

Contrary to our expectations, the total Sep-OTS assisted sfGFP-2TAG synthesis decreases upon stimulation of MiaA and TruB expression (Figure 5a). In BW25113, the mean fluorescence signal of the sfGFP-2TAG reporter decreases 1.3-fold in the case of MiaA and 2.1-fold for TruB overexpression relative to the cells expressing these enzymes solely from the chromosomal loci. However, homogeneity of Sep incorporation significantly improves upon overexpression of either MiaA or TruB, with Sep-GFP yields amounting to 81% and 88%, respectively, as analyzed by Phos-tag^{TM} (Figure 5b).

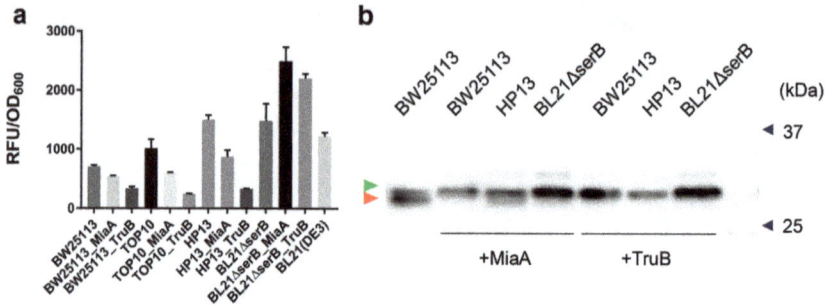

Figure 5. Overexpression of MiaA and TruB does not improve total yields of sfGFP-2TAG, but improves specific Sep incorporation markedly. (**a**) Stop codon read-through facilitated by Sep-OTS in the presence of overexpressed MiaA and TruB. Assay was executed in the strains BW25113 and TOP10, as well as the *serB* deletion strains BL21ΔserB and HP13. The values represent the mean ± S.D. derived from 4–8 biological replicates. (**b**) Phos-tag^{TM} mobility shift analysis of GFP-2TAG isolated from the corresponding strains (marked above the membrane). Overexpression of MiaA and TruB is indicated. Deleted genes are denoted above the wells, except for the parental BW25113 strain. Proteins were detected by Western blot using anti-GFP antibodies. The green arrow shows the position of the Sep-containing fraction, while the red one points to the position of nonphosphorylated, wild-type GFP. Control fraction containing GFP isolated from the BW25113 strain is also shown.

Sep is naturally synthesized in *E. coli* as part of the Ser metabolic pathway. Because Sep is effectively converted to Ser by the phosphoserine phosphatase SerB, its cellular concentration is low [45]. Thus, Sep-OTS-assisted read-through increases with Sep supplementation (Figure 3, Figure 4, and Figures S2–S4). Alternatively, the intracellular levels of Sep can be increased by deleting the *serB* gene [15,45]. However, in the *E. coli* strains HP13 (a TOP10 derivative) and BL21ΔserB, which lack the *serB* gene, the stimulation of Sep-OTS-aided sfGFP-2TAG read-through is markedly different (Figure 5a,b). This may be explained by the differences in metabolic fluxes between K12 and BL21 strains [51]. Compared with its parental TOP10 strain, HP13 allows a marginal (less than 1.5-fold) improvement of sfGFP-2TAG synthesis with MiaA overexpression. In the case of TruB overexpression, sfGFP-2TAG levels are comparably low in both cell strains. In terms of Sep-GFP homogeneity, the high purity of Sep-GFP isolated from the HP13-TruB overexpressing strain is preserved (94%), while purity decreases to 42% when MiaA is overexpressed in HP13 (Figure 5 and Figure S6). In the BL21ΔserB and wild-type BW25113 strains, sfGFP-2TAG synthesis significantly improved when either MiaA or TruB were overexpressed (4.6- and 4.1-fold improvement, respectively, Figure S6).

Based on the Phos-tag^{TM} analysis of GFP-2TAG isolated from the wild-type BW25113 strain, a considerable fraction of tRNA$^{Sep/G37A}$ is misacylated by *E. coli* aaRSs, which prevents the synthesis of homogenous protein samples. While orthogonality tests can estimate a tRNA's apparent orthogonality, in the absence of the cognate o-aaRS, the pool of deacylated o-tRNA increases, allowing it to compete for binding with endogenous aaRSs more easily. This phenomenon is exemplified by the *iscS* deletion strain, where apparent orthogonality decreases approximately twofold in the stop codon read-through assay, but analysis of the relative amounts of Sep-GFP in the mixture revealed that the relative misacylation is comparable to what is occurring in the wild-type BW25113 strain. While methods to accurately quantify ncAA incorporation in proteins are costly and less accessible, they are necessary in establishing the strength and efficiency of a particular OTS [52].

4. Conclusions

The efficiency of Sep-OTS—a translation system designed to synthesize proteins with Sep—was evaluated in a series of *E. coli* strains with deletions of single genes responsible for nucleotide modifications of tRNAs. Several *E. coli* enzymes were identified that positively affected the synthesis of a GFP reporter variant containing Sep. An *iscS* deletion strain enables more than eightfold higher production of this variant, while overexpression of the MiaA and TruB enzymes significantly improve the specificity of the Sep incorporation. This work provides new evidence highlighting the role of tRNA modification in efficient translation. This will help the design and construction of better o-tRNAs.

Supplementary Materials: The following are available online at www.mdpi.com/2306-5354/5/1/11/s1, Figure S1: Plasmid maps used in this study. Figure S2: Levels of near cognate suppression in selected Keio deletion strains. Figure S3: Levels of amber codon suppression efficiency in the selected Keio deletion in presence of Sep-OTS. Figure S4: Levels of amber codon suppression efficiency in the selected Keio deletion strains in presence of nonsense suppressor tRNA$^{Sep}_{CUA}$ G37A. Figure S5: Levels of wild-type sfGFP synthesis in the tested Keio collection strains. Figure S6: Quantification of the shifted bands corresponding to Sep-GFP yields observed in presence of increased amounts of MiaA and TruB. Table S1: List of Keio knockout strains employed in this study. Table S2: Plasmids used in this study. Table S3: Statistical analysis of the sfGFP-2TAG synthesis in the Keio deletion strains in presence of Sep-OTS. Table S4: Statistical analysis of the sfGFP-2TAG synthesis in the Keio deletion strains in presence of tRNA$^{Sep/G37A}$. Table S5: Statistical analysis of the sfGFP synthesis in the Keio deletion strains.

Acknowledgments: This work was supported by grants from the US National Institutes of Health (NIH) (R35GM122560) and from the Division of Chemical Sciences, Geosciences, and Biosciences, Office of Basic Energy Sciences of the Department of Energy (DE-FG02-98ER20311) to D.S. We thank all members of the Söll lab for enlightened discussions.

Author Contributions: A.C., O.V.-R. and D.S. conceived and designed the experiments; A.C. and A.M. performed the experiments; A.C. and O.V.-R. analyzed the data; all authors wrote the paper.

Conflicts of Interest: The authors declare no conflict of interest.

References

1. Gagner, J.E.; Kim, W.; Chaikof, E.L. Designing protein-based biomaterials for medical applications. *Acta Biomater.* **2014**, *10*, 1542–1557. [CrossRef] [PubMed]
2. Chin, J.W. Expanding and reprogramming the genetic code. *Nature* **2017**, *550*, 53–60. [CrossRef] [PubMed]
3. Dumas, A.; Lercher, L.; Spicer, C.D.; Davis, B.G. Designing logical codon reassignment—Expanding the chemistry in biology. *Chem. Sci.* **2015**, *6*, 50–69. [CrossRef] [PubMed]
4. Koole, C.; Reynolds, C.A.; Mobarec, J.C.; Hick, C.; Sexton, P.M.; Sakmar, T.P. Genetically encoded photocross-linkers determine the biological binding site of exendin-4 peptide in the N-terminal domain of the intact human glucagon-like peptide-1 receptor (GLP-1R). *J. Biol. Chem.* **2017**, *292*, 7131–7144. [CrossRef] [PubMed]
5. Voller, J.S.; Dulic, M.; Gerling-Driessen, U.I.; Biava, H.; Baumann, T.; Budisa, N.; Gruic-Sovulj, I.; Koksch, B. Discovery and Investigation of Natural Editing Function against Artificial Amino Acids in Protein Translation. *ACS Cent. Sci.* **2017**, *3*, 73–80. [CrossRef] [PubMed]
6. Tang, Y.; Tirrell, D.A. Biosynthesis of a highly stable coiled-coil protein containing hexafluoroleucine in an engineered bacterial host. *J. Am. Chem. Soc.* **2001**, *123*, 11089–11090. [CrossRef] [PubMed]
7. Melo Czekster, C.; Robertson, W.E.; Walker, A.S.; Söll, D.; Schepartz, A. In Vivo Biosynthesis of a beta-Amino Acid-Containing Protein. *J. Am. Chem. Soc.* **2016**, *138*, 5194–5197. [CrossRef] [PubMed]
8. Carrico, I.S.; Maskarinec, S.A.; Heilshorn, S.C.; Mock, M.L.; Liu, J.C.; Nowatzki, P.J.; Franck, C.; Ravichandran, G.; Tirrell, D.A. Lithographic patterning of photoreactive cell-adhesive proteins. *J. Am. Chem. Soc.* **2007**, *129*, 4874–4875. [CrossRef] [PubMed]
9. Hauf, M.; Richter, F.; Schneider, T.; Faidt, T.; Martins, B.M.; Baumann, T.; Durkin, P.; Dobbek, H.; Jacobs, K.; Moglich, A.; et al. Photoactivatable Mussel-Based Underwater Adhesive Proteins by an Expanded Genetic Code. *Chembiochem* **2017**, *18*, 1819–1823. [CrossRef] [PubMed]
10. Packer, M.S.; Liu, D.R. Methods for the directed evolution of proteins. *Nat. Rev. Genet.* **2015**, *16*, 379–394. [CrossRef] [PubMed]

11. Yang, A.; Ha, S.; Ahn, J.; Kim, R.; Kim, S.; Lee, Y.; Kim, J.; Söll, D.; Lee, H.Y.; Park, H.S. A chemical biology route to site-specific authentic protein modifications. *Science* **2016**, *354*, 623–626. [CrossRef] [PubMed]
12. Reynolds, N.M.; Vargas-Rodriguez, O.; Söll, D.; Crnkovic, A. The central role of tRNA in genetic code expansion. *Biochim. Biophys. Acta* **2017**, *1861*, 3001–3008. [CrossRef] [PubMed]
13. Lin, X.; Yu, A.C.; Chan, T.F. Efforts and Challenges in Engineering the Genetic Code. *Life* **2017**, *7*, 12. [CrossRef] [PubMed]
14. Krishnakumar, R.; Prat, L.; Aerni, H.R.; Ling, J.; Merryman, C.; Glass, J.I.; Rinehart, J.; Söll, D. Transfer RNA misidentification scrambles sense codon recoding. *Chembiochem* **2013**, *14*, 1967–1972. [CrossRef] [PubMed]
15. Park, H.S.; Hohn, M.J.; Umehara, T.; Guo, L.T.; Osborne, E.M.; Benner, J.; Noren, C.J.; Rinehart, J.; Söll, D. Expanding the genetic code of *Escherichia coli* with phosphoserine. *Science* **2011**, *333*, 1151–1154. [CrossRef] [PubMed]
16. Yu, A.C.; Yim, A.K.; Mat, W.K.; Tong, A.H.; Lok, S.; Xue, H.; Tsui, S.K.; Wong, J.T.; Chan, T.F. Mutations enabling displacement of tryptophan by 4-fluorotryptophan as a canonical amino acid of the genetic code. *Genome Biol. Evol.* **2014**, *6*, 629–641. [CrossRef] [PubMed]
17. El Yacoubi, B.; Bailly, M.; de Crecy-Lagard, V. Biosynthesis and function of posttranscriptional modifications of transfer RNAs. *Annu. Rev. Genet.* **2012**, *46*, 69–95. [CrossRef] [PubMed]
18. Baba, T.; Ara, T.; Hasegawa, M.; Takai, Y.; Okumura, Y.; Baba, M.; Datsenko, K.A.; Tomita, M.; Wanner, B.L.; Mori, H. Construction of *Escherichia coli* K-12 in-frame, single-gene knockout mutants: The Keio collection. *Mol. Syst. Biol.* **2006**, *2*. [CrossRef] [PubMed]
19. Ko, J.H.; Wang, Y.S.; Nakamura, A.; Guo, L.T.; Söll, D.; Umehara, T. Pyrrolysyl-tRNA synthetase variants reveal ancestral aminoacylation function. *FEBS Lett.* **2013**, *587*, 3243–3248. [CrossRef] [PubMed]
20. Englert, M.; Vargas-Rodriguez, O.; Reynolds, N.M.; Wang, Y.S.; Söll, D.; Umehara, T. A genomically modified *Escherichia coli* strain carrying an orthogonal *E. coli* histidyl-tRNA synthetase•tRNA^{His} pair. *Biochim. Biophys. Acta* **2017**, *1861*, 3009–3015. [CrossRef] [PubMed]
21. Schneider, C.A.; Rasband, W.S.; Eliceiri, K.W. NIH Image to ImageJ: 25 years of image analysis. *Nat. Methods* **2012**, *9*, 671–675. [CrossRef] [PubMed]
22. Väre, V.Y.; Eruysal, E.R.; Narendran, A.; Sarachan, K.L.; Agris, P.F. Chemical and Conformational Diversity of Modified Nucleosides Affects tRNA Structure and Function. *Biomolecules* **2017**, *7*, 29. [CrossRef] [PubMed]
23. Lorenz, C.; Lünse, C.E.; Mörl, M. tRNA modifications: Impact on structure and thermal adaptation. *Biomolecules* **2017**, *7*, 35. [CrossRef] [PubMed]
24. Jackman, J.E.; Alfonzo, J.D. Transfer RNA modifications: Nature's combinatorial chemistry playground. *Wiley Interdiscip. Rev. RNA* **2013**, *4*, 35–48. [CrossRef] [PubMed]
25. Giege, R.; Sissler, M.; Florentz, C. Universal rules and idiosyncratic features in tRNA identity. *Nucleic Acids Res.* **1998**, *26*, 5017–5035. [CrossRef] [PubMed]
26. Grosjean, H.; Westhof, E. An integrated, structure- and energy-based view of the genetic code. *Nucleic Acids Res.* **2016**, *44*, 8020–8040. [CrossRef] [PubMed]
27. Christian, T.; Hou, Y.M. Distinct determinants of tRNA recognition by the TrmD and Trm5 methyl transferases. *J. Mol. Biol.* **2007**, *373*, 623–632. [CrossRef] [PubMed]
28. Josefowicz, S.Z.; Shimada, M.; Armache, A.; Li, C.H.; Miller, R.M.; Lin, S.; Yang, A.; Dill, B.D.; Molina, H.; Park, H.S.; et al. Chromatin Kinases Act on Transcription Factors and Histone Tails in Regulation of Inducible Transcription. *Mol. Cell* **2016**, *64*, 347–361. [CrossRef] [PubMed]
29. Pirman, N.L.; Barber, K.W.; Aerni, H.R.; Ma, N.J.; Haimovich, A.D.; Rogulina, S.; Isaacs, F.J.; Rinehart, J. A flexible codon in genomically recoded *Escherichia coli* permits programmable protein phosphorylation. *Nat. Commun.* **2015**, *6*, 8130. [CrossRef] [PubMed]
30. Rogerson, D.T.; Sachdeva, A.; Wang, K.; Haq, T.; Kazlauskaite, A.; Hancock, S.M.; Huguenin-Dezot, N.; Muqit, M.M.; Fry, A.M.; Bayliss, R.; et al. Efficient genetic encoding of phosphoserine and its nonhydrolyzable analog. *Nat. Chem. Biol.* **2015**, *11*, 496–503. [CrossRef] [PubMed]
31. Lee, S.; Oh, S.; Yang, A.; Kim, J.; Söll, D.; Lee, D.; Park, H.S. A Facile Strategy for Selective Incorporation of Phosphoserine into Histones. *Angew. Chem. Int. Ed.* **2013**, *52*, 5771–5775. [CrossRef] [PubMed]
32. Zhang, C.M.; Liu, C.; Slater, S.; Hou, Y.M. Aminoacylation of tRNA with phosphoserine for synthesis of cysteinyl-tRNA^{Cys}. *Nat. Struct. Mol. Biol.* **2008**, *15*, 507–514. [CrossRef] [PubMed]

33. Cotlet, M.; Goodwin, P.M.; Waldo, G.S.; Werner, J.H. A comparison of the fluorescence dynamics of single molecules of a green fluorescent protein: One- versus two-photon excitation. *Chemphyschem* **2006**, *7*, 250–260. [CrossRef] [PubMed]

34. Hohn, M.J.; Park, H.S.; O'Donoghue, P.; Schnitzbauer, M.; Söll, D. Emergence of the universal genetic code imprinted in an RNA record. *Proc. Natl. Acad. Sci. USA* **2006**, *103*, 18095–18100. [CrossRef] [PubMed]

35. Gefter, M.L.; Russell, R.L. Role modifications in tyrosine transfer RNA: A modified base affecting ribosome binding. *J. Mol. Biol.* **1969**, *39*, 145–157. [CrossRef]

36. Nameki, N.; Tamura, K.; Asahara, H.; Hasegawa, T. Recognition of tRNA^{Gly} by three widely diverged glycyl-tRNA synthetases. *J. Mol. Biol.* **1997**, *268*, 640–647. [CrossRef] [PubMed]

37. Biddle, W.; Schmitt, M.A.; Fisk, J.D. Modification of orthogonal tRNAs: Unexpected consequences for sense codon reassignment. *Nucleic Acids Res.* **2016**, *44*, 10042–10050. [CrossRef] [PubMed]

38. Bon Ramos, A.; Bao, L.; Turner, B.; de Crecy-Lagard, V.; Iwata-Reuyl, D. QueF-Like, a Non-Homologous Archaeosine Synthase from the Crenarchaeota. *Biomolecules* **2017**, *7*, 36. [CrossRef] [PubMed]

39. Oliva, R.; Tramontano, A.; Cavallo, L. Mg^{2+} binding and archaeosine modification stabilize the G15–C48 Levitt base pair in tRNAs. *RNA* **2007**, *13*, 1427–1436. [CrossRef] [PubMed]

40. Waller, J.C.; Ellens, K.W.; Hasnain, G.; Alvarez, S.; Rocca, J.R.; Hanson, A.D. Evidence that the Folate-Dependent Proteins YgfZ and MnmEG Have Opposing Effects on Growth and on Activity of the Iron-Sulfur Enzyme MiaB. *J. Bacteriol.* **2012**, *194*, 362–367. [CrossRef] [PubMed]

41. Arifuzzaman, M.; Maeda, M.; Itoh, A.; Nishikata, K.; Takita, C.; Saito, R.; Ara, T.; Nakahigashi, K.; Huang, H.C.; Hirai, A.; et al. Large-scale identification of protein-protein interaction of *Escherichia coli* K-12. *Genome Res.* **2006**, *16*, 686–691. [CrossRef] [PubMed]

42. Helm, M.; Alfonzo, J.D. Posttranscriptional RNA Modifications: Playing metabolic games in a cell's chemical Legoland. *Chem. Biol.* **2014**, *21*, 174–185. [CrossRef] [PubMed]

43. Thiaville, P.C.; Iwata-Reuyl, D.; de Crecy-Lagard, V. Diversity of the biosynthesis pathway for threonylcarbamoyladenosine (t^{6}A), a universal modification of tRNA. *RNA Biol.* **2014**, *11*, 1529–1539. [CrossRef] [PubMed]

44. Cavuzic, M.; Liu, Y. Biosynthesis of Sulfur-Containing tRNA Modifications: A Comparison of Bacterial, Archaeal, and Eukaryotic Pathways. *Biomolecules* **2017**, *7*, 27. [CrossRef] [PubMed]

45. Steinfeld, J.B.; Aerni, H.R.; Rogulina, S.; Liu, Y.; Rinehart, J. Expanded cellular amino acid pools containing phosphoserine, phosphothreonine, and phosphotyrosine. *ACS Chem. Biol.* **2014**, *9*, 1104–1112. [CrossRef] [PubMed]

46. Mukai, T.; Hayashi, A.; Iraha, F.; Sato, A.; Ohtake, K.; Yokoyama, S.; Sakamoto, K. Codon reassignment in the *Escherichia coli* genetic code. *Nucleic Acids Res.* **2010**, *38*, 8188–8195. [CrossRef] [PubMed]

47. Kosako, H. Phos-tag Western blotting for detecting stoichiometric protein phosphorylation in cells. *Nature* **2009**. [CrossRef]

48. Laten, H.; Gorman, J.; Bock, R.M. Isopentenyladenosine deficient tRNA from an antisuppressor mutant of *Saccharomyces cerevisiae*. *Nucleic Acids Res.* **1978**, *5*, 4329–4342. [CrossRef] [PubMed]

49. Soderberg, T.; Poulter, C.D. *Escherichia coli* dimethylallyl diphosphate: tRNA dimethylallyltransferase: Essential elements for recognition of tRNA substrates within the anticodon stem-loop. *Biochemistry* **2000**, *39*, 6546–6553. [CrossRef] [PubMed]

50. Keffer-Wilkes, L.C.; Veerareddygari, G.R.; Kothe, U. RNA modification enzyme TruB is a tRNA chaperone. *Proc. Natl. Acad. Sci. USA* **2016**, *113*, 14306–14311. [CrossRef] [PubMed]

51. Waegeman, H.; Beauprez, J.; Moens, H.; Maertens, J.; De Mey, M.; Foulquie-Moreno, M.R.; Heijnen, J.J.; Charlier, D.; Soetaert, W. Effect of *iclR* and *arcA* knockouts on biomass formation and metabolic fluxes in *Escherichia coli* K12 and its implications on understanding the metabolism of *Escherichia coli* BL21 (DE3). *BMC Microbiol.* **2011**, *11*, 70. [CrossRef] [PubMed]

52. Ho, J.M.; Reynolds, N.M.; Rivera, K.; Connolly, M.; Guo, L.T.; Ling, J.; Pappin, D.J.; Church, G.M.; Söll, D. Efficient Reassignment of a Frequent Serine Codon in Wild-Type *Escherichia coli*. *ACS Synth. Biol.* **2016**, *5*, 163–171. [CrossRef] [PubMed]

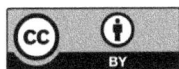

bioengineering

MDPI

Review

Progress in Integrative Biomaterial Systems to Approach Three-Dimensional Cell Mechanotransduction

Ying Zhang [1], Kin Liao [2], Chuan Li [3], Alvin C.K. Lai [4], Ji-Jinn Foo [5,*] and Vincent Chan [1,*]

[1] Department of Chemical Engineering, Khalifa University, Abu Dhabi 127788, UAE; chemicalbio@gmail.com
[2] Department of Aerospace Engineering, Khalifa University, Abu Dhabi 127788, UAE; kin.liao@kustar.ac.ae
[3] Department of Biomedical Engineering, National Yang Ming University, Taipei 11221, Taiwan; cli10@ym.edu.tw
[4] Department of Architecture and Civil Engineering, City University of Hong Kong, Tat Chee Avenue, Kowloon, Hong Kong; alvinlai@cityu.edu.hk
[5] School of Engineering, Monash University Malaysia, Jalan Lagoon Selatan, 46150 Bandar Sunway, Selangor, Malaysia
*   Correspondence: foo.ji.jinn@monash.edu (J.-J.F.); vincent.chan@kustar.ac.ae (V.C.)

Academic Editor: Gary Chinga Carrasco
Received: 1 May 2017; Accepted: 22 August 2017; Published: 24 August 2017

Abstract: Mechanotransduction between cells and the extracellular matrix regulates major cellular functions in physiological and pathological situations. The effect of mechanical cues on biochemical signaling triggered by cell–matrix and cell–cell interactions on model biomimetic surfaces has been extensively investigated by a combination of fabrication, biophysical, and biological methods. To simulate the in vivo physiological microenvironment in vitro, three dimensional (3D) microstructures with tailored bio-functionality have been fabricated on substrates of various materials. However, less attention has been paid to the design of 3D biomaterial systems with geometric variances, such as the possession of precise micro-features and/or bio-sensing elements for probing the mechanical responses of cells to the external microenvironment. Such precisely engineered 3D model experimental platforms pave the way for studying the mechanotransduction of multicellular aggregates under controlled geometric and mechanical parameters. Concurrently with the progress in 3D biomaterial fabrication, cell traction force microscopy (CTFM) developed in the field of cell biophysics has emerged as a highly sensitive technique for probing the mechanical stresses exerted by cells onto the opposing deformable surface. In the current work, we first review the recent advances in the fabrication of 3D micropatterned biomaterials which enable the seamless integration with experimental cell mechanics in a controlled 3D microenvironment. Then, we discuss the role of collective cell–cell interactions in the mechanotransduction of engineered tissue equivalents determined by such integrative biomaterial systems under simulated physiological conditions.

Keywords: mechanotransduction; soft lithography; cell-matrix interactions; cell–cell interactions; cell traction force microscopy; 3D tissue mechanics

---

1. Introduction

During tissue regeneration, the geometrical and mechanical cues of the surrounding microenvironment have been shown to regulate cellular responses, including migration, proliferation, differentiation, and apoptosis, etc. [1,2]. As such, tissue engineering traditionally refers to the development of various types of biomaterial scaffolds with specific bulk properties, such as porosity, microarchitecture, and compliance for extensive applications in cell therapy and tissue regeneration [3]. Although biomaterial scaffolding acts as a three-dimensional (3D) support for cell growth, it does not provide a highly engineered microenvironment with precise control in the location and morphology of various types of cells. Such spatial control is important for reestablishing the intricate organizations in the functional subunits of a typical organ. To overcome the limitations of biomaterial scaffolds, two-dimensional (2D) micropatterning of cells on various substrates has been exploited, with several techniques emerging, including microcontact printing [4], microfluidic patterning [5], photolithography [6,7], and plasma polymerization [8]. To date, surface features with spatial resolution of approximately 1 um can be fabricated by these techniques [9]. Increasingly, the 3D fabrication of precise microscale features which is not achievable with synthetic based approaches (e.g., hydrogel synthesis) is critical not only for controlling cell placement, but also for presenting spatially-controlled biological signals for the development of functional tissue constructs in vitro or in vivo [10]. In order to develop 3D micropatterned biomaterial scaffolds, several technical requirements in material selection, including mechanical properties, biocompatibility, and processability, must be thoroughly addressed for specific applications [11]. Recently, the advancement in 3D fabrication techniques has opened the possibility of attaining accurate spatial control of multiple cell types in engineered tissue equivalents. More importantly, such enabling technology facilitates the integration of cellular mechanical probes with a model microenvironment for studying intricate phenomena in mechanobiology [12]. Therefore, a timely review on the recent development of 3D cell patterning techniques in relation to the emerging investigations of 3D cellular mechanotransduction will highlight the importance of a generally ignored issue of mechanobiology for the design of tissue engineering products.

2. Cell Mechanotransduction

Mechanotransduction, which generally occurs at the cell–extracellular matrix (ECM) interface and cell–cell contacts, is the transmission of mechanical forces to biochemical signals and vice versa for the regulation of cellular physiology. Mechanical force fields in the 2D or 3D space containing cells and ECM, either in the form of externally applied forces or cellular traction forces produced by the cytoskeleton, have been intensely studied due to their important roles in maintaining homeostasis in tissues in vivo. Although the involvement of cell traction force (CTF) on cellular signaling and physiological function has been revealed, the precise mechanism of mechanotransduction in 3D systems remains to be elucidated [13]. In the physiological microenvironment, both cells and subcellular organelles can sense mechanical stresses from various sources, such as shear stress of flowing blood, mechanical stress from the surrounding ECM, and contractile forces from adjacent cells [13]. There are significant differences between external forces and cell-generated forces, which can be characterized from the differences in magnitude, direction, and distribution. However, certain indications on the existence of tight coupling between external applied forces and cell-generated forces have been highlighted [14,15]. For instance, biomacromolecules, such as carbohydrate-rich glycocalyx, which are found on the apical surface of vascular endothelial cells, have been shown to transmit fluid shear stress under blood flow to the cortical cytoskeleton [16]. In the mechanotransduction of the cardiovascular system, shear stress induced by flowing blood has been known to deform the endothelial cells at the inner wall of blood vessels and to trigger a cascade of cell signaling for the regulation of vascular physiology (Figure 1a). The endothelium mechanobiology, which leads to the generation of CTF (red arrows on Figure 1b indicate the direction of contractile forces), is actually governed by the highly synchronized interactions between external mechanical forces, cell–ECM adhesion, cytoskeletal protein binding, blood vessel stretching, cell–cell junction formation, and basal membrane mechanics, etc. (Figure 1b). Therefore, the mechanotransduction of cell layers will be thoroughly discussed herein by focusing on the feedback mechanisms of cell signaling with adjacent cells or ECM.

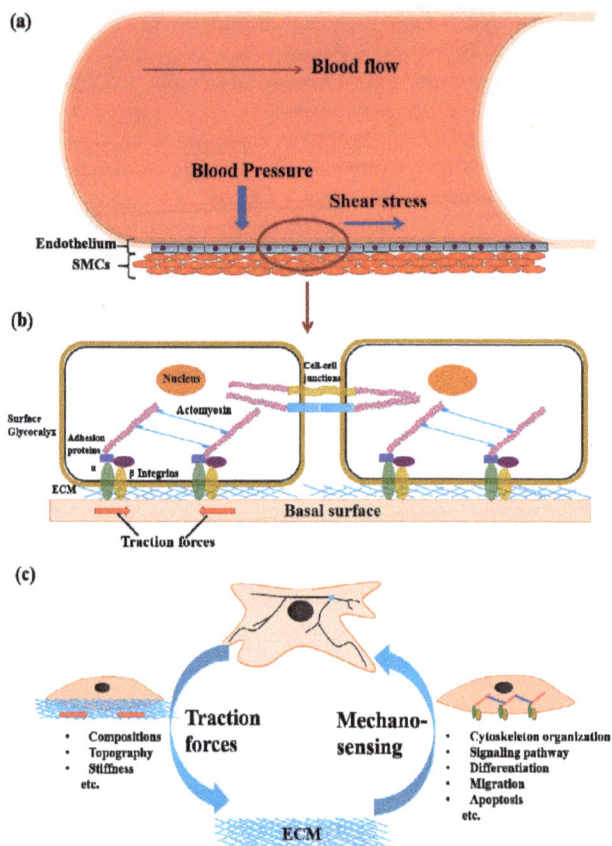

Figure 1. Schematic illustrations of (**a**) endothelial cells that form the interior surface of blood vessels subjected to stresses from the flowing blood; (**b**) The cell–cell junctions and cell–substrate tractions exerted by endothelial cells; (**c**) Positive feedback in cell–extracellular matrix (ECM) mechanotransduction. SMCs: smooth muscle cells.

In the first step of cell–ECM interaction, the binding between integrin and ECM protein triggers the assembly of focal adhesions (FAs) which in turn link the integrins to the actin filaments of the cytoskeleton with the help of adaptor proteins (e.g., talin, alpha actinin, vinculin) [17]. Moreover, FAs have been known to stabilize the adhesion sites by synergistic interactions of numerous signaling proteins (e.g., FAK, Ras, src) [18]. The biochemical processes involved in the generation of contractile force in cells after adhesion and spreading on the ECM or substrate are triggered by actomyosin interactions and actin polymerization [19,20]. These cell-generated forces, as mentioned above, are commonly known as CTF which are transmitted forward to the ECM through integrin, and then feed back to biochemical signals from ECM proteins to cytoskeletal proteins [21]. A series of molecular biology studies have revealed that CTF is associated with major cellular functions through their involvement in various signaling pathways. In smooth muscle cells (SMCs), CTF generation is mainly regulated by the Rho-kinase/ROCK pathway, which directly affects mitogen-induced DNA synthesis [22] and FA assembly [23]. As such, the presence of CTF plays a key role in modulating cell differentiation, migration, and apoptosis, and in maintaining cell homeostasis in the local microenvironment [24]. An emerging question on the intricate mechanisms of CTF regulations leading to various cellular responses needs to be better addressed. For instance, it has been demonstrated that the mechanotransduction response of cells towards principal substrate characteristics, such as stiffness and nanotopography, is linked to the talin-mediated mechanical regulation of the molecular clutch, integrin clustering, and FA dynamics [25,26].

Most anchorage-dependent cells, except endothelial cells and epithelial cells, are functional only in a 3D microenvironment in vivo. Thus, artificial 3D ECM networks have been developed as model systems for cell culture and bio-functional studies. In general, collagen in the form of a 3D network or a 2D gel has been widely used in various semi-quantitative assays of cell adhesion, biological functions, and chemotaxis. For instance, the phosphorylation level of focal adhesion kinase (FAK) in fibroblasts, which is associated with cell spreading, is reduced in 3D collagen gel matrix compared to that on 2D collagen gel, while the formation of FAs of fibroblasts in the 3D collagen gel matrix are triggered by the clustering of $\alpha_5\beta_1$ integrins instead of $\alpha_v\beta_3$ integrins found on the 2D collagen gel [27]. Comparing 3D to 2D collagen cultures of SMCs, an upregulation of p21 and transforming growth factor beta 1 (TGFβ1) expression, an upregulation of extracellular signal–regulated kinases (ERK) phosphorylation, and a downregulation of FAK phosphorylation have been found, which supports the role of geometrical factors of the microenvironment on cell proliferation and FA formation [28,29]. Similarly, an increase of matrix stiffness in 3D collagen network has been shown to promote the invasive phenotypes of mammalian epithelial cells, such as Rho-mediated contractility [30]. Also, primary dermal fibroblasts have switched from lamellipodia-based migration to lobopodia-based migration in response to the shift of the mechanics of 3D gel matrix from nonlinear elasticity to linear elasticity [31]. All results as mentioned above strongly suggest that the physical and mechanical properties of the ECM or biomaterial directly moderate the intricate mechanisms of cell adhesion and migration. Such influences have elicited the interplay between the mechanotransduction of adherent cells and molecular architecture of the biomaterial scaffold or ECM network.

The mechanotransduction of a single cell on 2D biomaterial has been extensively studied during the past two decades. CTF generated by the cytoskeletal remodeling of adherent cells is exerted to the ECM or material interfaces of the surrounding microenvironment through the anchoring of FAs. At the same time, the CTF of individual cells are influenced by both the surrounding ECM and neighboring cells. Under in vivo microenvironment, a cell migrates with the CTF generation on its surrounding ECM by synchronizing the protrusion and contraction at its leading edge and trailing edge, respectively. On the other hand, the collective mechanotransduction of multicellular aggregates in a 3D biomaterial, which has been studied to a lesser extent, likely influences major cellular physiology, including morphogenesis, wound healing, and embryogenesis. A recent study has reported the successful measurement of a CTF map exerted by an advancing epithelial cell sheet on a hydrogel matrix [32]. Moreover, CTF in relatively small cell colonies composed of 1–27 cells on 2D silicone gel has been found to be localized at the periphery of cell aggregate and is positively correlated with the colony size [33]. Interestingly, another group has demonstrated that CTF is generated from cells locating further behind the front edge of an advancing cell sheet instead of cells at the migrating front boundary during collective migration [34]. In comparison to the mechanotransduction of single cells, the maximal traction forces and stresses near the edge of the cell monolayer are significantly higher [35]. Furthermore, the higher responsiveness of a cell sheet towards a stiffness gradient on a planar substrate in comparison with a single cell suggests that cell–cell interaction enhances the collective cell migration of a cell sheet [36]. Recently, a key endocytic protein known as RAB5A has been shown to trigger collective migration of a cell population in originally stagnant epithelial monolayers [37].

In general, the mechanical properties of native tissues vary significantly according to the functional requirements of specific tissues or organs, and act as indicative parameters of the progression in certain disease, e.g., muscular dystrophy [38]. As the mechanotransduction of cells is related to cytoskeleton remodeling, ECM mechanics, and ECM protein composition, extensive studies have been focused on the fabrication of substrates with variable stiffness, adhesive ligands, and micropatterns in order to elicit the physiochemical factors for governing cell mechanics and function [39]. Cells exert CTF on the surrounding microenvironment, and at the same time moderate their cellular responses towards the mechanical feedback signals obtained from the surrounding ECM (Figure 1c). In detail, the interaction between individual cells and the ECM through interconnected pathways of receptor-mediated signal transductions, CTF generation, and external matrix mechanics dictate the expression of specific genes and phenotypes. At the same time, the elucidation of collective mechanics in cohesive cell layers as well as its feedforward-feedback responses with surrounding microenvironments are required for determining the working principle in tissue morphogenesis and regeneration. With the help of CTF measurements, the cell signaling pathways involved in many physiological functions and pathological processes of single cells have been revealed in more detail [15]. In addition to the mechanotransduction of individual cells, CTF measurement of cell populations will make the in vitro biophysical study of morphogenesis possible. It is believed that a thorough understanding of the intricate interplay between cell mechanics and cell–ECM interactions will facilitate the development of biofunctional and mechanoresponsive biomaterials for tissue regeneration and clinical diagnostics.

Mechanical stresses from the physiological microenvironment, including substrate, flowing fluid, ECM, and neighboring cells, directly influence the collective responses of cell layers, e.g., the regulation of the vasoactivity of blood vessels. A typical mechanosensing event in epithelial and endothelial tissues is triggered by the formation of cell–cell junctions, which contain adherens junctions, gap junctions, and tight junctions. For instance, adherens junction formation has been shown to induce actin polymerization in the cytoskeleton of adjacent cells through the interactions of various signaling proteins around the cytoplasmic domains of adherens junctions [40–42]. Moreover, cell–cell interaction has led to the inhibition of cell proliferation and migration which is known as "contact inhibition". In the 2D culture of epithelial cells, cells which are sparsely distributed on the substrate proliferate well, while the growth of a densely packed cell monolayer is impaired by the formation of cell–cell contacts [43,44]. The phenomenon of contact inhibition of cell proliferation in epithelial cells also exists in different types of cells [45,46]. Quantitative characterizations of contact inhibition dynamics in confluent cell monolayers with different cell densities have shown that the interfacial contact formation between adjacent cells is necessary but not sufficient for causing growth inhibition [47]. It has also been suggested that mechanical compression may provide an inhibitory signal for cell division [48].

In addition to the inhibition of cell proliferation, cell-cell junction formation between neighboring cells provides a cooperative effect to transmit appreciable normal stress, which guides the direction of cell monolayer migration along the course of minimal intercellular shear stress [49]. As epithelial cells require stable cell–cell adhesions and mesenchymal cells rely on transient and dynamic cell–cell contacts, the strategies of collective cell migration in various cell types are different based on their particular physiological functions [50]. A recent study has shown that the chase-run phenomenon between placode cells and neural crest cells was involved in both chemotaxis and *N*-cadherin signaling transduction, which in turn led to coordinated migration of different types of tissues [51]. With the hypothesized phenomena of mechanical coupling between neighboring cells, cell–cell interactions can be sufficient to guide the direction of collective cell migration, without the presence of a physical cue [52–54]. On the other hand, understanding the principles and mechanisms involved in collective cell migration remains a tremendous challenge, because the mechanical stresses of cell layers are difficult to probe by conventional experimental techniques. CTF, which is a known mechanical property, has been adopted as a model biophysical parameter for analyzing the intricate mechanotransduction of cell monolayers [55–57].

3. 3D Fabrications of Polymeric Biomaterials

In general, the most commonly used synthetic polymers for 3D fabrication of biomaterial scaffold include polyglycolic acid (PGA) [58], poly-caprolactone (PCL) [59], polydimethylsiloxane (PDMS) [60], and polyethylene glycol (PEG)-based hydrogels [61]. For example, PGA and its copolymers are widely used in the fabrication of various biomaterial scaffolds for tissue engineering applications because they are biodegradable and non-toxic [62]. However, the native surface of PGA does not provide the biological cues for direct cell attachment and regeneration. Thus, the modification of PGA with biologically active ligands is essential for cell culture applications, e.g., the addition of β-tricalcium phosphate (β-TCP) in porous 3D PGA scaffolds has been required for treating bone defects [63]. Moreover, polylactic-co-glycolic acid (PLG) copolymers have been used to design biomaterial scaffolds incorporated with controlled release capability of essential biomacromolecules, such as vascular endothelial growth factor, in vivo [62]. The PLG system mentioned above has facilitated blood vessel development and enhanced local vascularization during tissue regeneration [64]. Besides, microporous membrane composed of poly-D, Ł-lactide-co-glycolide (PLGA) has been applied for the 3D stacked culture of hepatic tissues [65].

In spite of the intense development of microporous polymeric scaffolds, there has been a lack of 3D biomaterial systems with precise microscale features for simultaneous cell culture and biomechanical measurement. As such, Shen et al. have developed a high-aspect ratio microchannel by UV embossing of an UV polymerizable biodegradable macromer in a liquid formulation composed of poly-e-caprolactone-r-Ł-lactide-r-glycolide diacrylate [66]. In detail, the master silicon (Si) mold is prepared from a lithography system which uniquely combines deep reactive ion etching (DRIE) with passivation treatments (Figure 2). After obtaining the daughter PDMS mold, an UV resin liquid formulation and a polyester film are successively loaded onto the PDMS mold. Lastly, the resin is polymerized under UV illumination and separated from the PDMS mold and polyester film [67,68]. The depth of the micropatterned biodegradable scaffold synthesized by this method can reach up to 70 μm. Furthermore, the layer-by-layer (LBL) process has been successfully applied to build multilayers of confluent SMCs on the micropatterned biodegradable scaffold as mentioned above, and to trigger the expression of the contractile phenotype of SMCs [69]. In addition to the formation of cell patterns, effective mass transfer of dissolved gas and essential nutrients to cells bound on the biodegradable scaffold are critical for maintaining cell viability and functionality. To address the limitation of mass transfer, Sarkar et al. [59] have developed a porous micropatterned PCL by combining soft lithography, melt molding, and PLGA micro/nanoparticles leaching. The group has further demonstrated that the diffusion rate of culture media into the PLGA-leached PCL scaffolds mentioned above was enhanced by six times in comparison with that through the non-porous PCL scaffolds. Later on, a biodegradable microstructured polycaprolactone construct functionalized with an adhesive layer of polyethylene glycol-diacrylate (PEG-DA) gel was incorporated into a 3D composite structure with a layer of vascular smooth cells with precisely controlled cell orientation and geometry [70]. Until now, most emerging techniques, as mentioned above, mainly focus on the precise 3D fabrication of microscale patterns in biomaterial scaffolds for facilitating the formation of tissue equivalents, instead of probing intricate cellular behavior in a controlled 3D microenvironment.

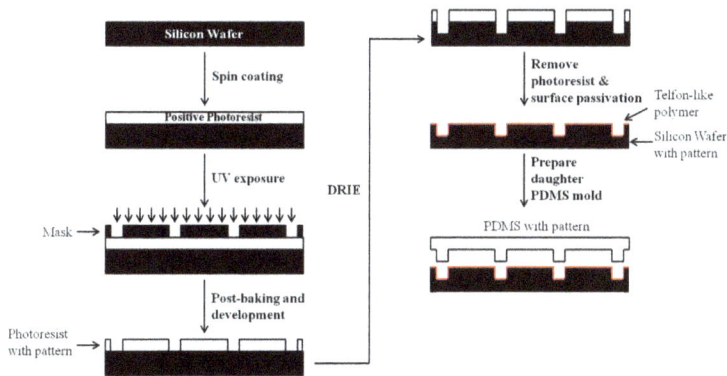

Figure 2. Schematic illustration on the fabrication process of a micropatterned polydimethylsiloxane (PDMS) scaffold by combining lithography and deep reactive ion etching (DRIE).

Interestingly, Deutsch et al. [60] have developed a new fabrication process for microgrooved topographical cues on a PDMS scaffold by combining photolithography and soft lithography. Briefly, the silicon wafer is spin-coated with a photoresist layer and exposed to UV light through a contact mask. The micropatterned PDMS scaffolds are created by casting and curing of siloxane oligomers and siloxane cross-linkers on the wafer surface. The fibronectin-coated PDMS scaffolds fabricated by this method have been shown to direct the spatial organization of cells and extracellular matrix [71]. Based on its ideal biocompatibility, polyacrylamide hydrogel has been used as a model system for studying the biophysics of cell migration, e.g., chemotaxis [34]. In another study, PEG-based hydrogel microstructures were fabricated on glass substrates by using photolithography-based patterning [61,72]. In detail, a glass substrate was first functionalized with 3-(trichlorosilyl)propyl methacrylate, then spin-coated with a PEG derivative and a photoinitiator, and finally exposed to UV light through a photomask for PEG crosslinking. Moreover, the PEG-based hydrogel was successfully fabricated into a cylindrical or cubic shape for the encapsulation of cells, detection of drug–drug interaction, and formation of tumor spheres [73–75]. Hahn et al. [76] have further developed confocal-based laser scanning lithography for 3D surface patterning (feature size ~5 µm) of PEG-based hydrogel substrates. The micropatterned PEG-based hydrogels embedded within independently fabricated PDMS housings are applied as a microfluidic device to study cell viability and metabolic activity, which contributes to the emerging applications for in vitro diagnostics and regenerative medicine [77]. At the same time, the PEG-based hydrogels can be further developed into a porous 3D structure to control spatial organization and enhance cell binding affinity for tissue morphogenesis and angiogenesis promotion [78,79]. In addition to lithographic patterning, other bottom-up approaches, such as electrospinning, nanoimprinting, anodization, and phase separation, have been applied to fabricate 3D patterns on biomaterials [80].

Naturally-derived polymers, such as proteins and polysaccharides, are ideal materials for the fabrication of biomimetic 3D scaffolds with superior biocompatibility compared to synthetic polymers. Collagen is one of the most important natural polymers widely found in most extracellular matrix (ECM) surrounding tissues in vivo as it serves as an adhesive ligand for major cell types [81]. Thus, phase change ink-jet printing and indirect 3D printing techniques have been applied to fabricate collagen scaffolds with micropatterns, such as internal channels and capillary networks [82,83]. For instance, indirect 3D printing of collagen involves three steps. Firstly, a negative mold is created by a solid freeform fabrication technique which produces freeform solid objects directly from computer-aided design without part-specific tooling or human intervention [84,85]. Secondly, a collagen solution is casted into the mold and solidified at low temperature. Lastly, the patterned collagen scaffold is recovered by the dissolution of the mold with ethanol, followed by critical point drying with liquid carbon dioxide. Another preferred method for fabricating collagen-based scaffolds with uniform pore structure is homogeneous freeze drying under a controlled freezing rate [86]. Cell attachment and viability on the freeze-dried 3D collagen scaffold are shown to be influenced by specific surface area and pore size of the resulted scaffold [87].

Besides protein, chitosan, which is formed from the deacetylation of chitin, is an important naturally-derived polysaccharide for fabricating biomaterial scaffolds in various applications of tissue engineering, such as hepatocyte regeneration [88,89]. In a pioneering study, a rapid prototyping robotic dispensing (RPBOD) system has been developed to fabricate 3D scaffolds of chitosan and chitosan-hydroxyapatite (HA) with reproducible macropore architecture by injecting chitosan and chitosan–HA solution (in acetic acid) into a mixture of sodium hydroxide solution and pure ethanol (in ratio of 7:3) [90]. Alternatively, a hydrogel with molecularly engineered filaments has been formed from the self-assembly of oligopeptides to mimic the ordered microporous structure of native ECM for 3D cell culture [91,92]. Recently, one self-assembly oligopeptide (SAP) designed with specific motifs for enhancing cell adhesion, cell differentiation, and bone marrow homing has been successfully developed into nanofibers for the functional maintenance of mouse adult neural stem cells in a 3D microenvironment. Also, SAP gels with high peptide concentration have been generated from a standard solid phase synthesis method for hosting cells inside their matrices. To date, the SAP gels have been further engineered with tunable physical properties such as nano-scale architecture and biological functionality for various applications in tissue engineering, such as vascular graft [93,94]. In spite of the recent advances in the 3D fabrication of natural materials, the quantitative correlation between scaffold properties and cellular responses for effective tissue regeneration remains to be elucidated. In general, a 3D biomaterial scaffold should mimic the physical microenvironment and biochemical cues of native ECM as closely as possible. Therefore, a better understanding of cell–biomaterial interaction and bidirectional mechanotransduction within the 3D microenvironment will simultaneously aid the design of superior biomaterial scaffolds for tissue regeneration and the development of a model experimental platform for the study of cell mechanotransduction.

4. Recent Progress in Cellular Biomechanics

It is now known that the bulk elasticity (ranging from rigid to soft material) and surface topography of a biomaterial directly modulates the contact mechanics of cells, while microfabrication technologies, such as soft lithography, provide the spatial control of cell populations on the biomaterial scaffold. Various types of cells, such as fibroblasts, SMCs, and hepatocytes, respond differently to substrates with a range of elasticity through intricate interplay between ligand–receptor binding, mechanotransduction, and cytoskeleton remodeling [95]. For instance, cell spreading and locomotion speed of normal rat kidney epithelial cells has been demonstrated to reduce and increase, respectively, on softer polyacrylamide gel substrates [96]. Moreover, 3T3 fibroblasts have demonstrated preferential migration, known as durotaxis, over an elasticity gradient from a soft region to a stiff region on a polyacrylamide gel substrate, but not vice versa on the same substrate [97]. Interestingly, a recent discovery has proven that the migration of multiple cell aggregates is responsive to certain perturbations of cell–cell adhesion, such as the downregulation of adherens junctions [98]. Recently, topographical cues such as micropillars [99] and nanoparticulates [100] have also been shown to effectively influence the contact mechanics and biological functions of adherent cells.

In general, the communication between cells and the apposing ECM or biomaterial scaffold leading to cell growth and motility is driven by intricate mechanotransduction through the active reorganization of the cytoskeletal network in the cytoplasm [101,102]. First of all, cell migration speed has been demonstrated to follow a biphasic dependence on the density of immobilized adhesive ligands, as predicted by a seminal mathematical model [103], and later on validated in experimental measurement [104]. At the same time, the increase of ECM stiffness has been shown to enhance cell motility as cells exert higher contractile forces towards stiffer substrate during cell body attachment, detachment, and displacement [105]. The geometry of the 2D biomaterial sub-region functionalized with adhesive islands can be precisely engineered with the use of microcontact printing techniques which are instrumental for studying the combined effects of geometrical constraint and biological recognition on cellular physiology. Several studies have shown that cell adhesion is not only triggered by the binding between membrane-bound integrin and adhesive ligands, but also related to the subsequent events, such as biochemical signal transduction and mechanical deformation of intracellular organelles in the adherent cells [106]. It has been revealed that both the formation of FAs and the emergence of actin stress fibers of adherent cells are dependent on ECM stiffness. Interestingly, the optimal value of substrate stiffness for supporting maximal migration is correlated with the concentration of ECM ligands covalently attached to the substrate [104]. Recently, a group has even demonstrated that nanotopographical features deposited on a planar glass substrate are sufficient to promote the maturation of neural networks [107].

Classical model systems for studying the mechanotransduction of cells at the cell–substrate interfaces have been made possible with the development of experimental biophysics since 1980. In the first report, the elastic distortion and wrinkling of a silicone substrate induced by the adherent cells through cytoskeleton remodeling during cell locomotion have been observed by optical microscopy [108], and can be further quantified through the variation of substrate elasticity [109,110].

Thereafter, Balaban et al. have combined the transparent micropatterned elastomer and FA characterization through the expression of green-fluorescent protein (GFP)-labeled vinculin in adherent cells for elucidating the relationship between the assembly dynamics of FAs and the alteration of CTF [111]. The method mentioned above mainly hinges on the use of a non-wrinkling substrate with micropatterns composed of dots or lines for the determination of cell-induced deformation of the material's surface.

In a seminal study, Tan et al. developed a microfabricated array of elastomeric microposts, each independently acting as a deformable structure to probe the mechanical transduction between the adherent cells and apposing substrates [112]. With the use of a micropost as the mechanical probe, the map of highly localized deformation caused by the CTF across the entire substrate can be determined from beam theory [113]. By changing the height of the micropost, a series of micropost arrays reported with a range of substrate rigidity further demonstrates the influence of microscale geometry and elasticity on cell morphology, FA organization, and global cell contractility [114]. By combining micropost array technology with ultrahigh-resolution cell imaging, the precision map of CTF with a sensitivity of 500 pN and the nanoscale resolution of individual force-bearing FAs have been simultaneously measured [115]. Moreover, the micropost array has been developed to probe the real-time mechanotransduction of entire cells through the integration with a cell stretching device, which provides a way of tuning the external force exerted on live cells [116,117]. Since microposts have been commonly fabricated on elastomeric polymers such as PDMS, the functionalization of the PDMS surface with ECM proteins is essential to create a more physiological relevant microenvironment for cell adhesion. In addition to PDMS, polymeric hydrogels have been used in the fabrication of micropost arrays [118]. In detail, the hydrogel monomers, such as hydroxyethyl methacrylate, were mixed with a photoinitiator, followed by replica molding and UV exposure in order to partially polymerize the precursors in solutions. Secondly, photo-crosslinking of the solutions, as mentioned above, with ethylene glycol dimethacrylate leads to the formation of a stabilized hydrogel micropost array. Moreover, the stability and surface clustering of a range of high-aspect-ratio hydrogel microarrays under capillary forces have been studied by controlling the geometry and elastic moduli of individual microposts [119].

Another popular substratum for studying cell–substrate mechanotransduction is polyacrylamide-based hydrogel (Figure 3), a microporous material which has been proven to be an ideal experimental system for various cell types due to its tunable chemical and mechanical properties [120,121]. Firstly, polyacrylamide-based hydrogel can be easily tuned from an extremely soft to stiff material with a distinct elastic modulus by adjusting the concentration ratio of acrylamide and bis-acrylamide before the initiation of polymerization. Secondly, the polyacrylamide-based hydrogel can be loaded with fluorescently labeled microbeads which serve as positional markers for the detection of local deformation in selected regions of interest [122]. More importantly, polyacrylamide-based hydrogel can be linearly deformed in response to the applied biological forces and can be fully recovered to its original state upon the removal of force. Thirdly, the low thickness and transparent nature of polyacrylamide-based hydrogel ensures the detection of small displacements of the fluorescent beads with conventional fluorescence microscopy. Furthermore, the polyacrylamide-based gels are naturally non-adhesive for mammalian cells unless specific ECM molecules (e.g., type I collagen) are covalently coupled onto the surface.

In addition to the micropost array and polymeric hydrogel, the microelectromechanical systems (MEMS) with on-line force transducers have determined the contractile force of adherent cells from the measured deflection and the spring constant in the enclosed microbeams [123]. In one typical MEMS design, the cell contraction force was measured from the deflections of micron-sized pads connected to a cantilever [124]. A substrate composed of an array of closely packed cantilevers has been designed with different tip geometry and spatial distribution for probing the local mechanical forces at the cell adhesion contact [125]. At the same time, the control of the geometric pattern of a cell population on planar MEMS can be achieved by using microcontact printing, as mentioned earlier.

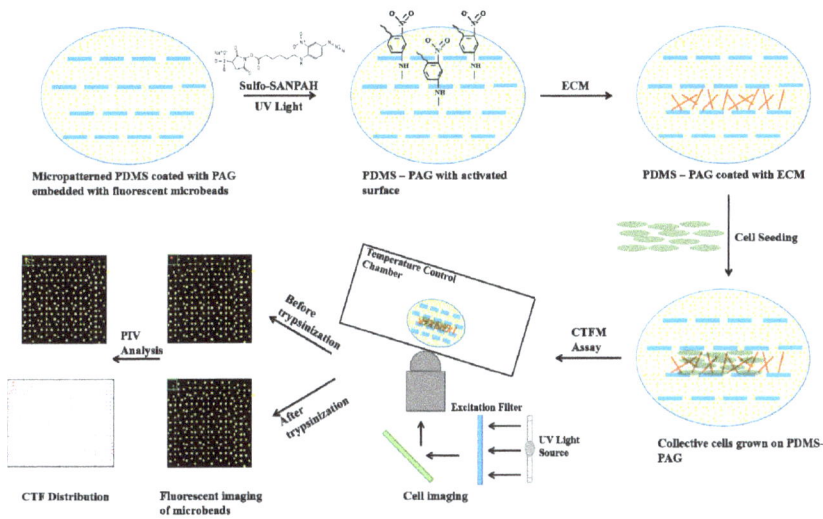

Figure 3. The schematic illustration for the making of PDMS microchannels with a polyacrylamide gel (PAG) coating for cell traction force microscopy measurement (Top views). The micropatterned PDMS is coated with PAG embedded with a thin layer of fluorescent microbeads. A UV-activated heterobifunctional cross linker, sulfo-SANPAH, is applied for ECM coupling. Cells are then seeded onto the activated surface for further study with cell traction force microscopy. After obtaining a pair of fluorescent images of the same frame before and after trypsinization, the deformation of the elastic substrate is determined and used for the CTF computation.

It is known that cell spreading and migration within 3D microenvironment is highly dependent on the topological properties [126] and mechanical stiffness [127,128] of the surrounding ECM or biomaterial scaffold. The stiffness of a 3D collagen gel matrix has been engineered with different degrees of crosslinking under the same collagen concentration in solution for probing the effect of gel matrix stiffness on cellular behavior. The result indicates that the increase of gel matrix stiffness enhanced the spreading of endothelial cells [129]. When cells are partially or completely embedded within a 3D matrix, the cellular responses are quite different from those observed in a 2D culture dish, e.g., FAs become smaller, more diffusively distributed, and changed in FAK composition in the cell cytoplasm [130,131]. Moreover, FA-associated proteins regulate the migration speed of live cells embedded in a 3D matrix through their distinctive roles in driving protrusion activity and matrix deformation, which are unimportant in 2D cell migration [132,133]. In contrast to individual cells, the spatial organization of FAs within multicellular aggregates cultured inside a 3D matrix remains to be fully elucidated.

5. Cell Traction Force Measurement

Mechanotransduction is an emerging research area which requires the knowledge from several disciplines. A variety of methods have been developed to measure the CTF of both individual cells and collective cell populations during the past few years [118], including cell-populated collagen gel (CPCG) [119], thin silicone membrane [108], force sensor array [123], and improved micropost force sensor [112]. The reported force and spatial resolution of major force sensing techniques mentioned above have been summarized in Table 1 [134]. Currently, the most reliable and comprehensive method primarily developed for CTF measurement is the cell traction force microscopy (CTFM) assay, which was developed by Dembo and Wang in 1999 [135].

Table 1. Force Sensitivity of Cellular Forces Measured with Selective Cell Mechanics Techniques

TECHNIQUE	FORCE SENSITIVITY
Optical Tweezers	1–100 pN
Atomic Force Microscope	$10-10^5$ pN
Magnetic Tweezers	$10-10^3$ pN
Gel Wrinkling Method	10–100 nN
Micropost Deformation	1–100 nN
Cell Traction Force Microscope	$10-10^6$ pN

In CTFM, the fluorescent microbeads embedded in the substrate serve as positional markers to record and track the deformation caused by CTFs (Figure 3). By taking a pair of 'force loaded' and 'null force' images in the same region of interest, the deformation of the elastic substrate is determined and used for the CTF computation. By dividing images into overlapped windows with a constant distance, a pair of small windows respectively from 'force loaded' and 'null force' images are obtained and applied to calculate the displacements. There are two other versions of CTFM techniques that have been developed by Butler et al. [19] and Yang et al. [136]. Both methods rely on the setting window, and conduct the correlation computation by using Fourier transform. On the other hand, the bead displacement calculation used in the Dembo and Wang [135] method is not fixed to the paired windows as mentioned above. Butler et al. have developed explicit formulas for transforming the traction and displacement fields of microbeads to cell mechanotransduction parameters, such as the contraction moments and strain energy at cell-substrate interfaces [19]. While other approaches based on pixel windows ignore the local rotational displacements of microbeads, the method developed by Yang et al. incorporates a pattern recognition technique to track microbead movements for estimating the displacement field of the elastic substrate [136]. Most importantly, all CTFM associated methods need to overcome the challenge of the accurate measurement of the small displacements of fluorescent microbeads. In addition, all methods of data analysis mentioned above are limited to the positional mapping on a 2D substrate. The CTFM method can achieve a broader application if the CTF characterizations can be extended to 3D matrices.

Recently, more efforts have been devoted to the development of novel experimental and numerical methods for probing 3D CTFs, which have similar elastic moduli and physiological features to in vivo situations. By combining laser scanning confocal microscopy with digital volume (3D) correlation, 3D full field traction can be computed by the cross-correlation function and displacement-gradient technique [126,137–139]. In this method, the 3D CTFs of single cells are mapped over the 2D surface between cell and polyacrylamide gel, and the dynamic CTFs during cell migration and locomotion are calculated. Similarly, Hur et al. have developed 3D CTFM techniques to probe the cell–matrix interaction of live bovine aortic endothelial cells (BAECs) on a polyacrylamide deformable substrate in real time [140]. Moreover, Delanoë-Ayari et al. have presented the temporal map of CTFs during the crawling of Dictyostelium cells on a soft hydrogel surface [141]. The differences among the two methods mentioned above are the maximum limit of bead displacement in the computation algorithms [142]. In comparison to the traditional linear deformation framework used in traditional CTFM, a large deformation formulation for characterizing the cellular displacement field in conjunction with the high resolution digital volume correction technique has been recently developed [143].

For 3D CTF measurements, i.e., for cells completely immersed within ECM, collagen rather than synthetic hydrogel is used as a model system. The challenges of using a naturally-derived 3D scaffold hinge on the difficulty in the control of its mechanical properties and in the limitation of its fabrication process [93]. Legant et al. have successfully encapsulated GFP (EGFP)-expressing cells in well-defined PEG hydrogel matrices, tracked the displacement of embedded fluorescent beads, and calculated the CTFs exerted by the entrapped live cells [144]. They have applied linear elastic theory and the finite element method to analyze the bead displacement map generated from confocal microscopy of hydrogels. Their results indicate that the stiffer the hydrogels is, the stronger CTF the cells exert on the surrounding 3D ECM. Strong inward forces have been revealed to locate predominantly near the long extensions of the encapsulated cell, while the shear tractions are the main type of CTF produced by the cells encapsulated in 3D hydrogel [144]. By applying a 3D type I collagen network for cell encapsulation, Gjorevski et al. [145] and Koch et al. [146] have obtained the 3D CTF mapping of single cells throughout the surrounding hydrogel matrix. One challenge of this method is the interpretation of the traction field from the cell types, like fibroblasts and certain tumor cells which can degrade surrounding collagen matrix and subsequently change the mechanical properties of the surrounding hydrogel during the CTFM assay [131].

Various external mechanical stimulations acting on cells from the surrounding microenvironment take the form of shape, topology, and rigidity, which trigger the cycles of mechanosensing, mechanotransduction, and mechanoresponse [147]. The exact mechanisms of mechanochemical signaling from extracellular mechanical forces to intracellular molecular recognitions remain unclear. To date, fluorescence resonance energy transfer (FRET)-based single-molecule spectroscopy of mechanosensory molecular beacons has been validated with the high sensitivity required for probing forces in the piconewton scale [148]. Such a technique opens up the new possibility for tracking the propagation of molecular forces within cells during mechanotransduction. By incorporating FRET into CTFM, valuable information connecting the cascade of mechanical stimuli propagations to the identification of mechanosensitive proteins can be gathered conveniently. One of the possible exploitations of the study of cell mechanics is to elucidate the developmental processes of mesenchymal stem cells in response to external matrices of different underlying rigidities. For instance, the differentiation into various cell lineages ranging from neurogenic cells on a softer matrix, myogenic cells that resemble muscle tissues on a stiffer matrix, to the osteogenic cells on the most rigid matrix, are identified on various crosslinked-collagen matrices [100].

By combining soft lithography with CTFM techniques, recent work focusing on confluent cell monolayers cultured on a micropatterned polymeric substrate has been carried out to elucidate the cell–cell interactions and intracellular mechanics, such as the collective CTF distribution of SMC layers during the emergence of contractile phenotypes under a controlled 3D microenvironment (Figure 4) [149]. In the vascular physiology of the endothelium, the effect of confluency of an endothelial cell monolayer on the tensions at adherens junctions and the cytoplasm under both static and shear flow conditions has been revealed [150]. A few groups have also shown that the spatial distribution of CTFs exerted by cohesive cell colonies is significantly concentrated at the periphery of the colony [33,151]. A similar homogeneous zone of lower CTF or von Mises stress was observed in the center of a circumferentially aligned SMC sheet, as shown in our recent study (Figure 4). In other words, collective CTF is strongly influenced by the shape of the adhesive zone prescribed on the micropatterned substrate. For better understanding of collective cell activities, novel CTFM has been developed to show the dynamic traction domains and the compressions among cell clusters [152]. To quantify the cell-generated mechanical stress in situ within living tissues, an emerging technique based on 3D functionalized fluorocarbon microdroplets has been developed for studying the mechanical properties of aggregates of mammary epithelial cells [153]. Moreover, the shape deformation of the microdroplets (with similar size to individual cells) which are microinjected into the tissue of mouse embryo can be used to calculate the anisotropic stresses generated by epithelial cell colonies via fluorescent imaging and computerized analysis.

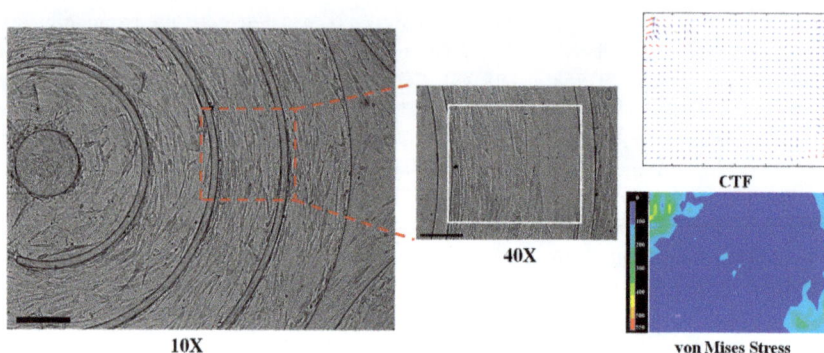

Figure 4. The distributions of CTFs and von Mises stresses of a confluent SMC sheet aligned in the circumferential direction. Scale bars are 250 μm and 100 μm in the 10X and 40X images, respectively.

Although 3D CTFM has attracted much attention, the techniques are still immature and not applicable to various experimental systems. Several challenges, including the fabrication and understanding of the 3D matrix, the influences of nanotopography, the techniques of high resolution 3D imaging, and the necessity for complex computational algorithms, need to be overcome for promoting the general adaptations of this potentially powerful technique [154]. In addition, various methods for probing the collective cell traction field are affected by the intricate mechano-sensing mechanisms of cells within a 3D microenvironment. Considering that multiple-cell sheets instead of single cells participate in most physiological processes, there is an essential need to develop measurement methods based on biomaterial innovations for 3D CTF that result from cell populations.

6. Conclusions

In order to study cell/tissue mechanotransduction under physiological conditions, a transition from 2D to 3D biomaterial systems with prescribed microscale features is necessary. 3D micropatterning tools for biomaterial fabrication can improve our knowledge about the influence of microenvironments, like the composition, topography, stiffness, etc., on cellular functions, physiological regulations, and pathophysiological progressions. While the general principles of the design for an appropriate 3D scaffold have been formulated, the better understanding of the mechanosensory responses of cells within 3D microenvironments will in turn facilitate better scaffold design. Since cells undergo complex mechanotransduction when they attach to and spread on a substrate surface, new advances in the development of integrative biomaterial systems for probing the CTFs of single cells as well as cell layers have been recently achieved. Given CTF as an ideal model to analyze the complex mechanotransduction of multiple cells, 3D CTFM and derived techniques for the measurement of collective CTF will become increasingly important.

Acknowledgments: The work described in this paper was partly supported by a General Research Fund from the Research Grants Council of Hong Kong Special Administrative Region of China [CityU 11210015] and the National Science Foundation China [51378447].

Conflicts of Interest: The authors declare no conflict of interest.

References

1. Chen, C.S.; Mrksich, M.; Huang, S.; Whitesides, G.M.; Ingber, D.E. Geometric control of cell life and death. *Science* **1997**, *276*, 1425–1428. [CrossRef] [PubMed]
2. Dike, L.E.; Chen, C.S.; Mrksich, M.; Tien, J.; Whitesides, G.M.; Ingber, D.E. Geometric control of switching between growth, apoptosis, and differentiation during angiogenesis using micropatterned substrates. *Vitro Cell Dev. Biol.* **1999**, *35*, 441–448. [CrossRef] [PubMed]

3. Hogrebe, N.J.; Reinhardt, J.W.; Gooch, K.J. Biomaterial microarchitecture: A potent regulator of individual cell behavior and multicellular organization. *J. Biomed. Mater. Res. A* **2016**, *105*, 640–661. [CrossRef] [PubMed]
4. Singhvi, R.; Kumar, A.; Lopez, G.P.; Stephanopoulos, G.N.; Wang, D.I.C.; Whitesides, G.M.; Ingber, D.E. Engineering Cell-Shape and Function. *Science* **1994**, *264*, 696–698. [CrossRef] [PubMed]
5. Delamarche, E.; Bernard, A.; Schmid, H.; Bietsch, A.; Michel, B.; Biebuyck, H. Microfluidic networks for chemical patterning of substrate: Design and application to bioassays. *J. Am. Chem. Soc.* **1998**, *120*, 500–508. [CrossRef]
6. Michel, R.; Lussi, J.W.; Csucs, G.; Reviakine, I.; Danuser, G.; Ketterer, B.; Hubbell, J.A.; Textor, M.; Spencer, N.D. Selective molecular assembly patterning: A new approach to micro- and nanochemical patterning of surfaces for biological applications. *Langmuir* **2002**, *18*, 3281–3287. [CrossRef]
7. Falconnet, D.; Koenig, A.; Assi, T.; Textor, M. A combined photolithographic and molecular-assembly approach to produce functional micropatterns for applications in the biosciences. *Adv. Funct. Mater.* **2004**, *14*, 749–756. [CrossRef]
8. Goessl, A.; Bowen-Pope, D.F.; Hoffman, A.S. Control of shape and size of vascular smooth muscle cells in vitro by plasma lithography. *J. Biomed. Mater. Res.* **2001**, *57*, 15–24. [CrossRef]
9. Falconnet, D.; Csucs, G.; Grandin, H.M.; Textor, M. Surface engineering approaches to micropattern surfaces for cell-based assays. *Biomaterials* **2006**, *27*, 3044–3063. [CrossRef] [PubMed]
10. Desai, T.A. Micro- and nanoscale structures for tissue engineering constructs. *Med. Eng. Phys.* **2000**, *22*, 595–606. [CrossRef]
11. Sachlos, E.; Czernuszka, J.T. Making tissue engineering scaffolds work. Review: The application of solid freeform fabrication technology to the production of tissue engineering scaffolds. *Eur. Cells Mater.* **2003**, *5*, 29–39. [CrossRef]
12. Shin, H. Fabrication methods of an engineered microenvironment for analysis for cell-biomaterial interactions. *Biomaterials* **2007**, *28*, 126–133. [CrossRef] [PubMed]
13. Lammerding, J.; Hsiao, J.; Schulze, P.C.; Kozlov, S.; Stewart, C.L.; Lee, R.T. Abnormal nuclear shape and impaired mechanotransduction in emerin-deficient cells. *J. Cell Biol.* **2005**, *170*, 781–791. [CrossRef] [PubMed]
14. Zhao, X.H.; Laschinger, C.; Arora, P.; Szaszi, K.; Kapus, A.; McCulloch, C.A. Force activates smooth muscle alpha-actin promoter activity through the Rho signaling pathway. *J. Cell Sci.* **2007**, *120*, 1801–1809. [CrossRef] [PubMed]
15. Choquet, D.; Felsenfeld, D.P.; Sheetz, M.P. Extracellular matrix rigidity causes strengthening of integrin-cytoskeleton linkages. *Cell* **1997**, *88*, 39–48. [CrossRef]
16. Hahn, C.; Schwartz, M.A. Mechanotransduction in vascular physiology and atherogenesis. *Nat. Rev. Mol. Cell Biol.* **2009**, *10*, 53–62. [CrossRef] [PubMed]
17. Plopper, G.; Ingber, D.E. Rapid induction and isolation of focal adhesion complexes. *Biochem. Biophys. Res. Commun.* **1993**, *193*, 571–578. [CrossRef] [PubMed]
18. Miyamoto, S.; Akiyama, S.K.; Yamada, K.M. Synergistic roles for receptor occupancy and aggregation in integrin transmembrane function. *Science* **1995**, *267*, 883–885. [CrossRef] [PubMed]
19. Butler, J.P.; Tolic-Norrelykke, I.M.; Fabry, B.; Fredberg, J.J. Traction fields, moments, and strain energy that cells exert on their surroundings. *Am. J. Phys.* **2002**, *282*, C595–C605. [CrossRef] [PubMed]
20. Chicurel, M.E.; Chen, C.S.; Ingber, D.E. Cellular control lies in the balance of forces. *Curr. Opin. Cell Biol.* **1998**, *10*, 232–239. [CrossRef]
21. Fouchard, J.; Bimbard, C.; Bufi, N.; Durand-Smet, P.; Proag, A.; Richert, A.; Cardoso, O.; Asnacios, A. Three-dimensional cell body shape dictates the onset of traction force generation and growth of focal adhesions. *Proc. Natl. Acad. Sci. USA* **2014**, *111*, 13075–13080. [CrossRef] [PubMed]
22. Pirone, D.M.; Liu, W.F.; Ruiz, S.A.; Gao, L.; Raghavan, S.; Lemmon, C.A.; Romer, L.H.; Chen, C.S. An inhibitory role for FAK in regulating proliferation: A link between limited adhesion and RhoA-ROCK signaling. *J. Cell Biol.* **2006**, *174*, 277–288. [CrossRef] [PubMed]
23. Watanabe, N.; Kato, T.; Fujita, A.; Ishizaki, T.; Narumiya, S. Cooperation between mDia1 and ROCK in Rho-induced actin reorganization. *Nat. Cell Biol.* **1999**, *1*, 136–143. [PubMed]
24. Sun, Y.; Chen, C.S.; Fu, J. Forcing Stem cells to behave: A biophysical perspective of the cellular microenvironment. *Ann. Rev. Biophys.* **2012**, *41*, 519–542. [CrossRef] [PubMed]

25. Elosegui-Artola, A.; Oria, R.; Chen, Y.; Kosmalska, A.; Pérez-González, C.; Castro, N.; Zhu, C.; Trepat, X.; Roca-Cusachs, P. Mechanical regulation of a molecular clutch defines force transmission and transduction in response to matrix rigidity. *Nat. Cell Biol.* **2016**, *18*, 540–548. [CrossRef] [PubMed]

26. Schulte, C.; Rodighiero, S.; Cappelluti, M.A.; Puricelli, L.; Maffioli, E.; Borghi, F.; Negri, A.; Sogne, E.; Galluzzi, M.; Piazzoni, C.; et al. Conversion of nanoscale topographical information of cluster-assembled zirconia surfaces into mechanotransductive events promotes neuronal differentiation. *J. Nanobiotechnol.* **2016**, *14*, 18. [CrossRef] [PubMed]

27. Cukierman, E.; Pankov, R.; Yamada, K.M. Cell interactions with three-dimensional matrices. *Curr. Opin. Cell Biol.* **2002**, *14*, 633–639. [CrossRef]

28. Li, S.; Lao, J.; Chen, B.P.; Li, Y.S.; Zhao, Y.; Chu, J.; Chen, K.D.; Tsou, T.C.; Peck, K.; Chien, S. Genomic analysis of smooth muscle cells in 3-dimensional collagen matrix. *Faseb. J.* **2003**, *17*, 97–99. [CrossRef] [PubMed]

29. Hong, H.; McCullough, C.M.; Stegemann, J.P. The role of ERK signaling in protein hydrogel remodeling by vascular smooth muscle cells. *Biomaterials* **2007**, *28*, 3824–3833. [CrossRef] [PubMed]

30. Provenzano, P.P.; Inman, D.R.; Eliceiri, K.W.; Keely, P.J. Matrix density-induced mechanoregulation of breast cell phenotype, signaling and gene expression through a FAK-ERK linkage. *Oncogene* **2009**, *28*, 4326–4343. [CrossRef] [PubMed]

31. Petrie, R.J.; Gavara, N.; Chadwick, R.S.; Yamada, K.M. Nonpolarized signaling reveals two distinct modes of 3D cell migration. *J. Cell Biol.* **2012**, *197*, 439–455. [CrossRef] [PubMed]

32. Li, C.Y.; Stevens, K.R.; Schwartz, R.E.; Alejandro, B.S.; Huang, J.H.; Bhatia, S.N. Micropatterned Cell-Cell Interactions Enable Functional Encapsulation of Primary Hepatocytes in Hydrogel Microtissues. *Tissue Eng. Part A* **2014**, *20*, 2200–2212. [CrossRef] [PubMed]

33. Mertz, A.F.; Banerjee, S.; Che, Y.L.; German, G.K.; Xu, Y.; Hyland, C.; Marchetti, M.C.; Horsley, V.; Dufresne, E.R. Scaling of Traction Forces with the Size of Cohesive Cell Colonies. *Phys. Rev. Lett.* **2012**, *108*, 198101. [CrossRef] [PubMed]

34. Trepat, X.; Wasserman, M.R.; Angelini, T.E.; Millet, E.; Weitz, D.A.; Butler, J.P.; Fredberg, J.J. Physical forces during collective cell migration. *Nat. Phys.* **2009**, *5*, 426–430. [CrossRef]

35. Serra-Picamal, X.; Conte, V.; Sunyer, R.; Muñoz, J.J.; Trepat, X. Mapping forces and kinematics during collective cell migration. *Methods Cell Biol.* **2015**, *125*, 309–330. [PubMed]

36. Sunyer, R.; Conte, V.; Escribano, J.; Elosegui-Artola, A.; Labernadie, A.; Valon, L.; Navajas, D.; García-Aznar, J.M.; Muñoz, J.J.; Roca-Cusachs, P.; Trepat, X. Collective cell durotaxis emerges from long-range intercellular force transmission. *Science* **2016**, *353*, 1157–1161. [CrossRef] [PubMed]

37. Malinverno, C.; Corallino, S.; Giavazzi, F.; Bergert, M.; Li, Q.; Leoni, M.; Disanza, A.; Frittoli, E.; Oldani, A.; Martini, E.; et al. Endocytic reawakening of motility in jammed epithelia. *Nat. Mater.* **2017**, *16*, 587–596. [CrossRef] [PubMed]

38. Guilak, F.; Butler, D.L.; Goldstein, S.A.; Baaijens, F.P.T. Biomechanics and mechanobiology in functional tissue engineering. *J. Biomech.* **2014**, *47*, 1933–1940. [CrossRef] [PubMed]

39. Chin, L.; Xia, Y.; Discher, D.E.; Janmey, P.A. Mechanotransduction in cancer. *Curr. Opin. Chem. Eng.* **2016**, *11*, 77–84. [CrossRef] [PubMed]

40. Vasioukhin, V.; Fuchs, E. Actin dynamics and cell-cell adhesion in epithelia. *Curr. Opin. Cell Biol.* **2001**, *13*, 76–84. [CrossRef]

41. Dejana, E. Endothelial cell-cell junctions: Happy together. *Nat. Rev. Mol. Cell Biol.* **2004**, *5*, 261–270. [CrossRef] [PubMed]

42. Leckband, D.E.; le Duc, Q.; Wang, N.; de Rooij, J. Mechanotransduction at cadherin-mediated adhesions. *Curr. Opin. Cell Biol.* **2011**, *23*, 523–530. [CrossRef] [PubMed]

43. Abercrombie, M. Contact inhibition: The phenomenon and its biological implications. *Natl. Cancer Inst. Monogr.* **1967**, *26*, 249–277.

44. Castor, L.N. Contact regulation of cell division in an epithelial-like cell line. *J. Cell Phys.* **1968**, *72*, 161–172. [CrossRef] [PubMed]

45. Abercrombie, M. Contact inhibition in tissue culture. *Vitro* **1970**, *6*, 128–142. [CrossRef]

46. Martz, E.; Steinberg, M.S. The role of cell-cell contact in "contact" inhibition of cell division: A review and new evidence. *J. Cell Phys.* **1972**, *79*, 189–210. [CrossRef] [PubMed]

47. Puliafito, A.; Hufnagel, L.; Neveu, P.; Streichan, S.; Sigal, A.; Fygenson, D.K.; Shraiman, B.I. Collective and single cell behavior in epithelial contact inhibition. *Proc. Natl. Acad. Sci. USA* **2012**, *109*, 739–744. [CrossRef] [PubMed]

48. Shraiman, B.I. Mechanical feedback as a possible regulator of tissue growth. *Proc. Natl. Acad. Sci. USA* **2005**, *102*, 3318–3323. [CrossRef] [PubMed]

49. Tambe, D.T.; Hardin, C.C.; Angelini, T.E.; Rajendran, K.; Park, C.Y.; Serra-Picamal, X.; Zhou, E.H.H.; Zaman, M.H.; Butler, J.P.; Weitz, D.A.; et al. Collective cell guidance by cooperative intercellular forces. *Nat. Mater.* **2011**, *10*, 469–475. [CrossRef] [PubMed]

50. Theveneau, E.; Mayor, R. Collective cell migration of epithelial and mesenchymal cells. *Cell. Mol. Life Sci.* **2013**, *70*, 3481–3492. [CrossRef] [PubMed]

51. Theveneau, E.; Steventon, B.; Scarpa, E.; Garcia, S.; Trepat, X.; Streit, A.; Mayor, R. Chase-and-run between adjacent cell populations promotes directional collective migration. *Nat. Cell Biol.* **2013**, *15*, 763–772. [CrossRef] [PubMed]

52. Szabo, B.; Szollosi, G.J.; Gonci, B.; Juranyi, Z.; Selmeczi, D.; Vicsek, T. Phase transition in the collective migration of tissue cells: Experiment and model. *Phys. Rev. E* **2006**, *74*, 061908. [CrossRef] [PubMed]

53. Szabo, A.; Unnep, R.; Mehes, E.; Twal, W.O.; Argraves, W.S.; Cao, Y.; Czirok, A. Collective cell motion in endothelial monolayers. *Phys. Biol.* **2010**, *7*, 046007. [CrossRef] [PubMed]

54. Kabla, A.J. Collective cell migration: Leadership, invasion and segregation. *J. R. Soc. Interf.* **2012**, *9*, 3268–3278. [CrossRef] [PubMed]

55. Maruthamuthu, V.; Sabass, B.; Schwarz, U.S.; Gardel, M.L. Cell-ECM traction force modulates endogenous tension at cell-cell contacts. *Proc. Natl. Acad. Sci. USA* **2011**, *108*, 4708–4713. [CrossRef] [PubMed]

56. Jasaitis, A.; Estevez, M.; Heysch, J.; Ladoux, B.; Dufour, S. E-Cadherin-Dependent Stimulation of Traction Force at Focal Adhesions via the Src and PI3K Signaling Pathways. *Biophys. J.* **2012**, *103*, 175–184. [CrossRef] [PubMed]

57. Mertz, A.F.; Che, Y.; Banerjee, S.; Goldstein, J.M.; Rosowski, K.A.; Revilla, S.F.; Niessen, C.M.; Marchetti, M.C.; Dufresne, E.R.; Horsley, V. Cadherin-based intercellular adhesions organize epithelial cell-matrix traction forces. *Proc. Natl. Acad. Sci. USA* **2013**, *110*, 842–847. [CrossRef] [PubMed]

58. Giordano, R.A.; Wu, B.M.; Borland, S.W.; Cima, L.G.; Sachs, E.M.; Cima, M.J. Mechanical properties of dense polylactic acid structures fabricated by three dimensional printing. *J. Biomater. Sci. Polym. E* **1996**, *8*, 63–75. [CrossRef]

59. Sarkar, S.; Lee, G.Y.; Wong, J.Y.; Desai, T.A. Development and characterization of a porous micro-patterned scaffold for vascular tissue engineering applications. *Biomaterials* **2006**, *27*, 4775–4782. [CrossRef] [PubMed]

60. Deutsch, J.; Motiagh, D.; Russell, B.; Desai, T.A. Fabrication of microtextured membranes for cardiac myocyte attachment and orientation. *J. Biomed. Mater. Res.* **2000**, *53*, 267–275. [CrossRef]

61. Hahn, M.S.; Taite, L.J.; Moon, J.J.; Rowland, M.C.; Ruffino, K.A.; West, J.L. Photolithographic patterning of polyethylene glycol hydrogels. *Biomaterials* **2006**, *27*, 2519–2524. [CrossRef] [PubMed]

62. Athanasiou, K.A.; Niederauer, G.G.; Agrawal, C.M. Sterilization, toxicity, biocompatibility and clinical applications of polylactic acid polyglycolic acid copolymers. *Biomaterials* **1996**, *17*, 93–102. [CrossRef]

63. Cao, H.; Kuboyama, N. A biodegradable porous composite scaffold of PGA/beta-TCP for bone tissue engineering. *Bone* **2010**, *46*, 386–395. [CrossRef] [PubMed]

64. Peters, M.C.; Polverini, P.J.; Mooney, D.J. Engineering vascular networks in porous polymer matrices. *J. Biomed. Mater. Res.* **2002**, *60*, 668–678. [CrossRef] [PubMed]

65. Kasuya, J.; Sudo, R.; Tamogami, R.; Masuda, G.; Mitaka, T.; Ikeda, M.; Tanishita, K. Reconstruction of 3D stacked hepatocyte tissues using degradable, microporous poly(D,L-lactide-co-glycolide) membranes. *Biomaterials* **2012**, *33*, 2693–2700. [CrossRef] [PubMed]

66. Shen, J.Y.; Chan-Park, M.B.; Zhu, A.P.; Zhu, X.; Beuerman, R.W.; Yang, E.B.; Chen, W.; Chan, V. Three-dimensional microchannels in biodegradable polymeric films for control orientation and phenotype of vascular smooth muscle cells. *Tissue Eng.* **2006**, *12*, 2229–2240. [CrossRef] [PubMed]

67. Shen, J.Y.; Chan-Park, M.B.E.; Feng, Z.O.; Chan, V.; Feng, Z.W. UV-embossed microchannel in biocompatible polymeric film: Application to control of cell shape and orientation of muscle cells. *J. Biomed. Mater. Res. B* **2006**, *77B*, 423–430. [CrossRef] [PubMed]

68. Chan-Park, M.B.; Yan, Y.H.; Neo, W.K.; Zhou, W.X.; Zhang, J.; Yue, C.Y. Fabrication of high aspect ratio poly(ethylene glycol)-containing microstructures by UV embossing. *Langmuir* **2003**, *19*, 4371–4380. [CrossRef]

69. Feng, J.; Chan-Park, M.B.; Shen, J.Y.; Chan, V. Quick layer-by-layer assembly of aligned multilayers of vascular smooth muscle cells in deep microchannels. *Tissue Eng.* **2007**, *13*, 1003–1012. [CrossRef] [PubMed]

70. Sarkar, S.; Isenberg, B.C.; Hodis, E.; Leach, J.B.; Desai, T.A.; Wong, J.Y. Fabrication of a layered microstructured polycaprolactone construct for 3-D tissue engineering. *J. Biomater. Sci. Polym. E* **2008**, *19*, 1347–1362. [CrossRef] [PubMed]

71. Sarkar, S.; Dadhania, M.; Rourke, P.; Desai, T.A.; Wong, J.Y. Vascular tissue engineering: Microtextured scaffold templates to control organization of vascular smooth muscle cells and extracellular matrix. *Acta Biomater.* **2005**, *1*, 93–100. [CrossRef] [PubMed]

72. Revzin, A.; Russell, R.J.; Yadavalli, V.K.; Koh, W.G.; Deister, C.; Hile, D.D.; Mellott, M.B.; Pishko, M.V. Fabrication of poly(ethylene glycol) hydrogel microstructures using photolithography. *Langmuir* **2001**, *17*, 5440–5447. [CrossRef] [PubMed]

73. Koh, W.G.; Revzin, A.; Pishko, M.V. Poly(ethylene glycol) hydrogel microstructures encapsulating living cells. *Langmuir* **2002**, *18*, 2459–2462. [CrossRef] [PubMed]

74. Jiang, Z.; Xia, B.; McBride, R.; Oakey, J. A microfluidic-based cell encapsulation platform to achieve high long-term cell viability in photopolymerized PEGNB hydrogel microspheres. *J. Mater. Chem. B* **2017**, *5*, 173–180. [CrossRef] [PubMed]

75. Yang, X.M.; Sarvestani, S.K.; Moeinzadeh, S.; He, X.Z.; Jabbari, E. Three-Dimensional-Engineered Matrix to Study Cancer Stem Cells and Tumorsphere Formation: Effect of Matrix Modulus. *Tissue Eng. Part A* **2013**, *19*, 669–684. [CrossRef] [PubMed]

76. Hahn, M.S.; Miller, J.S.; West, J.L. Laser scanning lithography for surface micropatterning on hydrogels. *Adv. Mater.* **2005**, *17*. [CrossRef]

77. Cuchiara, M.P.; Allen, A.C.B.; Chen, T.M.; Miller, J.S.; West, J.L. Multilayer microfluidic PEGDA hydrogels. *Biomaterials* **2010**, *31*, 5491–5497. [CrossRef] [PubMed]

78. Zhu, J.M.; Tang, C.; Kottke-Marchant, K.; Marchant, R.E. Design and Synthesis of Biomimetic Hydrogel Scaffolds with Controlled Organization of Cyclic RGD Peptides. *Bioconj. Chem.* **2009**, *20*, 333–339. [CrossRef] [PubMed]

79. Oliviero, O.; Ventre, M.; Netti, P.A. Functional porous hydrogels to study angiogenesis under the effect of controlled release of vascular endothelial growth factor. *Acta Biomater.* **2012**, *8*, 3294–3301. [CrossRef] [PubMed]

80. Chen, W.; Shao, Y.; Li, X.; Zhao, G.; Fu, J. Nanotopographical surfaces for stem cell fate control: Engineering mechanobiology from the bottom. *Nano Today* **2014**, *9*, 759–784. [CrossRef] [PubMed]

81. Chevallay, B.; Herbage, D. Collagen-based biomaterials as 3D scaffold for cell cultures: Applications for tissue engineering and gene therapy. *Med. Biol. Eng. Comput.* **2000**, *38*, 211–218. [CrossRef] [PubMed]

82. Liu, C.Z.; Xia, Z.D.; Han, Z.W.; Hulley, P.A.; Triffitt, J.T.; Czernuszka, J.T. Novel 3D collagen scaffolds fabricated by indirect printing technique for tissue engineering. *J. Biomed. Mater. Res. B* **2008**, *85B*, 519–528. [CrossRef] [PubMed]

83. Sachlos, E.; Reis, N.; Ainsley, C.; Derby, B.; Czernuszka, J.T. Novel collagen scaffolds with predefined internal morphology made by solid freeform fabrication. *Biomaterials* **2003**, *24*, 1487–1497. [CrossRef]

84. Hutmacher, D.W.; Sittinger, M.; Risbud, M.V. Scaffold-based tissue engineering: Rationale for computer-aided design and solid free-form fabrication systems. *Trends Biotechnol.* **2004**, *22*, 354–362. [CrossRef] [PubMed]

85. Taboas, J.M.; Maddox, R.D.; Krebsbach, P.H.; Hollister, S.J. Indirect solid free form fabrication of local and global porous, biomimetic and composite 3D polymer-ceramic scaffolds. *Biomaterials* **2003**, *24*, 181–194. [CrossRef]

86. O'Brien, F.J.; Harley, B.A.; Yannas, I.V.; Gibson, L. Influence of freezing rate on pore structure in freeze-dried collagen-GAG scaffolds. *Biomaterials* **2004**, *25*, 1077–1086. [CrossRef]

87. O'rien, F.J.; Harley, B.A.; Yannas, I.V.; Gibson, L.J. The effect of pore size on cell adhesion in collagen-GAG scaffolds. *Biomaterials* **2005**, *26*, 433–441. [CrossRef] [PubMed]

88. Chung, T.W.; Yang, J.; Akaike, T.; Cho, K.Y.; Nah, J.W.; Kim, S.I.; Cho, C.S. Preparation of alginate/galactosylated chitosan scaffold for hepatocyte attachment. *Biomaterials* **2002**, *23*, 2827–2834. [CrossRef]

89. Zhao, F.; Yin, Y.J.; Lu, W.W.; Leong, J.C.; Zhang, W.J.; Zhang, J.Y.; Zhang, M.F.; Yao, K.D. Preparation and histological evaluation of biomimetic three-dimensional hydroxyapatite/chitosan-gelatin network composite scaffolds. *Biomaterials* **2002**, *23*, 3227–3234. [CrossRef]

90. Ang, T.H.; Sultana, F.S.A.; Hutmacher, D.W.; Wong, Y.S.; Fuh, J.Y.H.; Mo, X.M.; Loh, H.T.; Burdet, E.; Teoh, S.H. Fabrication of 3D chitosan-hydroxyapatite scaffolds using a robotic dispensing system. *Mater. Sci. Eng. C* **2002**, *20*, 35–42. [CrossRef]

91. Zhang, S.; Holmes, T.C.; DiPersio, C.M.; Hynes, R.O.; Su, X.; Rich, A. Self-complementary oligopeptide matrices support mammalian cell attachment. *Biomaterials* **1995**, *16*, 1385–1393. [CrossRef]

92. Gelain, F.; Bottai, D.; Vescovi, A.; Zhang, S. Designer self-assembling peptide nanofiber scaffolds for adult mouse neural stem cell 3-dimensional cultures. *PLoS ONE* **2006**, *1*, e119. [CrossRef] [PubMed]

93. Tsutsumi, H.; Mihara, H. Soft materials based on designed self-assembling peptides: From design to application. *Mol. Biol. Syst.* **2013**, *9*, 609–617. [CrossRef] [PubMed]

94. Davis, M.E.; Motion, J.P.; Narmoneva, D.A.; Takahashi, T.; Hakuno, D.; Kamm, R.D.; Zhang, S.; Lee, R.T. Injectable self-assembling peptide nanofibers create intramyocardial microenvironments for endothelial cells. *Circulation* **2005**, *111*, 442–450. [CrossRef] [PubMed]

95. Discher, D.E.; Janmey, P.; Wang, Y.L. Tissue cells feel and respond to the stiffness of their substrate. *Science* **2005**, *310*, 1139–1143. [CrossRef] [PubMed]

96. Pelham, R.J.; Wang, Y.L. Cell locomotion and focal adhesions are regulated by substrate flexibility. *Proc. Natl. Acad. Sci. USA* **1997**, *94*, 13661–13665. [CrossRef] [PubMed]

97. Lo, C.M.; Wang, H.B.; Dembo, M.; Wang, Y.L. Cell movement is guided by the rigidity of the substrate. *Biophys. J.* **2000**, *79*, 144–152. [CrossRef]

98. Bazellières, E.; Conte, V.; Elosegui-Artola, A.; Serra-Picamal, X.; Bintanel-Morcillo, M.; Roca-Cusachs, P.; Muñoz, J.J.; Sales-Pardo, M.; Guimerà, R.; Trepat, X. Control of cell-cell forces and collective cell dynamics by the intercellular adhesome. *Nat. Cell Biol.* **2015**, *17*, 409–420. [CrossRef] [PubMed]

99. Mann, J.M.; Lam, R.H.W.; Weng, S.N.; Sun, Y.B.; Fu, J.P. A silicone-based stretchable micropost array membrane for monitoring live-cell subcellular cytoskeletal response. *Lab Chip* **2012**, *12*, 731–740. [CrossRef] [PubMed]

100. Engler, A.J.; Sen, S.; Sweeney, H.L.; Discher, D.E. Matrix elasticity directs stem cell lineage specification. *Cell* **2006**, *126*, 677–689. [CrossRef] [PubMed]

101. Bidone, T.C.; Jung, W.; Maruri, D.; Borau, C.; Kamm, R.D.; Kim, T. Morphological Transformation and Force Generation of Active Cytoskeletal Networks. *PLoS Comput. Biol.* **2017**, *13*, e1005277. [CrossRef] [PubMed]

102. Iskratsch, T.; Wolfenson, H.; Sheetz, M.P. Appreciating force and shape: The rise of mechanotransduction in cell biology. *Nat. Rev. Mol. Cell Biol.* **2014**, *15*, 825–833. [CrossRef] [PubMed]

103. Dimilla, P.A.; Barbee, K.; Lauffenburger, D.A. Mathematical model for the effects of adhesion and mechanics on cell migration speed. *Biophys. J.* **1991**, *60*, 15–37. [CrossRef]

104. Peyton, S.R.; Putnam, A.J. Extracellular matrix rigidity governs smooth muscle cell motility in a biphasic fashion. *J. Cell Phys.* **2005**, *204*, 198–209. [CrossRef] [PubMed]

105. Lauridsen, H.M.; Gonzalez, A.L. Biomimetic, ultrathin and elastic hydrogels regulate human neutrophil extravasation across endothelial-pericyte bilayers. *PLoS One* **2017**, *12*, e0171386. [CrossRef] [PubMed]

106. Paul, R.; Heil, P.; Spatz, J.P.; Schwarz, U.S. Propagation of mechanical stress through the actin cytoskeleton toward focal adhesions: Model and experiment. *Biophys. J.* **2008**, *94*, 1470–1482. [CrossRef] [PubMed]

107. Schulte, C.; Ripamonti, M.; Maffioli, E.; Cappelluti, M.A.; Nonnis, S.; Puricelli, L.; Lamanna, J.; Piazzoni, C.; Podestà, A.; Lenardi, C.; et al. Scale invariant disordered nanotopography promotes hippocampal neuron development and maturation with involvement of mechanotransductive pathways. *Front. Cell Neurosci.* **2016**, *10*, 267. [CrossRef] [PubMed]

108. Harris, A.K.; Wild, P.; Stopak, D. Silicone rubber substrata: A new wrinkle in the study of cell locomotion. *Science* **1980**, *208*, 177–179. [CrossRef] [PubMed]

109. Oliver, T.; Jacobson, K.; Dembo, M. Design and use of substrata to measure traction forces exerted by cultured cells. *Method Enzymol.* **1998**, *298*, 497–521.

110. Oliver, T.; Dembo, M.; Jacobson, K. Traction Forces in Locomoting Cells. *Cell Motil. Cytoskel.* **1995**, *31*, 225–240. [CrossRef] [PubMed]

111. Balaban, N.Q.; Schwarz, U.S.; Riveline, D.; Goichberg, P.; Tzur, G.; Sabanay, I.; Lamanna, J.; Piazzoni, C.; Podestà, A.; Lenardi, C.; et al. Force and focal adhesion assembly: A close relationship studied using elastic micropatterned substrates. *Nat. Cell Biol.* **2001**, *3*, 466–472. [CrossRef] [PubMed]

112. Tan, J.L.; Tien, J.; Pirone, D.M.; Gray, D.S.; Bhadriraju, K.; Chen, C.S. Cells lying on a bed of microneedles: An approach to isolate mechanical force. *Proc. Natl. Acad. Sci. USA* **2003**, *100*, 1484–1489. [CrossRef] [PubMed]

113. Cesa, C.M.; Kirchgessner, N.; Mayer, D.; Schwarz, U.S.; Hoffmann, B.; Merkel, R. Micropatterned silicone elastomer substrates for high resolution analysis of cellular force patterns. *Rev. Sci. Instrum.* **2007**, *78*. [CrossRef] [PubMed]

114. Fu, J.P.; Wang, Y.K.; Yang, M.T.; Desai, R.A.; Yu, X.A.; Liu, Z.J.; Chen, C.S. Mechanical regulation of cell function with geometrically modulated elastomeric substrates. *Nat. Methods* **2010**, *7*. [CrossRef] [PubMed]

115. Van Hoorn, H.; Harkes, R.; Spiesz, E.M.; Storm, C.; van Noort, D.; Ladoux, B.; Schmidt, T. The Nanoscale Architecture of Force-Bearing Focal Adhesions. *Nano Lett.* **2014**, *14*, 4257–4262. [CrossRef] [PubMed]

116. Bendell, A.C.; Williamson, E.K.; Chen, C.S.; Burkhardt, J.K.; Hammer, D.A. The Arp2/3 complex binding protein HS1 is required for efficient dendritic cell random migration and force generation. *Integr. Biol.* **2017**, *9*, 695–708. [CrossRef] [PubMed]

117. Lam, R.H.W.; Weng, S.N.; Lu, W.; Fu, J.P. Live-cell subcellular measurement of cell stiffness using a microengineered stretchable micropost array membrane. *Integr. Biol. UK* **2012**, *4*, 1289–1298. [CrossRef] [PubMed]

118. Chandra, D.; Taylor, J.A.; Yang, S. Replica molding of high-aspect-ratio (sub-)micron hydrogel pillar arrays and their stability in air and solvents. *Soft Matter.* **2008**, *4*, 979–984. [CrossRef]

119. Chandra, D.; Yang, S. Stability of High-Aspect-Ratio Micropillar Arrays against Adhesive and Capillary Forces. *Accounts Chem. Res.* **2010**, *43*, 1080–1091. [CrossRef] [PubMed]

120. Wang, Y.L.; Pelham, R.J. Preparation of a flexible, porous polyacrylamide substrate for mechanical studies of cultured cells. *Method Enzymol.* **1998**, *298*, 489–496.

121. Kandow, C.E.; Georges, P.C.; Janmey, P.A.; Beningo, K.A. Polyacrylamide hydrogels for cell mechanics: Steps toward optimization and alternative uses. *Method Cell Biol.* **2007**, *83*. [CrossRef]

122. Beningo, K.A.; Lo, C.M.; Wang, Y.L. Flexible polyacrylamide substrata for the analysis of mechanical interactions at cell-substratum adhesions. *Methods Cell Matrix Adhes.* **2002**, *69*, 325–339.

123. Lin, G.; Pister, K.S.J.; Roos, K.P. Surface micromachined polysilicon heart cell force transducer. *J. Microelectromech. S* **2000**, *9*, 9–17. [CrossRef]

124. Galbraith, C.G.; Sheetz, M.P. A micromachined device provides a new bend on fibroblast traction forces. *Proc. Natl. Acad. Sci. USA* **1997**, *94*, 9114–9118. [CrossRef] [PubMed]

125. Petronis, S.; Gold, J.; Kasemo, B. Microfabricated force-sensitive elastic substrates for investigation of mechanical cell-substrate interactions. *J. Micromech. Microeng.* **2003**, *13*, 900–913. [CrossRef]

126. Even-Ram, S.; Yamada, K.M. Cell migration in 3D matrix. *Curr. Opin. Cell Biol.* **2005**, *17*, 524–532. [CrossRef] [PubMed]

127. Zaman, M.H.; Trapani, L.M.; Sieminski, A.L.; Mackellar, D.; Gong, H.; Kamm, R.D.; Wells, A.; Lauffenburger, D.A.; Matsudaira, P. Migration of tumor cells in 3D matrices is governed by matrix stiffness along with cell-matrix adhesion and proteolysis. *Proc. Natl. Acad. Sci. USA* **2006**, *103*, 10889–10894. [CrossRef] [PubMed]

128. Critser, P.J.; Kreger, S.T.; Voytik-Harbin, S.L.; Yoder, M.C. Collagen matrix physical properties modulate endothelial colony forming cell-derived vessels in vivo. *Microvasc. Res.* **2010**, *80*, 23–30. [CrossRef] [PubMed]

129. Ehrbar, M.; Sala, A.; Lienemann, P.; Ranga, A.; Mosiewicz, K.; Bittermann, A.; Rizzi, S.C.; Weber, F.E.; Lutolf, M.P. Elucidating the role of matrix stiffness in 3D cell migration and remodeling. *Biophys. J.* **2011**, *100*, 284–293. [CrossRef] [PubMed]

130. Mason, B.N.; Starchenko, A.; Williams, R.M.; Bonassar, L.J.; Reinhart-King, C.A. Tuning three-dimensional collagen matrix stiffness independently of collagen concentration modulates endothelial cell behavior. *Acta Biomater.* **2013**, *9*, 4635–4644. [CrossRef] [PubMed]

131. Cukierman, E.; Pankov, R.; Stevens, D.R.; Yamada, K.M. Taking cell-matrix adhesions to the third dimension. *Science* **2001**, *294*, 1708–1712. [CrossRef] [PubMed]

132. Goreczny, G.J.; Ouderkirk-Pecone, J.L.; Olson, E.C.; Krendel, M.; Turner, C.E. Hic-5 remodeling of the stromal matrix promotes breast tumor progression. *Oncogene* **2017**, *36*, 2693–2703. [CrossRef] [PubMed]

133. Fraley, S.I.; Feng, Y.F.; Krishnamurthy, R.; Kim, D.H.; Celedon, A.; Longmore, G.D.; Wirtz, D. A distinctive role for focal adhesion proteins in three-dimensional cell motility. *Nat. Cell Biol.* **2010**, *12*. [CrossRef] [PubMed]

134. Rodriguez, M.L.; Mcgarry, P. Review on cell mechanics: Experimental and modeling approaches. *Appl. Mech. Rev.* **2013**, *65*, 60801. [CrossRef]

135. Dembo, M.; Wang, Y.L. Stresses at the cell-to-substrate interface during locomotion of fibroblasts. *Biophys. J.* **1999**, *76*, 2307–2316. [CrossRef]

136. Yang, Z.C.; Lin, J.S.; Chen, J.X.; Wang, J.H.C. Determining substrate displacement and cell traction fields—a new approach. *J. Theor. Biol.* **2006**, *242*, 607–616. [CrossRef] [PubMed]

137. Franck, C.; Hong, S.; Maskarinec, S.A.; Tirrell, D.A.; Ravichandran, G. Three-dimensional full-field measurements of large deformations in soft materials using confocal microscopy and digital volume correlation. *Exp. Mech.* **2007**, *47*, 427–438. [CrossRef]

138. Franck, C.; Maskarinec, S.A.; Tirrell, D.A.; Ravichandran, G. Three-dimensional traction force microscopy: A new tool for quantifying cell-matrix interactions. *PLoS ONE* **2011**, *6*, e17833. [CrossRef] [PubMed]

139. Maskarinec, S.A.; Franck, C.; Tirrell, D.A.; Ravichandran, G. Quantifying cellular traction forces in three dimensions. *Proc. Natl. Acad. Sci. USA* **2009**, *106*, 22108–22113. [CrossRef] [PubMed]

140. Hur, S.S.; Zhao, Y.; Li, Y.S.; Botvinick, E.; Chien, S. Live Cells Exert 3-Dimensional Traction Forces on Their Substrata. *Cell Mol. Bioeng.* **2009**, *2*, 425–436. [CrossRef] [PubMed]

141. Delanoe-Ayari, H.; Rieu, J.P.; Sano, M. 4D traction force microscopy reveals asymmetric cortical forces in migrating Dictyostelium cells. *Phys. Rev. Lett.* **2010**, *105*, 248103. [CrossRef] [PubMed]

142. Hall, M.S.; Long, R.; Feng, X.Z.; Huang, Y.L.; Hui, C.Y.; Wu, M.M. Toward single cell traction microscopy within 3D collagen matrices. *Exp. Cell Res.* **2013**, *319*, 2396–2408. [CrossRef] [PubMed]

143. Toyjanova, J.; Bar-Kochba, E.; Lopez-Fagundo, C.; Reichner, J.; Hoffman-Kim, D.; Franck, C. High resolution, large deformation 3D traction force microscopy. *PLoS ONE* **2014**, *9*, e90976. [CrossRef] [PubMed]

144. Legant, W.R.; Miller, J.S.; Blakely, B.L.; Cohen, D.M.; Genin, G.M.; Chen, C.S. Measurement of mechanical tractions exerted by cells in three-dimensional matrices. *Nat. Methods* **2010**, *7*, 969–971. [CrossRef] [PubMed]

145. Gjorevski, N.; Nelson, C.M. Mapping of mechanical strains and stresses around quiescent engineered three-dimensional epithelial tissues. *Biophys. J.* **2012**, *103*, 152–162. [CrossRef] [PubMed]

146. Koch, T.M.; Munster, S.; Bonakdar, N.; Butler, J.P.; Fabry, B. 3D Traction forces in cancer cell invasion. *PLoS ONE* **2012**, *7*, e33476. [CrossRef] [PubMed]

147. Vogel, V.; Sheetz, M. Local force and geometry sensing regulate cell functions. *Nat. Rev. Mol. Cell Biol.* **2006**, *7*, 265–275. [CrossRef] [PubMed]

148. Freikamp, A.; Mehlich, A.; Klingner, C.; Grashoff, C. Investigating piconewton forces in cells by FRET-based molecular force microscopy. *J. Struct. Biol.* **2017**, *197*, 37–42. [CrossRef] [PubMed]

149. Zhang, Y.; Ng, S.S.; Wang, Y.L.; Feng, H.X.; Chen, W.N.; Chan-Park, M.B.; Li, C.; Chan, V. Collective cell traction force analysis on aligned smooth muscle cell sheet between three-dimensional microwalls. *Interf. Focus* **2014**, *4*. [CrossRef] [PubMed]

150. Hur, S.S.; del Alamo, J.C.; Park, J.S.; Li, Y.S.; Nguyen, H.A.; Teng, D.; Wang, K.C.; Flores, L.; Alonso-Latorre, B.; Lasheras, J.C.; et al. Roles of cell confluency and fluid shear in 3-dimensional intracellular forces in endothelial cells. *Proc. Natl. Acad. Sci. USA* **2012**, *109*, 11110–11115. [CrossRef] [PubMed]

151. Du Roure, O.; Saez, A.; Buguin, A.; Austin, R.H.; Chavrier, P.; Siberzan, P.; Ladoux, B. Force mapping in epithelial cell migration (vol 102, pg 2390, 2005). *Proc. Natl. Acad. Sci. USA* **2005**, *102*, 14122.

152. Tang, X.; Tofangchi, A.; Anand, S.V.; Saif, T.A. A novel cell traction force microscopy to study multi-cellular system. *PLoS Comput. Biol.* **2014**, *10*, e1003631. [CrossRef] [PubMed]

153. Campas, O.; Mammoto, T.; Hasso, S.; Sperling, R.A.; O'Connell, D.; Bischof, A.G.; Maas, R.; Weitz, D.A.; Mahadevan, L.; Ingber, D.E. Quantifying cell-generated mechanical forces within living embryonic tissues. *Nat. Methods* **2014**, *11*. [CrossRef]

154. Kim, D.H.; Provenzano, P.P.; Smith, C.L.; Levchenko, A. Matrix nanotopography as a regulator of cell function. *J. Cell Biol.* **2012**, *197*, 351. [CrossRef] [PubMed]

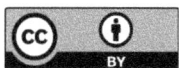

üü *bioengineering*

MDPI

Opinion
Safety Aspects of Bio-Based Nanomaterials

Julia Catalán [1,2,]* and Hannu Norppa [1]

[1] Work Environment, Occupational Safety, Finnish Institute of Occupational Health,
    FI-00250 Helsinki, Finland; hannu.norppa@ttl.fi
[2] Department of Anatomy, Embryology and Genetics, University of Zaragoza, 50013 Zaragoza, Spain
*   Correspondence: julia.catalan@ttl.fi; Tel.: +358-438251541

Academic Editor: Gary Chinga Carrasco
Received: 31 October 2017; Accepted: 29 November 2017; Published: 1 December 2017

Abstract: Moving towards a bio-based and circular economy implies a major focus on the responsible and sustainable utilization of bio-resources. The emergence of nanotechnology has opened multiple possibilities, not only in the existing industrial sectors, but also for completely novel applications of nanoscale bio-materials, the commercial exploitation of which has only begun during the last few years. Bio-based materials are often assumed not to be toxic. However, this pre-assumption is not necessarily true. Here, we provide a short overview on health and environmental aspects associated with bio-based nanomaterials, and on the relevant regulatory requirements. We also discuss testing strategies that may be used for screening purposes at pre-commercial stages. Although the tests presently used to reveal hazards are still evolving, regarding modifications required for nanomaterials, their application is needed before the upscaling or commercialization of bio-based nanomaterials, to ensure the market potential of the nanomaterials is not delayed by uncertainties about safety issues.

Keywords: nanosafety; bio-based nanomaterials; toxicity testing; hazard assessment; regulations

1. Introduction

The movement of our society towards a bio-based and circular economy implies a major focus on the responsible and sustainable utilization of bio-resources [1,2]. Pressure on biological resources should be reduced, and a circular economy needs to be realized by utilizing bio-waste as a resource and ensuring sustainable biomass production [3]. Renewable resources will play a key role in the production of novel bio-based materials, contributing to improving the environmental profile of polymer systems and composites currently produced from petroleum-based sources [2,4].

The forests constitute a major source of lignocellulosic biomass, a sustainable resource that, in addition, is not competing with food production [5]. Lignocellulosic materials have long been used in the paper and packing industrial sector, in healthcare products, such as wound healing materials, dialysis membranes, and excipients in tablets, and as rheology modifiers in food products and cosmetic formulations [6,7]. However, the emergence of nanotechnology has opened new and multiple possibilities, not only in the existing industrial sectors, but also for completely novel applications, such as biofuels, aerogels for insulation, vehicles' components, electronics, or tissue engineering [2,4,6,7]. The commercial exploitation of nanoscale bio-materials has only begun during the last few years, and although it is currently at pilot-scale for many applications, large-scale commercialization is anticipated [4,6]. Therefore, companies have a unique chance of being proactive by demonstrating the safety of the emerging bio-based nanomaterials in advance of their commercialization, ensuring that their market potential is not delayed by uncertainties about safety issues [4,7].

2. Toxicity of Bio-Based Nanomaterials

Due to their natural origin, bio-based materials are often assumed not to be toxic. In the middle of last century, the recognition of byssinosis as an occupational lung disease, observed in workers of the textile industry exposed to cotton dust, led to several studies investigating the possible health risks associated with cellulosic materials. An excellent review of these studies has been published by Endes et al. [6]. Whereas toxicological findings were contradictory among studies, all of them showed an extremely high biopersistence of cellulose fibers. Biopersistent long and thin high-aspect-ratio fibers have been postulated to have the potential to be carcinogenic, and lead to mesothelioma and lung cancer, according to the fiber pathogenicity paradigm [8]. Nanoscale features may impart novel material properties and biological behavior, as compared with conventional materials. A decrease in particle size is associated with improved penetration through biological barriers, resulting in increased doses of materials within cellular compartments or translocation to new localizations (e.g., the brain) [9]. On the other hand, the large surface area of nanomaterials may result in enhanced interaction with their biological surroundings [10–12], leading in some cases to an accelerated formation of reactive oxygen species [9,12]. In light of these findings, it is necessary to address the human health and environmental safety aspects of lignocellulosic nanomaterials before scaling up their production [6,7,13,14].

Currently, little is known about the potential adverse biological impact of lignocellulose nanomaterials, which comprise a broad spectrum of different structures from cellulose nanocrystals and different types of nanofibrillated celluloses to lignin nanomaterials (see, e.g., reviews by Shatkin et al. [4], Endes et al. [6] and Roman [13]; as well as summaries of more recent articles included in Shvedova et al. [15] and Catalán et al. [16]). The scarce toxicological data are interpreted in different ways by researchers. Whereas several authors think that the available results suggest that nanocelluloses have a limited associated toxic potential [4,6,17], conflicting conclusions are reached, especially for inhalation results and cytotoxicity [13,16]. However, all authors agree on assuming an association between the hazard profile of lignocellulosic nanomaterials and their physicochemical characteristics. It is well-recognized that the physicochemical features of nanomaterials can affect their toxicity [18]. For instance, the interaction of nanofibrillated cellulose and dendritic cells depended on the thickness and length of the material [19]. Therefore, differences in production technique, which can dramatically affect the physicochemical characteristics of cellulosic nanomaterials [20], may also affect their hazard features. That is the case for surface chemistry, which has been reported to drive the inflammatory response to nanofibrillated cellulose [21]. Although most toxicological studies have focused on unmodified materials [4], for many applications, such as uses in healthcare products and food packaging, nanocellulose may be surface functionalized, imparting new properties to the material [6]. However, far from being an obstacle, the possibility of moderating biological responses by introducing surface modifications opens up the option of safe-by-design for these materials [21].

The route of exposure may also determine the toxicological responses of bio-based nanomaterials. The main portals of entry to the human body include the gastrointestinal tract, skin, systemic circulation, and the lung, through inhalation [6]. The latter is considered the primary route of exposure for humans for any nanoparticle released into the environment, especially in the case of occupational exposure [22], as also confirmed by a life cycle risk assessment of nanocelluloses [23]. In addition, nanocelluloses are expected to be biopersistent, as indicated by in vitro experiments with artificial lung airway lining and macrophage phagolysosomal fluids [24], and in vivo evidence [14,15]. As previously mentioned, biopersistence of fibers has been identified as a key factor governing the biological response following chronic inhalation exposures [8]. Therefore, the release and inhalation of cellulose/polymer particles during processing steps, such as drilling, cutting, and sanding of polymer nanocomposites [6], in addition to possible liquid aerosols in wet operations, might be a concern.

Although inhalation has been pointed out as the main route for human exposure to nanomaterials, little is known about exposure concentrations or doses [25]. Few studies have reported measurements of cellulose nanomaterials in occupational environments [17,26]. This means that there is not enough data on occupational exposure or inhalation toxicity exist for cellulose nanomaterials to determine material-specific occupational exposure limits (OELs) for airborne dusts [4]. As for other nanomaterials, lower exposure levels may be expected to be harmful for nanosized, than bulk forms. Applying the pre-cautionary principle, Stockmann-Juvala et al. [27] recommended an OEL for nanocelluloses of 0.01 fibers/cm^3, which is the same value as suggested for other biopersistent fibrous nanomaterials, e.g., carbon nanofibers. As pointed out by these authors, the comparison of air sample concentrations with the suggested OEL is difficult at the moment, due to the lack of reliable methods for quantitative measurement. Therefore, a minimization of the exposure is recommended, as long as these methods are not available [27].

3. Regulatory Requirements and Testing Strategies

The identification of material-posed hazards is required under several international regulations (e.g., Registration, Evaluation, Authorization and Restriction of Chemicals—REACH, biocides, pharmaceuticals, medical devices, food additives, cosmetics, etc.) dealing with the safe use of chemical substances, products or devices (including nanomaterials-enabled ones). The corresponding regulations under which the bio-based nanomaterial will need to be evaluated in connection with scaling up of production or commercialization will depend on the uses and applications of the materials, and the countries where they apply [7]. For instance, in the European Union, approval of medical devices is addressed by three different European Commission directives [28], whereas different directives apply to pharmaceuticals [29]. In addition, commercialization of chemical substances is regulated by REACH [9,30], which aims at ensuring the protection of workers, downstream users, consumers and the environment. Furthermore, the United Nations' Globally Harmonized System (GHS), which harmonizes the classification and communication of hazardous properties of chemicals worldwide [31], has been adopted in several international regulations (e.g., in Europe). In an interesting article, Shatkin et al. [4] identified the data gaps needed for cellulose nanomaterials to comply with the requirements of this system.

Although there is a broad range of regulations, most of them agree on some basic human health and environmental effects that should be addressed [7]. In general, hazard assessment relies on several endpoints (e.g., cytotoxicity, sensitization, genotoxicity, etc.) that are assessed using validated assays, most of them still requiring animal experiments. It is, however, expected that new alternative methods, in accordance with the 3 Rs principles, will substitute them in the future [32]. Therefore, the commercialization of bio-based materials will have to comply with the corresponding regulatory requirements, depending on the intended final use of the products. Nevertheless, a first screening of the toxic potential of the materials can be done at the pre-commercialization or pre-clinical stages using in vitro assays.

During the last few years, several approaches and frameworks have proposed a testing strategy suitable for nanomaterials [33–36]. Most toxicological studies on nanomaterials assess cytotoxic potential in different human or mammalian cell systems. Cytotoxicity is one of the endpoints requested for medical device biocompatibility testing to obtain regulatory approval in most markets [37]. It is also required as a pre-test for establishing the range of doses to be evaluated in more specific endpoints, such as genotoxicity. However, although cytotoxicity assays may allow a way to rank nanomaterials [38], differentiating between partly soluble and poorly soluble metal-based nanoparticles, they do not indicate which doses are toxic in vivo, or if the effect is organ-specific. Cytotoxicity neither provides information on the type of hazardous event and the possible mechanism of action. The latter two can be assessed by a battery of assays that, in addition to cytotoxicity in a relevant cell system for the route of exposure, also include more specific endpoints. Furthermore, the lack of cytotoxicity does not mean the lack of hazardous effects [39]. For instance, the woodderived nanofibrillated celluloses studied by Lopes et al. [21] did not impair the cell viability of dermal cells, lung cells, or macrophages. However, the unmodified nanofibrils promoted an inflammatory response in macrophages.

Genotoxicity is a key endpoint in the toxicity testing of nanomaterials [33,34,36,40]. It has important consequences to human health, because mutations play a crucial role in the initiation and progression of carcinogenesis, and in reproductive and developmental abnormalities [41,42]. Genotoxicity is a hazard endpoint required in all product regulations (REACH, biocides, pharmaceuticals, medical devices, food additives, cosmetics, etc.), as well as one of the categories considered within the GHS for Hazard Communication [31]. The assessment of genotoxicity is based on validated in vitro assays, which can be followed up by validated in vivo assays, depending on the in vitro outcome and the regulation involved. Therefore, genotoxicity assessment at an early stage of pre-commercialization is highly advised.

Inflammation is one of the initial steps that may give rise to lung fibrosis, secondary genotoxic effects, and carcinogenesis after inhaling biopersistent nanofibers. In addition, most of the nanomaterials administrated intravenously (e.g., nanomedicines) end up in immune-related organs containing cells of the mononuclear phagocytic system [43]. Furthermore, all new human pharmaceuticals should be evaluated for potential immunotoxic activity [44]. Therefore, immunotoxicity testing should be included in a testing strategy [34,36].

Oxidative stress has been suggested to be a mechanism often underlying the possible toxicity of nanomaterials, causing both immunotoxic and genotoxic effects [36,45]. Therefore, this endpoint is included in most of the testing strategies proposed for nanomaterials. For instance, the in vitro testing strategy suggested by Endes et al. [46] to mimic the inhalation of high aspect ratio nanoparticles includes the assessment of cytotoxicity, oxidative stress, and pro-inflammatory responses in a 3D lung model.

Bacterial lipopolysaccharides (LPS, also termed endotoxin) are common contaminators of naturally derived materials [47]. Endotoxins are known to trigger inflammation, and they may induce oxidative stress and subsequently other toxic effects (e.g., DNA damage) [16]. The absence of endotoxin in nanomaterial test samples is considered important, and should be reported in toxicity studies [48], especially in the case of immunotoxicity testing for biomedical applications [47,49]. However, endotoxin testing of nanomaterials is not straightforward, due to the interference of nanomaterials with the endotoxin assays [49]. Polymyxin B is sometimes used in parallel immunotoxicity experiments to inhibit the potential effects of any endotoxin present in the samples [21]. Nevertheless, producing and handling of the nanomaterials in an environment as much endotoxin-free as possible is highly advised [49]. For instance, Nordli et al. [47] have described an updated method to produce ultrapure cellulose nanofibrils suitable for wound dressings.

It is worth emphasizing that there are few legislations specifically dealing with nanomaterials (e.g., the European biocidal products and cosmetics regulations). Instead, nanomaterial safety evaluation is based on the existing regulatory frameworks and, hence, on validated standard toxicological assays. However, the ability of some of these assays to detect the potential hazards of nanomaterials has not well been established [35,43], and recommendations for assay modifications have been suggested [48]. Furthermore, an important question in toxicological testing of nanomaterials is the limited ability of the present in vitro assays to deal with secondary toxic mechanisms and organ specificity that are fully present only in a whole organism in vivo. Co-culture of e.g., inflammatory and target cells may provide a simple system for detecting secondary effects, such as secondary genotoxicity [40], although such approaches have not widely been evaluated. 3D tissue models have received increased attention in toxicology, but only a limited number of studies utilizing these techniques has thus far been carried out with nanomaterials [50]. The integration of new technologies (e.g., "omics") may in the future allow researchers to elucidate mechanistic pathways involved in toxicological responses of nanomaterials [40]. In the meantime, assay limitations should be taken into account when using conventional in vitro tests for the hazard identifications of bio-based nanomaterials.

4. Environmental Issues

Finally, effects on the environment are also part of safety evaluation. Bio-based materials are assumed to be environmentally friendly [51,52]. In fact, wood-based feedstocks have much shorter carbon cycle and lower greenhouse gas emissions than fossil-based feedstocks [2]. In addition, the use of wood-based materials can represent a bio-based alternative that does not compete with food production, since forest areas are usually unsuitable for food production [2]. However, the ecotoxicological data available by now are not adequate to allow the environmental hazard classification of cellulose nanomaterials [4] or bio-based materials in general. Many bio-based materials are regarded as readily biodegradable [4], but this is not true for all of them. For instance, some plastics are not really biodegraded, but they break down into very small fragments that accumulate in the environment [2]. Even for completely biodegradable materials, there are limited data regarding their bioaccumulative potential and soil mobility [4], which prevents the exclusion of environmental concerns.

5. Conclusions

Although legislation specifically concerning the safety of nanomaterials is still rare, existing regulations governing the risks of chemical substances, biocides, pharmaceuticals, medical devices, food additives, cosmetics, etc. are in effect, and also apply to bio-based nanomaterials. Despite the tests presently used to reveal hazards to human health and the environment are still evolving, regarding modifications required for nanomaterials, their application is needed before the upscaling or commercialization of bio-based nanomaterials.

Acknowledgments: This paper was funded by the Finnish Work Environment Fund (grant No. 117146).

Author Contributions: Both authors equally contributed to writing the paper.

Conflicts of Interest: The authors declare no conflict of interest.

References

1. Ronzon, T.; Santini, F.; M'Barek, R. *The Bioeconomy in the European Union in Numbers. Facts and Figures on Biomass, Turnover and Employment*; European Commission, Joint Research Centre, Institute for Prospective Technological Studies: Seville, Spain, 2015; p. 4.
2. Brodin, M.; Vallejos, M.; Opedal, M.T.; Area, M.C.; Chinga-Carrasco, G. Lignocellulosics as sustainable resources for production of bioplastics—A review. *J. Clean. Prod.* **2017**, *162*, 646–664. [CrossRef]
3. Bell, J.; Paula, L.; Dodd, T.; Németh, S.; Nanou, C.; Mega, V.; Campos, P. EU ambition to build the world's leading bioeconomy-Uncertain times demand innovative and sustainable solutions. *New Biotechnol.* **2018**, *40*, 25–30. [CrossRef] [PubMed]
4. Shatkin, J.A.; Ong, K.J.; Ede, J.D.; Wegner, T.H.; Goergen, M. Toward cellulose nanomaterial commercialization: Knowledge gap analysis for safety data sheets according to the globally harmonized system. *Tappi J.* **2016**, *15*, 425–437.
5. Broeren, M. Production of Bio-Ethylene. *IEA-ETSAP and IRENA*© *Technology-Policy Brief* **2013**, *13*. Available online: https://iea-etsap.org/E-TechDS/PDF/I13IR_Bioethy_MB_Jan2013_final_GSOK (accessed on 28 October 2017).
6. Endes, C.; Camarero-Espinosa, S.; Mueller, S.; Foster, E.J.; Petri-Fink, A.; Rothen-Rutishauser, B.; Weder, C.; Clift, M.J. A critical review of the current knowledge regarding the biological impact of nanocellulose. *J. Nanobiotechnol.* **2016**, *14*, 78. [CrossRef] [PubMed]
7. Ong, K.J.; Shatkin, J.A.; Nelson, K.; Ede, J.D.; Retsina, T. Establishing the safety of novel bio-based cellulose nanomaterials for commercialization. *NanoImpact* **2017**, *6*, 19–29. [CrossRef]
8. Donaldson, K.; Poland, C.A. Nanotoxicology: New insights into nanotubes. *Nat. Nanotechnol.* **2009**, *4*, 708–710. [CrossRef] [PubMed]
9. Schwirn, K.; Tietjen, L.; Beer, I. Why are nanomaterials different and how can they be appropriately regulated under REACH? *Environ. Sci. Eur.* **2014**, *26*, 4. [CrossRef]
10. Zhang, L.; Webster, T.J. Nanotechnology and nanomaterials: Promises for improved tissue regeneration. *Nano Today* **2009**, *4*, 66–80. [CrossRef]
11. Braakhuis, H.M.; Park, M.V.; Gosens, I.; De Jong, W.H.; Cassee, F.R. Physicochemical characteristics of nanomaterials that affect pulmonary inflammation. *Part. Fibre Toxicol.* **2014**, *11*, 18. [CrossRef] [PubMed]

12. Padmanabhan, J.; Kyriakides, T.R. Nanomaterials, inflammation and tissue engineering. *Wiley Interdiscip. Rev. Nanomed. Nanobiotechnol.* **2015**, *7*, 355–370. [CrossRef] [PubMed]

13. Roman, M. Toxicity of cellulose nanocrystals: A review. *Ind. Biotechnol.* **2015**, *11*, 25–33. [CrossRef]

14. Lindberg, H.K.; Catalán, J.; Aimonen, K.J.; Wolff, H.; Wedin, I.; Nuopponen, M.; Savolainen, K.M.; Norppa, H. Evaluation of the genotoxic potential of different types of nanofibrillated celluloses. *TechConnect Briefs* **2017**, 229–232.

15. Shvedova, A.A.; Kisin, E.R.; Yanamala, N.; Farcas, M.T.; Menas, A.L.; Williams, A.; Fournier, P.M.; Reynolds, J.S.; Gutkin, D.W.; Star, A.; et al. Gender differences in murine pulmonary responses elicited by cellulose nanocrystals. *Part. Fibre Toxicol.* **2016**, *13*, 28. [CrossRef] [PubMed]

16. Catalán, J.; Rydman, E.; Aimonen, K.; Hannukainen, K.S.; Suhonen, S.; Vanhala, E.; Moreno, C.; Meyer, V.; Perez, D.D.; Sneck, A.; et al. Genotoxic and inflammatory effects of nanofibrillated cellulose in murine lungs. *Mutagenesis* **2017**, *32*, 23–31. [CrossRef] [PubMed]

17. Vartiainen, J.; Pohler, T.; Sirola, K.; Pylkkänen, L.; Alenius, H.; Hokkinen, J.; Tapper, U.; Lahtinen, P.; Kapanen, A.; Putkisto, K.; et al. Health and environmental safety aspects of friction grinding and spray drying of microfibrillated cellulose. *Cellulose* **2011**, *18*, 775–786. [CrossRef]

18. Lynch, I.; Weiss, C.; Valsami-Jones, E. A strategy for grouping of nanomaterials based on key physico-chemical descriptors as a basis for safer-by-design nanomaterials. *Nano Today* **2014**, *9*, 266–270. [CrossRef]

19. Tomić, S.; Kokol, V.; Mihajlović, D.; Mirčić, A.; Čolić, M. Native cellulose nanofibrills induce immune tolerance in vitro by acting on dendritic cells. *Sci. Rep.* **2016**, *6*, 31618. [CrossRef] [PubMed]

20. Sacui, I.A.; Nieuwendaal, R.C.; Burnett, D.J.; Stranick, S.J.; Jorfi, M.; Weder, C.; Foster, E.J.; Olsson, R.T.; Gilman, J.W. Comparison of the properties of cellulose nanocrystals and cellulose nanofibrils isolated from bacteria, tunicate, and wood processed using acid, enzymatic, mechanical and oxidative methods. *ACS Appl. Mater. Interfaces* **2014**, *6*, 6127–6138. [CrossRef] [PubMed]

21. Lopes, V.R.; Sanchez-Martinez, C.; Strømme, M.; Ferraz, N. In vitro biological responses to nanofibrillated cellulose by human dermal, lung and immune cells: Surface chemistry aspect. *Part. Fibre Toxicol.* **2017**, *14*, 1. [CrossRef] [PubMed]

22. Stone, V.; Miller, M.R.; Clift, M.J.D.; Elder, A.; Mills, N.L.; Møller, P.; Schins, R.P.F.; Vogel, U.; Kreyling, W.G.; Jensen, K.A.; et al. Nanomaterials versus ambient ultrafine particles: An opportunity to exchange toxicology knowledge. *Environ. Health Perspect.* **2017**, *125*, 106002. [CrossRef] [PubMed]

23. Shatkin, J.A.; Kim, B. Cellulose nanomaterials: Life cycle risk assessment, and environmental health and safety roadmap. *Environ. Sci. Nano* **2015**, *2*, 477. [CrossRef]

24. Stefaniak, A.B.; Seehra, M.S.; Fix, N.R.; Leonard, S.S. Lung biodurability and free radical production of cellulose nanomaterials. *Inhal. Toxicol.* **2014**, *26*, 733–749. [CrossRef] [PubMed]

25. Donaldson, K.; Schinwald, A.; Murphy, F.; Cho, W.S.; Duffin, R.; Tran, L.; Poland, C. The biologically effective dose in inhalation nanotoxicology. *Acc. Chem. Res.* **2013**, *46*, 723–732. [CrossRef] [PubMed]

26. O'Connor, B.; Berry, R.; Goguen, R. Commercialization of Cellulose Nanocrystal (NCC™) Production: A Business Case Focusing on the Importance of Proactive EHS Management. In *Nanotechnology Environmental Health and Safety*, 2nd ed.; Hull, M., Bowman, D., Eds.; Elsevier Inc.: Oxford, UK, 2014; Chapter 10; pp. 225–246. ISBN 978-1-4557-3188-6.

27. Stockmann-Juvala, H.; Taxell, P.; Santonen, T. *Formulating Occupational Exposure Limits Values (OELs) (Inhalation & Dermal)*; Finnish Institute of Occupational Health: Helsinki, Finland, 2014. Available online: http://scaffold.eu-vri.eu/filehandler.ashx?file=13717 (accessed on 28 October 2017).

28. Van Norman, G.A. Drugs and devices. Comparison of European and U.S. approval processes. *JACC Basic Transl. Sci.* **2016**, *1*, 399–412. [CrossRef]

29. Scholz, N. Medicinal products in the European Union. *Eur. Parliam. Res. Serv.* **2015**. Available online: http://www.europarl.europa.eu/RegData/etudes/IDAN/2015/554174/EPRS_IDA(2015)554174_EN (accessed on 28 October 2017). [CrossRef]

30. Regulation, Evaluation, Authorization and Restriction of Chemicals (REACH), 2006. Available online: http://eur-lex.europa.eu/legal-content/EN/TXT/PDF/?uri=CELEX:32006R1907&from=EN (accessed on 28 October 2017).

31. United Nations (UN). Globally Harmonized System of Classification and Labelling of Chemicals (GHS). 2011. Available online: https://www.unece.org/fileadmin/DAM/trans/danger/publi/ghs/ghs_rev04/English/ST-SG-AC10--30-Rev4e (accessed on 28 October 2017).

32. Worth, A.; Barroso, J.; Bremer, S.; Burton, J.; Casati, S.; Coecke, S.; Corvi, R.; Desprez, B.; Dumont, C.; Gouliarmou, V.; et al. *Alternative Methods for Regulatory Toxicology—A State-Of-The-Art Review*; JRC Science and Policy Reports, European Union: Luxemburg, 2014; ISBN 978-92-79-39651-9.

33. Stone, V.; Pozzi-Mucelli, S.; Tran, L.; Aschberger, K.; Sabella, S.; Vogel, U.; Poland, C.; Balharry, D.; Fernandes, T.; Gottardo, S.; et al. ITS-NANO—Prioritizing nanosafety research to develop a stakeholder driven intelligent testing strategy. *Part. Fibre Toxicol.* **2014**, *11*, 9. [CrossRef] [PubMed]

34. Dekkers, S.; Oomen, A.G.; Bleeker, E.A.; Vandebriel, R.J.; Micheletti, C.; Cabellos, J.; Janer, G.; Fuentes, N.; Vázquez-Campos, S.; Borges, T.; et al. Towards a nanospecific approach for risk assessment. *Regul. Toxicol. Pharmacol.* **2016**, *80*, 46–59. [CrossRef] [PubMed]

35. Dusinska, M.; Boland, S.; Saunders, M.; Juillerat-Jeanneret, L.; Tran, L.; Pojana, G.; Marcomini, A.; Volkovova, K.; Tulinska, J.; Knudsen, L.E.; et al. Towards an alternative testing strategy for nanomaterials used in nanomedicine: Lessons from NanoTEST. *Nanotoxicology* **2015**, *9*, 118–132. [CrossRef] [PubMed]

36. Dusinska, M.; Tulinska, J.; El Yamani, N.; Kuricova, M.; Liskova, A.; Rollerova, E.; Rundén-Pran, E.; Smolkova, B. Immunotoxicity, genotoxicity and epigenetic toxicity of nanomaterials: New strategies for toxicity testing? *Food Chem. Toxicol.* **2017**, *109*, 797–811. [CrossRef] [PubMed]

37. Food and Drug Administration (FDA). Use of International Standard ISO 10993-1, Biological Evaluation of Medical Devices—Part 1: Evaluation and Testing within a Risk Management Process. 2016. Available online: https://www.fda.gov/downloads/medicaldevices/deviceregulationandguidance/guidancedocuments/ucm348890 (accessed on 28 October 2017).

38. Farcal, L.; Torres Andón, F.; Di Cristo, L.; Rotoli, B.M.; Bussolati, O.; Bergamaschi, E.; Mech, A.; Hartmann, N.B.; Rasmussen, K.; Riego-Sintes, J.; et al. Comprehensive in vitro toxicity testing of a panel of representative oxide nanomaterials: First steps towards an intelligent testing strategy. *PLoS ONE* **2015**, *10*, e0127174. [CrossRef] [PubMed]

39. Xia, T.; Hamilton, R.F.; Bonner, J.C.; Crandall, E.D.; Elder, A.; Fazlollahi, F.; Girtsman, T.A.; Kim, K.; Mitra, S.; Ntim, S.A.; et al. Interlaboratory evaluation of in vitro cytotoxicity and inflammatory responses to engineered nanomaterials: The NIEHS Nano GO Consortium. *Environ. Health Perspect.* **2013**, *121*, 683–690. [CrossRef] [PubMed]

40. Catalán, J.; Stockmann-Juvala, H.; Norppa, H. A theoretical approach for a weighted assessment of the mutagenic potential of nanomaterials. *Nanotoxicology* **2017**, *18*, 1–14. [CrossRef] [PubMed]

41. Alenius, H.; Catalán, J.; Lindberg, H.; Norppa, H.; Palomäki, J.; Savolainen, K. Nanomaterials and human health. In *Handbook of Nanosafety—Measurement, Exposure and Toxicology*; Vogel, U., Savolainen, K., Wu, Q., van Tongeren, M., Brouwer, D., Berges, M., Eds.; Elsevier Inc.: Oxford, UK, 2014; Chapter 3; pp. 59–133. ISBN 978-0-12-416604-2.

42. Doak, S.H.; Manshian, B.; Jenkins, G.J.; Singh, N. In vitro genotoxicity testing strategy for nanomaterials and the adaptation of current OECD guidelines. *Mutat Res.* **2012**, *745*, 104–111. [CrossRef] [PubMed]

43. Giannakou, C.; Park, M.V.; de Jong, W.H.; van Loveren, H.; Vandebriel, R.J.; Geertsma, R.E. A comparison of immunotoxic effects of nanomedicinal products with regulatory immunotoxicity testing requirements. *Int. J. Nanomed.* **2016**, *11*, 2935–2952. [CrossRef] [PubMed]

44. European Medicines Agency (EMA). 2006—Committee for Medicinal Products for Human Use (CHMP). ICH Topic S8 Immunotoxicity Studies for Human Pharmaceuticals. London CHMP/167235/2004. Available online: http://www.ema.europa.eu/docs/en_GB/document_library/Scientific_guideline/2009/09/WC500002851 (accessed on 28 October 2017).

45. Donaldson, K.; Poland, C.A. Inhaled nanoparticles and lung cancer—What we can learn from conventional particle toxicology. *Swiss Med. Wkly.* **2012**, *142*, w13547. [CrossRef] [PubMed]

46. Endes, C.; Schmid, O.; Kinnear, C.; Mueller, S.; Camarero-Espinosa, S.; Vanhecke, D.; Foster, E.J.; Petri-Fink, A.; Rothen-Rutishauser, B.; Weder, C.; et al. An in vitro testing strategy towards mimicking the inhalation of high aspect ratio nanoparticles. *Part. Fibre Toxicol.* **2014**, *11*, 40. [CrossRef] [PubMed]

47. Nordli, H.R.; Chinga-Carrasco, G.; Rokstad, A.M.; Pukstad, B. Producing ultrapure wood cellulose nanofibrils and evaluating the cytotoxicity using human skin cells. *Carbohydr. Polym.* **2016**, *150*, 65–73. [CrossRef] [PubMed]

48. European Chemicals Agency (ECHA). Guidance on Information Requirements and Chemical Safety Assessment. Appendix R7-1 Recommendations for Nanomaterials Applicable to Chapter R7a Endpoint Specific Guidance, Version 2.0, May 2017. Available online: https://echa.europa.eu/documents/10162/13632/appendix_r7a_nanomaterials_en.pdf/1bef8a8a-6ffa-406a-88cd-fd800ab163ae (accessed on 28 October 2017).

49. Giannakou, C.; Geertsma, R.E.; de Jong, W.H.; van Loveren, H.; Vandebriel, R.J.; Park, M.V.D.Z. Immunotoxicity testing of nanomedicinal products: Possible pitfalls in endotoxin determination. *Curr. Bionanotechnol.* **2016**, *2*, 95–102. [CrossRef]

50. Evans, S.J.; Clift, M.J.; Singh, N.; de Oliveira Mallia, J.; Burgum, M.; Wills, J.W.; Wilkinson, T.S.; Jenkins, G.J.; Doak, S.H. Critical review of the current and future challenges associated with advanced in vitro systems towards the study of nanoparticle (secondary) genotoxicity. *Mutagenesis* **2017**, *32*, 233–241. [CrossRef] [PubMed]

51. Kimura, K.; Horikoshi, Y. Bio-based polymers. *Fujitsu Sci. Tech. J.* **2005**, *41*, 173–180.

52. Narayan, R. Biobased and biodegradable plastics: Rationale, drivers, and technology exemplars. In *Degradable Polymers and Materials: Principles and Practice*, 2nd ed.; Khemani, K., Scholz, C., Eds.; American Chemical Society: Washington, DC, USA, 2012; Chapter 2; pp. 13–31.

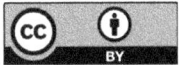

MDPI

St. Alban-Anlage 66

4052 Basel

Switzerland

Tel. +41 61 683 77 34

Fax +41 61 302 89 18

www.mdpi.com

Bioengineering Editorial Office

E-mail: bioengineering@mdpi.com

www.mdpi.com/journal/bioengineering

MDPI

St. Alban-Anlage 66

4052 Basel

Switzerland

Tel. +41 61 683 77 34

Fax +41 61 302 89 18

www.mdpi.com

Bioengineering Editorial Office

E-mail: bioengineering@mdpi.com

www.mdpi.com/journal/bioengineering

www.ingramcontent.com/pod-product-compliance
Lightning Source LLC
Chambersburg PA
CBHW051845210326
41597CB00033B/5782